VETs

Complete Preparation for the Veterinary Entrance Tests

The Science of Review™

VETs

Complete Preparation for the Veterinary Entrance Tests

The Science of Review™

2000 Edition

Aftab S. Hassan, Ph.D.

Contributing Authors

Leon Anderson, Jr., D.M.D.
Jesse Blankenship, B.S.
Ruth E. Lowe Gordon, B.S.
Frank Kessler, M.A.
Dana Mitchell, B.A.
Emily Meyer Naegali, M.A.
Jeffrey D. Zubkowski, Ph.D.

LIPPINCOTT WILLIAMS & WILKINS
A **Wolters Kluwer** Company
Philadelphia • Baltimore • New York • London
Buenos Aires • Hong Kong • Sydney • Tokyo

351 West Camden Street
Baltimore, Maryland 21201-2436 USA

227 East Washington Square
Philadelphia, PA 19106

Printed in the United States of America

ISBN: 0-683-30783-5

99 00 01 02 03
2 3 4 5 6 7 8 9 10

Contents

CHAPTER 2
Developing Verbal Ability for the VETs

CHAPTER 3
Reading Comprehension for the VETs

CHAPTER 5
Developing Quantitative Reasoning Skills for the VETs

CHAPTER 6

Preparing for the VETs Chemistry Test

CHAPTER 7

Test-Taking Skills

CHAPTER 8

Model Test

List of Figures

CHAPTER 6

Preparing for the VETs Chemistry Test

List of Tables

CHAPTER 1

Study Skills for the VETs

CHAPTER 2

Developing Verbal Ability for the VETs

CHAPTER 3

Reading Comprehension for the VETs

CHAPTER 4

Preparing for the VETs Biology Test

CHAPTER 5
Developing Quantitative Reasoning Skills for the VETs

CHAPTER 6
Preparing for the VETs Chemistry Test

CHAPTER 7
Test-Taking Skills

CHAPTER 8
Model Test

Foreword

Roscoe M. Moore, Jr., D.V.M., Ph.D., D.Sc.
Assistant Surgeon General
United States Public Health Service

You are to be commended for embarking on this critical first step in preparing for entrance into the profession of veterinary medicine. Entrance into veterinary medicine is highly competitive, and you have spent the last few years of your undergraduate curriculum preparing to meet the challenge. It is a pleasure to share your early interest in veterinary medicine and surgery as a career goal.

This unique and comprehensive guide is published by a company that for many years has been a leader in test preparation for the health professions. It emphasizes problem-solving and self-managed learning skills along with content review. By choosing this guide, not only will you improve your test performance but you will also acquire skills that will serve you throughout veterinary school and your professional life. Also, as you journey through your career as a veterinary student and a professional, Lippincott Williams & Wilkins offers resources to assist you right through board certification and into your professional career.

Veterinary medical education encompasses extensive instruction in multiple clinical as well as scientific disciplines, including epidemiology, pathology, microbiology, physiology, and biochemistry. The clinical training of veterinarians provides them with substantial experience in a number of fields, ranging from private practice to the management of zoonotic diseases within state and federal public health agencies.

The scientific knowledge and clinical and surgical skills of the veterinarian benefit society through the protection of animal health, the relief of animal suffering, the conservation of livestock resources, the promotion of public health, and the advancement of medical knowledge.

There are approximately 60,174 graduate veterinarians in the United States, and entry into highly competitive colleges/schools of veterinary medicine is a worthy accomplishment. Doctors of veterinary medicine possess extensive knowledge in disease and disease processes and are capable of managing disease and injury in affected animal populations. I look forward to your joining the ranks of professional veterinarians in the next century.

Good luck. I trust that you are prepared for the future.

Dr. Roscoe M. Moore, Jr., is a career officer within the Commissioned Corps of the United States Public Health Service. Dr. Moore attained the rank of Assistant Surgeon General (Rear Admiral, USPHS) in January 1995. As Rear Admiral, Dr. Moore is the highest ranking veterinarian in the United States. Dr. Moore presently serves as the Associate Director for Development Support and African Affairs for the Department of Health and Human Services.

Dr. Moore received his undergraduate and D.V.M. degrees from Tuskegee Institute, his M.P.H. degree in Epidemiology from the University of Michigan, and his Ph.D. in Epidemiology from Johns Hopkins University. Among his many affiliations, Dr. Moore is Assistant Professor and Advisor of Medicine in the Department of Community Health and Family Practice at Howard University. He is an Affiliate Associate Professor of Environmental Health for the University of Washington, Seattle. Dr. Moore serves as a consultant to the School of Veterinary Medicine, Tuskegee University. He has served as President of Friends of the National Zoo in Washington, D.C.

Preface

Complete Preparation for the Veterinary Entrance Tests (formerly known as *The Betz Guide*) is written in an easy-to-understand format as a joint effort of Aftab S. Hassan, Frank Kessler, and Emily Meyer Naegali. The book is based on the teaching experiences of the authors and their perception of verbal reasoning as it relates to verbal ability.

Complete Preparation for the Veterinary Entrance Tests is structured according to a publishing project for the Dental Admission Test (DAT) to help students to understand the level of skills and knowledge required to achieve a high score on the DAT. Leon Anderson, Jr., a professor, DAT preparation teacher, and advisor, joined with Aftab S. Hassan, Ruth Lowe Gordon, and Jeffrey D. Zubkowski to develop the first edition of *Dental College Admission Test: The Betz Guide.*

HOW TO USE THIS GUIDE

This book is designed to help students prepare for entrance into a school of veterinary medicine. It emphasizes practice in reading, quantitative, and study skills; natural science content review; and finally, the test-taking experience.

Chapter 1 includes information for undergraduate or preveterinary students preparing to take the VETs. It emphasizes study skills, time management, memorization techniques, and problem-solving strategies.

Chapters 2, 3, and 5 focus on verbal ability, reading comprehension, and quantitative reasoning, respectively. The sample questions are designed to help students determine how much time they must spend to prepare for the VETs. Developing skills often takes longer than developing a good science knowledge base. Many students underestimate the level of reading skill that is required for a major admission test such as the Veterinary College Admission Test (VCAT) or the Graduate Record Examination (GRE) and overestimate their skills. A mathematics review section is provided in Chapter 5 because mathematics skills decline if they are not used. Practice restores these skills to the level required for the test.

Chapters 4 and 6, respectively, outline the biology and chemistry concepts required for the VETs. Science textbooks should be consulted as necessary.

Chapter 7 describes test-taking skills and strategies for attaining the highest possible score. Finally, Chapter 8 contains a model test.

Organized preparation will help you to prepare for veterinary school. The most effective overall strategy is to learn all of the sections as thoroughly as possible and then to practice what you have learned until your performance is almost automatic. The skills and the science concepts emphasized in this guide are essential for high achievement on the VETs.

ABOUT THE AUTHORS

Leon Anderson, Jr., D.M.D., is an assistant professor of restorative dentistry at the University of Mississippi School of Dentistry. Dr. Anderson earned bachelor and master of science degrees in biology from Jackson State University and a doctor of pharmacy medicine degree from the University of Mississippi School of Dentistry. Dr. Anderson is an attending dentist in restorative dentistry at the University of Mississippi Medical Center and also the director of minority student affairs. He has worked with many allied health professionals in dental hygiene, surgical technology, and laboratory research. For many years, he taught biology in the Jackson public school system. He has written numerous publications and abstracts and serves on the Medical and Pharmacy School Admissions Committee at the University of Mississippi.

Jesse Blankenship, B.S., is a faculty research assistant at the University of Maryland, College Park. Mr. Blankenship earned a bachelor of science degree in biology from the University of South Carolina, Columbia. Mr. Blankenship also worked as a trauma technician at the Maryland Institute for Emergency Medical Services Systems in Baltimore and as the assistant trauma coordinator at the Sinai Hospital of Baltimore. He has received several scholarships and awards for advanced training in cellular and molecular biology and for the laboratory animal science technologist program. He was trained as a veterinary technician at Michigan State University College of Veterinary Medicine and completed the Laboratory Animal Science Technologist training course at New York.

Ruth E. Lowe Gordon, B.S., is an assistant director/education specialist in the Office of Minority Student Affairs, University of Mississippi Medical Center. Ms. Gordon earned a bachelor of science degree in mathematics and science from Alabama State University and did her graduate study at the University of Illinois. Ms. Gordon has been a mathematics teacher in the United States, Ghana, and Scotland. She has worked with premedical and predental training programs and has developed and implemented MCAT and other preprofessional health preparation workshops at undergraduate schools.

Aftab S. Hassan, Ph.D., has a doctorate degree in water resources and hydraulics from Columbia Pacific University (UCLA program). He is also a doctoral scientist in ocean, coastal, and environmental engineering at George Washington University. Dr. Hassan is an education specialist in the health and life sciences and supports active learning and problem-based teaching. He also specializes in hydrodynamics, pollutant transport, and coastal engineering. He was formerly affiliated with George Washington University School of Engineering and Applied Science and with the Department of Community and Family Medicine at Georgetown University, Washington, DC. He has been actively involved in MCAT and DAT teaching for students at Georgetown University and at Charles R. Drew University of Medicine and Science, Los Angeles, California. He has administered active learning workshops, including physician assistant programs, for approximately 20 other schools across the United States. In addition, he has taught, tutored, and advised premedical, medical, and engineering students for more than 20 years.

Frank Kessler, M.A., earned a master's degree in history at Eastern Michigan University. Formerly an assistant professor in history at Virginia State University, Petersburg, Mr. Kessler entered the graduate program in American history at the University of North Carolina. He is currently a reading instructor at the Academic Learning Skills Center, preparing students entering the health professions at the University of North Carolina, Chapel Hill. He has advised international students and has worked as an allied health professional.

Dana Mitchell, B.A., is a natural history instructor and curator at the Center for Educational Achievement at Charles R. Drew University of Medicine and Science, Los Angeles, California. Ms. Mitchell received her bachelor of arts degree in zoology from the University of Minnesota. She taught invertebrate and vertebrate zoology and microbiology at Chaffey College, Rancho Cucamonga, California. She has helped to improve educational opportunities for disadvantaged students by teaching active learning of complex health science courses to elementary and middle school students. Because of her work in teaching, she received the Franklin Hicks Award for Biology and the Chaffey College Life Science Division Award for Excellence. She is also the academic coordinator for the Summer Science Camp and the Saturday Science Academy at Drew Medical School.

Emily Meyer Naegeli, M.A., is an art historian. Ms. Naegeli has bachelor degrees in English and art history from Vanderbilt University and a master of arts degree in art history from Northwestern University. She is involved in the appraisal, cataloging, and research of several private collections. Ms. Naegeli also serves on the Board of the Center for American Archeology. While at Block Gallery, Northwestern University, she worked as an exhibit and catalog researcher and as a lecturer on Chinese ceramics at an exhibition in Chicago.

Jeffrey D. Zubkowski, Ph.D., is an associate professor of chemistry at Jackson State University. Dr. Zubkowski has a bachelor of science degree in chemistry from the University of Pittsburgh and a doctor of philosophy degree in chemistry from Indiana University. He is an associate professor of chemistry at Jackson State University. He has helped students prepare for chemistry (general and organic) requirements for almost all health professions programs. Dr. Zubkowski was a postdoctoral fellow at the University of Toronto, Ontario, Canada, and has written several scientific publications.

ABOUT THE SCIENCE OF REVIEW

Williams & Wilkins is a world-wide leader in medical publishing, offering thousands of publications to keep medical students and professionals informed, educated, and prepared throughout their careers. With the purchase of your first Science of Review product, you join a long tradition of excellence. We are the experts in presenting medical information. No other test preparation company has this focus or expertise. Simply put, we know what you need for success on the VETs, throughout your years in medical school, and in your medical career.

ACKNOWLEDGMENTS

The authors thank third-year medical students Clyde Brown, Rhonda Thigpen, and Ervin Fox, who tested the mathematics problems and evaluated other portions of the manuscript; they also thank Bruttie Jean Allen, Sandra Michael, Kathy Beys, and Susan Kimner, who prepared the manuscript.

1

CHAPTER

Study Skills for the VETs

1.0 INTRODUCTION TO PREVETERINARY PREPARATION

The veterinary entrance tests (VETs), including the Graduate Record Examination (GRE) General Test, GRE Biology Test, Veterinary College Admission Test (VCAT), and Medical College Admission Test (MCAT), require good reading, data interpretation, and scientific reasoning skills. These skills take a long time to develop and cannot be acquired in a month or two of test preparation. For this reason, what students learn in college, high school, and even elementary school classes helps them to prepare for the VETs and the veterinary profession as much as any review manual or review course. In college, it is important to select courses that demand interpretive and inferential reading (e.g., literature, philosophy, history) as well as science courses that require understanding and application of principles and interpretation of data rather than those that demand only memorization. Many schools offer courses to improve study skills.

Read outside your assigned texts, especially newspapers, news magazines, and scientific journals. When you read, practice drawing conclusions, interpreting graphs and charts, predicting trends in data, and evaluating the limitations and errors of the data or opinions stated. When studying biology, apply what you have learned in chemistry or even physics. Humans understand and learn best in complex webs of information, not in isolated facts.

1.1 THE ROLE OF THE VETs IN THE ADMISSION PROCESS

The most widely used VETs are standardized tests designed to measure the cognitive skills and scientific knowledge that are important for veterinary education. As an objective measure, these scores can be reviewed and compared with more lengthy recommendations and the personal interview. Requirements for entrance examinations differ. The entrance requirements for specific schools are listed in the *Veterinary Medical School Admission Requirements* (VMSAR), published by the Association of American Veterinary Medical Colleges.

1.2 VETERINARY ADMISSION PATHWAYS

Admission to veterinary school is usually based on performance on a standardized test (e.g.,GRE General Test, GRE Biology Subject Test, MCAT) coupled with grade point average (GPA). Table 1-1

TABLE 1-1. ***Scores of Students Admitted to Veterinary School***

Test or Measure	Score
Cumulative or overall GPA	2.5–3.5
Average GPA	3.2–3.49
Science GPA or GPA in major	3.0–3.3
GRE General Test score	
Verbal	497–636
Quantitative	517–675
Analytical	594–689
GRE Biology Subject Test score	556–723
MCAT score	
Verbal Reasoning	Above average (> 8)
Physical Sciences	Above average (> 8)
Biological Sciences	Above average (> 8)
Writing Sample	O through T
VCAT score	
Average for all sciences	52–75
Scaled score average	50th percentile

Adapted with permission from Association of American Veterinary Medical Colleges: *Veterinary Medical School Admission Requirements.* Baltimore, Williams & Wilkins, 1996.

shows the general ranges for standardized scores and GPAs of students who were admitted to veterinary school in the last 5 years.

1.3 STUDY SKILLS FOR THE VETs

The best background for taking the VETs is good preparation in high school and college. However, a well-planned review can improve your performance. Test preparation is an opportunity to master the skills and concepts that will provide the solid foundation that you will need as a veterinary student and a practicing veterinarian.

The study strategies provided below can be applied to all portions of the tests. Chapter 7 discusses strategies for managing your preparation time immediately before the test and offers suggestions for the test day.

1.3.1 Make a Study Schedule

Make a realistic, well-planned schedule that allows adequate time to study all natural science subjects. If you dislike a subject, plan to study it first. Make a schedule for each day with a checklist of things to do and a list of tasks completed. If you do not complete an item one day, be sure to complete it the next day. After a few days, evaluate how realistically you estimated your time. Figure 1-1 shows sample checklists.

Course content outlines can be found in the candidate information booklets of the tests that you plan to take. Use these outlines to create your daily schedules. Block out available time for study, and list as specifically as you can what you plan to study during each session. Whenever possible, link your lecture or laboratory class time to test preparation. For example, if you are taking organic chemistry, review while you study for class. Many questions in the organic chemistry subtest integrate laboratory experience with lecture material (e.g., nuclear mangnetic resonance spectroscopy).

THINGS TO DO TODAY

1. Read TIME magazine article on biofeedback instruments.
2. Learn probability concepts.
3. What are orthographic projections? Do library research.
4. Review carboxylic acids and their stereochemistry.
5. Learn differences between virus, viron, bacteriophage and bacteria.
6. Take GRE test for reading comprehension.

THINGS DONE TODAY

1. Read TIME magazine article in a hurry; didn't understand it.
2. Learned probability concepts.
3. Found two references on orthographic projections and 3-D drawings.
4. Took + graded GRE test for reading comprehension.
5. Did some probability problems.
6. Skipped 4+5 on Things To Do Today list due to lack of time, interest + resources.

Figure 1-1 Scheduling with daily checklists.

Even if the time is theoretically available, do not schedule a 12-hour test preparation day. Allow a maximum of 6–8 hours per day for test preparation. If you complete all of the items on your list, practice reading comprehension, science, and mathematics word problems. Improve your verbal abilities by reviewing antonyms, synonyms, and analogies, and building your vocabulary.

Reading comprehension is often the most difficult skill to improve. The best way to improve your reading abilities is to spend more time reading and to read a variety of scientific and technical materials and laboratory reports.

It is best not to schedule study time later than 10:00 P.M., even if you consider yourself a "night person." People learn best when they are fresh, and it is difficult to absorb new information when you are tired.

1.3.2 Develop a Disciplined Approach

Use a disciplined approach when studying scientific concepts. Many students dislike organic chemistry and may not allow adequate time to study this subject. On the day of the test, they may spend too much time on other sections and hurry through the organic chemistry section. This approach will not lead to the highest possible score. Problem-solving and reasoning skills are mastered by repetition and practice.

1.3.3 Use Test Items Efficiently and Effectively

Practice on a small number of items at a time (e.g., one reading passage and follow-up questions, ten test items). To improve your performance, analyze your errors and try to remember the reasoning you used as you worked the problems.

When analyzing your errors, use the answer key first. If you do not understand an answer, refer to the answer analysis section for help.

Keep a record of your errors. Errors can be classified in a number of ways. For example, specific content areas (e.g., genetics problems in biology) as well as specific question formats (e.g., multiple choice) cause some students trouble. A record of your errors can help you to focus on subject areas that need further study and skills that need practice.

As you answer questions, note the emphasis of the test. The outline in the application brochure can provide useful information. For example, you may find that genetics is an important topic, so time spent reviewing mendelian genetics and the application of the Hardy-Weinberg principle would be worthwhile. However, taking a course so that you can answer a single obscure question would not be.

1.3.4 Prepare for the Skills Requirements

Short daily practice sessions in the skills areas of the tests (i.e., reading comprehension, quantitative and scientific reasoning) are better than long, infrequent blocks of sustained practice. Plan to spend 30–45 minutes daily on skills development, perhaps alternating daily among reading comprehension, quantitative reasoning, and verbal ability. Spend more time on the skills that you find difficult.

If you have forgotten the basic mathematics skills used in quantitative reasoning, schedule additional time to review these skills. Scholastic Aptitude Tests (SATs) may be used for additional practice. Old tests are available from bookstores or from the College Board in New York, in books of five and ten tests. It is also good practice to learn how to estimate a reasonable answer. If you usually work with a calculator, stop using it while you are preparing for the VETs.

If the concept of verbal ability as a problem-solving skill is new to you, practice working with antonyms and analogies. When you make an error on the practice material, create similar questions for additional practice.

The easiest way to improve reading skills is simply to read more and pay attention to the underlying assumptions, hypotheses, inferences, and conclusions. In addition to practicing test items, read at least one of the following publications daily: *Time,* the *New York Times* (especially the Tuesday edition, which regularly has a science and education section), *Discover, USA Today, Science,* and veterinary journals such as the *Journal of the American Veterinary Association.* After you read an article, summarize it. For example, explain the author's main points to a friend, form a reading group to discuss articles, or write a 5-minute critical summary. Collect lists of antonyms and analogies.

You can answer questions for the reading comprehension, quantitative reasoning, and verbal ability sections of the test as though they were "warm-up" exercises, or you can use this practice as a break from your science review.

1.3.5 Review the Natural Sciences

After you have assessed your skill levels in reading comprehension, quantitative reasoning, and verbal ability and determined how much time you need to sharpen these skills, you are ready to review biology and general and organic chemistry.

Review at least one topic in each of the three science content areas every day, even if you spend most of your time on only one topic. Do not schedule a week for biology, a week for general chemistry, and a week for organic chemistry, and do not schedule a full day to study one subject. Instead, spend at least some time on each subject each day. You need to commit basic information to long-term memory, and the best technique for developing long-term memory is constant review.

Most people like to work on what they do best and tend to review what they already know. In preparing for the entrance tests, develop strategies to compensate for these natural tendencies. For the most efficient review, study your least favorite subject first. If you schedule a 4-hour block of study time for a given day, divide the time as follows: older content review, new skills review, new content review, and older skills review.

It is essential to divide your study time between content review and skills development. Also, remember that you will be tested on what you review at the beginning of your preparation period as well as on what you review in the weeks immediately before the test; therefore, spend some time each day reviewing the material that you studied earlier as well as new material.

1.3.6 Anticipate Examination-Type Questions: Conceptual Learning

When you study or read, try to formulate examination-type questions and possible responses. For example, for each test item and the corresponding responses, think about what is false, or the exception,

D	Define or describe the concept. [What is molarity? Define molarity and its relation to concentration measurements.]
E	Example of the concept. [Prepare a 0.5 M solution for NaCl, HCl, or NaOH and determine the pH value of the solution.]
F	Find a formula, equation, or sketch for the concept. [Is there an equation for molarity? Is there a formula to find molarity? Can you draw molarity on a volume diagram? Yes, molarity is defined as moles/liter. It can also be drawn as shown.]
IN	Investigate the concept in detail. [Compare and contrast molarity, molality, pH, normality, etc. Relate your findings to usage on the VCAT.]
E	Expand your conceptual horizon by application. [Apply the concept of molarity applied to titration problems; also review acids, bases, and salts.]

Molarity drawing

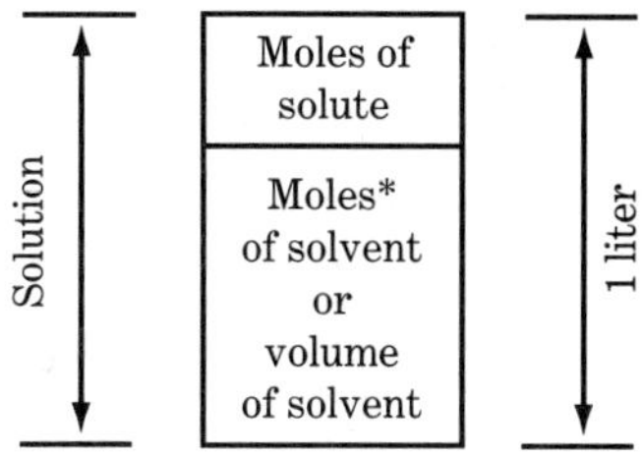

* Density of solvent is required to determine moles.

Figure 1-2 Components of a science concept: D-E-F-IN-E.

and memorize what is true. This approach is especially important when the text provides a concept and one or two examples. The examples are important for understanding, but not for memorization, because the test is not likely to include the same items. Instead, the test will evaluate whether you can understand new examples by applying what you have learned in textbooks or in class. The entire review can be grouped into concepts. Each concept can be learned by identifying and using its five analytical components (Figure 1-2).

1.3.7 Look for Patterns of Error

In an ideal multiple-choice question, student errors are spread evenly across all of the distracters, or incorrect responses. Each distracter ideally represents a typical error that students make. In addition, most people tend to repeat patterns of errors unless they use an intervention strategy.

When you make an error, note your reaction. Many students react with a statement such as, "I always have trouble with Boyle's law." This type of statement is usually followed by a rationalization, such as, "It's not that I don't know it; it's just that the wording of the test item confuses me." It is easy to confuse recognition with knowing or understanding. If you cannot explain a concept clearly to someone who knows it well and can therefore check your reasoning and accuracy, you really do not know it. Use graphic or visual strategies to reinforce each concept.

The first step in correcting error patterns is to recognize them. The second step is to develop a mnemonic, or memory device, that you apply every time you see a related term. For example, it may help you to remember Boyle's law by thinking of a car. As the driver steps on the accelerator, the piston is depressed; as the volume decreases, the pressure increases. If necessary, you can draw a picture in the margin to remind yourself of this concept. It is important to use the mnemonic consistently. Patterns of error tend to be well developed, and they usually cannot be corrected by rote memorization alone.

1.3.8 Develop Your Ability to Concentrate

Taking the VETs requires a full morning of concentrated problem solving involving knowledge and reasoning. Practice applying yourself without a break for an entire morning. Without practice, concentrating on problem solving can be unexpectedly difficult. During the test, the demands for problem solving increase and your concentration may decrease.

To increase your ability to concentrate, begin with an honest self-assessment. Work with a clock in view. Note the time that you begin to work and the time that you would normally take a break. A break can be either conscious or unconscious. Getting a cup of coffee is an example of a conscious break; reading a page or more without knowing what you have read is an unconscious break.

The second step in improving your ability to concentrate is to recognize the need for breaks. Conscious breaks are more productive than unconscious breaks. Commercial television, among other influences, has shortened the concentration span for viewers to brief episodes that fit between advertisements. If you can concentrate for only 15 minutes at a time, then 15 minutes is the baseline from which you can build.

The third step is to increase your ability to concentrate gradually. If you start with 15 minutes, increase to 20 minutes, then 25 minutes, and so on, soon you will be able to work without losing concentration for 2 full hours.

The fourth step is to recognize your strengths and weaknesses. Which subjects are the most difficult for you? What time of day do you concentrate best? When do you find it especially difficult to concentrate? Does the food that you eat affect your ability to concentrate? Do you work better with or without background noise? Does the stress you experience in school or at work affect your level of concentration? Does your study area affect your ability to concentrate?

Concentration requires both endurance and discipline. It helps to limit the time that you plan to work. Avoid scheduling open-ended study sessions (e.g., I'm going to work on this organic chemistry until I've finished it, all night if necessary.). Open-ended study sessions encourage daydreaming. Instead, set a time limit (e.g., I'll allow 2 hours to finish this organic chemistry. If it isn't finished by then, I'll stop for the day.). When the allotted time is up, stop. Limitless sessions encourage a lack of focus, but limiting the time you spend on specific material encourages you to manage your time and concentrate more effectively.

1.3.9 Work With a Study Partner

Find a study partner who is strong in your weak subjects and weak in your strong subjects. If your study partner is having difficulty, you can act as a critical listener. It is the job of the critical listener to make sure that what the speaker says is accurate, complete, and to the point. The student who is weaker in a given topic cannot act as a critical listener for the student who is stronger in that topic. The stronger student should use a textbook, class notes, or course outlines to evaluate his understanding.

1.3.10 Develop Your Long-Term Memory

Compared with students in many other societies, the ability of some American students to memorize information is poor. The American educational system relies heavily on the written word to build information cumulatively. High school science courses build a basis for college courses, and both provide a foundation for veterinary or other professional school. However, little attention is given to developing memory in school. Some students acquire useful strategies accidentally or by trial and error, but there is no formal instruction or guidance.

A cumulative information model of memory distinguishes between long-term memory and short-term, or operational, memory. An example of short-term memory is scheduling a dental appointment. Once you have kept the appointment, you erase the date and time from your memory. When you memorize material without conceptualizing it (e.g., when studying for a test the next day), the information tends to be stored in short-term memory. Immediately after the test, the memory of this information is erased, just as the memory of the date and time of the appointment is erased. Rote memorization alone is a short-term memory technique.

Long-term memory is based on understanding what is read or learned. People tend to retain information that they clearly understand. This understanding forms the basis for subsequent learning. Information that is not fully understood is probably handled by rote memorization and stored in short-term memory.

People also remember best what they enjoy, and they tend to like what they understand. A student who says that he never liked mathematics is really saying that he never fully understood it. This student may have had a poor teacher or a bad classroom experience. Mathematics, science, and Shakespeare are topics that are too broad and important to dismiss with a statement such as, "I never liked it."

Understanding a topic contributes to liking it, and liking it contributes to remembering key concepts. If you dislike a subject, find an area or application that interests you. Connect the topic with a subject that you like. Stating that you dislike a given subject makes learning that subject more difficult.

Understanding information also helps you to build a complex web of information. The most difficult memory task is memorizing a list of discrete and unconnected statements or items. The more connections that can be made between items in a list, the easier it is to memorize. Look for connections or pathways to enhance your ability to learn.

Long-term memory is also enhanced by increasing the ways in which you can absorb and express information. For example, when a student enjoys a course, she tends to discuss it. By talking about the subject, the student reinforces what she has learned, clarifies her conceptual understanding, and increases the precision of her use of details. You can develop these skills by reading difficult material and expressing the information in a simpler way in a letter to a friend.

Immediate review is important for developing long-term memory. Research shows that unless you review what you have read or heard before you go to sleep at night, you will forget more than 90% of it 24 hours later. High school is structured to take advantage of this tendency, because most classes are held each day. However, college classes are held less frequently. Therefore, it is important to review your class notes every night. If you are preparing for the VETs, the same principle applies. Unless you review what you studied each day, you will not remember it. You will still remember the topics that you like and understand, but you may not remember any new information.

Finally, constant use of information contributes to long-term memory. A chemistry teacher knows a great deal about chemistry and can refer to a remarkable amount of information easily without consulting notes or books. She probably works with this material every day, both in lectures and in the laboratory. If she took a break from teaching chemistry for several months, some of this information would fade from her memory. While preparing for the VETs, it is helpful to work with various subject areas every day and to apply this information to solving complex problems.

1.3.11 Distinguish Short-Term From Long-Term Memory Tasks

Ideally, most learning would be long term. For example, learning the function of the circulatory system is a long-term memory task. It requires the student to understand what happens at each step as the blood enters and leaves various chambers of the heart. As the student talks about this process and explains it to his study partner, he is storing it in his long-term memory. Drawing a flow diagram also helps. If the student goes to a grocery store and purchases animal organs, such as a heart and kidneys, he can learn still more. He can hold each organ under a water faucet in the kitchen or bathroom and fill the organ with water. Then the student can observe the shape, size, and texture of the organ and its various parts by cutting it and observing the flow of water. In this way, the student is making a model for blood or fluid circulation. This type of activity can strengthen visual skills, which aid in long-term memory.

When you visit a drugstore and look at the labels of prescription and nonprescription drugs, try to remember the chemical names, symbols, and units of measure for chemical compounds. This exercise will give you real-life experience with chemicals and a basic preparation in stoichiometry. For example, what are the ingredients in aspirin? Can you draw the molecules of the ingredients?

Different approaches to the same topic help you to retain details and understand related concepts. Explaining biologic concepts and repeating review material, along with drawings and observation, improves long-term memory. Repetition and conceptual drawing are keys to long-term learning. Organic chemistry may sound like a difficult subject, but buying plastic model molecules and observing changes in their structure by changing single atoms or groups of atoms is a useful way to learn about it. Three-dimensional perception can be improved tremendously with these organic molecular structures. The concepts of organic chemistry then can become a part of your long-term memory.

Items stored in short-term, or operational, memory are forgotten as soon as they are used. Do not waste time memorizing short-term memory information, such as seldom-used equations or a chart comparing smooth, skeletal, and cardiac muscles, 3 months before the test.

During the last few days of study time, memorize what you have identified as short-term memory tasks. On the test day, take a few minutes to write out short-term memory items so that you can use them without having to concentrate on storing them in your memory.

1.4 REASONING SKILLS FOR TEST PREPARATION

Reasoning skills are needed for the examination subtests, including Reading Comprehension, Verbal and Quantitative Ability, Biology, and Chemistry. The diagramming and reasoning approaches described in this section will help you to prepare for these tests.

1.4.1 Venn Diagrams

Venn, or association, diagrams help to improve the ability to concentrate and focus on important concepts. They help you to recognize and represent the difference between *some* and *all,* and help you to think about what is not as well as what is. A Venn diagram is a visual representation of an outline. Deciding what information belongs in the diagram helps you to understand and conceptualize the important concepts. It is especially important to check what each space represents.

For example: The statement "All roses are red" can be diagrammed as shown in Figure 1-3.

- things that are red
- roses (all red)
- things that are red, but are not roses

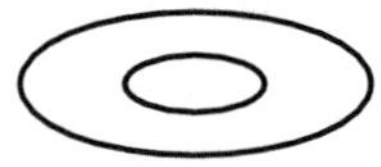

Figure 1-3 Venn diagram.

In a Venn diagram, a circle entirely contained within another circle indicates that all of the members of the inner group belong in the outer group as well. Circles, ovals, or squares may be used to construct Venn diagrams. In Figure 1-3, the inner circle denotes roses (all red), and the outer circle denotes things that are red. In a Venn diagram, only the relation given in the statement is important; for the purpose of the diagram, it does not matter that in real life not all roses are red.

For example: The statement "Some roses are red" can be diagrammed as shown in Figure 1-4.

- roses
- red things

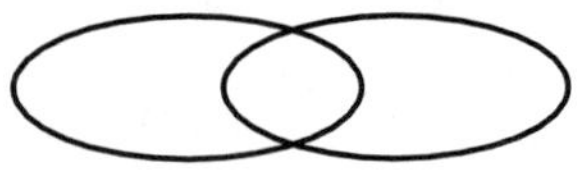

Figure 1-4 Venn diagram.

The lines of the ovals show the relation between red things and roses, only some of which are red. However, the spaces, rather than the lines, show the relations among three categories:

- roses that are not red (the space on the left)
- some roses that are red (the space in the middle)
- red things that are not roses (the space on the right)

For example: The statement "No roses are red" can also be diagrammed as shown in Figure 1-5.

- roses (none of which are red)
- red things (which include no roses)

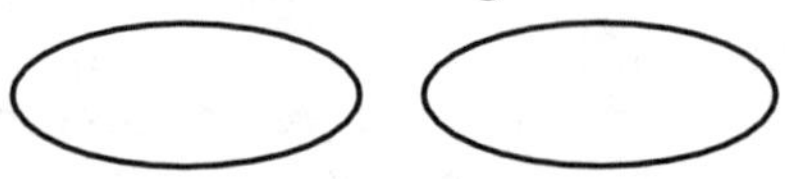

Figure 1-5 Venn diagram.

1.4.2 Exercises

The following exercises can help to strengthen reasoning skills. The more you work with these problems, the more proficient you will become. After you complete the exercises, check the solutions shown in Figures 1-6, 1-7, and 1-8.

Exercise 1. Draw a Venn diagram to illustrate the relations between the following words:

(A) mothers
daughters
grandmothers
aunts

(B) animals
dogs
cats
domestic animals

Note: Exercise 1(A) is not an easy relation to diagram. It is easiest to start with mothers and daughters. Any circle contained within another circle indicates that all of its members belong to both groups. After that relation is represented by a Venn diagram, a circle is added for grandmothers; then one is added for aunts.

Exercise 2. Read the following passage, and draw a Venn diagram to illustrate the relations between the words listed at the end of the passage.

Passage 1

Carbohydrates have the general formula $C_n(H_2O)_m$, where n and m are whole numbers. Monosaccharides are the basic units of carbohydrates. They are classified by the number of carbons they contain, i.e., hexoses (C_6), pentoses (C_5). Hexoses and pentoses exist in predominantly ring forms called pyranoses (six-membered rings) or furanoses (five-membered rings) in equilibrium with the open-chain forms. Ring forms are hemiacetals; open-chain forms are polyhydroxyl aldehydes. In the ring forms, a (alpha) or b (beta) anomers are possible. The pyranoses exist in the stable chair conformation with most, if not all, of the hydroxyls in equatorial positions. When two monosaccharides differ by the configuration of one hydroxyl group, they are called epimers. If n is the number of asymmetric carbons, then 2^n is the number of optical isomers (based on an open-chain form).

Hexoses usually have $n = 4$, and pentoses usually have $n = 3$. Sugars are given a relative configuration on the basis of the orientation of the next to last carbon's hydroxyl group as compared to D-glyceraldehyde. Most naturally occurring sugars have the D configuration. A ketose is a carbohydrate with a ketone group; an aldose has an aldehyde group.

Monosaccharides bond to form disaccharides. The new bond is called a glycosidic bond and is between the hemiacetal carbon and a hydroxyl group of the other sugar; water is released when the bond is formed. Hydrolysis (breaking) of the bond requires water. The glycosidic bond is an acetal grouping. Sucrose (common sugar) is made of glucose and fructose. Lactose (milk sugar) is made of galactose and glucose. Maltose (a-1,4 bond) is made of two glucose units and is a hydrolysis product of starch or glycogen. Cellobiose (b-1,4 bond) is also made of two glucoses, and it is the breakdown product of the cellulose.

Polysaccharides are many monosaccharides joined by glycosidic bonds; they may also be branched. Starch (plant energy storage), glycogen (animal short-term energy storage), and cellulose (plant structural component) are all made from glucose. Cellulose has b-1,4 bonds not found in the other two. Starch and glycogen both have a-1,4 bonds, but differ in the frequency and position of branch points (alpha-1,6 bond).

Insulin is a polymer of fructose.

Adapted with permission from *A Complete Preparation for the MCAT*. Baltimore, Williams & Wilkins, 1995.

- carbohydrates
- monosaccharides
- disaccharides
- starch

- glucose
- polysaccharides
- fructose
- sucrose
- lactose
- maltose
- cellobiose
- glycogen
- cellulose

Exercise 3. The following exercises offer additional practice in constructing Venn diagrams. Check your answers in reference books.

(A) Draw a Venn diagram to illustrate the characteristics of eukaryotic and prokaryotic cells.
(B) Draw a Venn diagram to illustrate the relations between isomers, stereoisomers, and enantiomers.
(C) Draw a Venn diagram to illustrate the relation between diasteromers and meso compounds.

1.5 REASONING SKILLS

Developing reasoning skills can improve your understanding of the material you study and can improve test performance.

1.5.1 Analytical Reasoning

Analysis is breaking something down into its components. This concept applies to chemical analysis as well as textual analysis. Taking notes in class is one way to use analytical reasoning. An effective note taker identifies the main points and the supporting details and uses an outline to indicate the relation between the two. Underlining is also a tool for analyzing text. A good student selectively underlines key words. At the same time, she makes notes in the margin or uses numbers to indicate the relations between the components. Analysis identifies significant terms, often nouns, or pieces of information, but the work is incomplete unless the relation of the part to the whole is recognized.

If analysis involves identifying key nouns as indicators of primary and secondary information, reasoning often requires focusing on words that a careless or hurried reader may overlook. These are qualifying words, such as *always, some, for example, most likely, probably, however, consequently, as a result of,* and *or,* as distinguished from *and.* These words are the traffic lights and road signs for reading. As you work practice test items, circle these qualifying words and think about what they tell you (e.g., how to proceed, what to look for, which stored information is relevant).

Two books are recommended to strengthen your analytical skills: *Problem Solving and Comprehension* and *How to Study in College.* To build your reasoning skills, you can use the practice items in any manual that prepares students to take the Law School Admission Test (LSAT) or the GRE.

1.5.2 Synthetic Reasoning

Learning is incomplete unless analysis is followed by synthesis. Can you summarize the main points in a textbook chapter? Can you write class notes in complete sentences? Can you clearly explain a concept (e.g., entropy) to a friend who may not understand it? These activities require you to synthesize what you have learned. Synthesis is the test, or proof, of your learning. In addition, you can synthesize facts from various subjects to construct new possibilities (e.g., human physiology may be seen in light of what you know about physics, chemistry, and biology). When memorizing concepts, try to link key words. Thus, the words *synapse, axon, neuron, dendrite, effector organ,* and *neurotransmitter* belong together and should be associated in your memory to provide an interrelated web of information. For practice, make a list of words to memorize in association with *pancreatic duct,* and check the accuracy of your list in reference books.

1.5.3 Associative Reasoning

Associative reasoning is a tool used to improve memory by considering similar, or analogous, situations. For example, it is easier to remember the items on a list if you associate them with something you know well, such as the rooms in your house.

By comparing an unfamiliar concept with a familiar idea, associative reasoning allows students to transfer concepts from one subject to another, as in learning biology principles within a chemistry framework. For example, does the movement of blood inside veins and arteries relate to the chemical structure of hemoglobin in organic chemistry? Can you create an analogy between biologic cells and chemical cells?

Scientists often use analogies to enhance their understanding of new or unfamiliar ideas. It is not by accident that the discovery of the structure of DNA occurred as a dream of two snakes coiled around each other.

1.5.4 Comparative Reasoning

Associative reasoning leads naturally to comparison and contrast. Normally, people compare things that are similar in some ways and dissimilar in others. For example, no one compares an orange and a truck, but textbooks compare smooth and skeletal muscles or afferent and efferent nerves. When two items are compared and contrasted, the information must be organized so that the features of the items are not confused (e.g., the functions of the liver and the spleen).

Many students find comparison and contrast questions difficult. Part of the reason for this difficulty is the tendency to read textbooks passively. One way to develop the skills needed to compare and contrast items or ideas effectively is to read actively, for example, by constructing a chart whenever a textbook compares and contrasts two or more items (e.g., liquids, solids,and gases; eukaryotic and prokaryotic cells).

Exercise 4. List the similarities and differences between the items listed in each group. Check your answers against information in a reference book or textbook.

(A) electrolytic, galvanic, and concentration cells
(B) heterozygous and homozygous genes
(C) period and group for the atomic table
(D) entropy and enthalpy

1.5.5 Intuitive Reasoning

Using imagination, or intuitive reasoning, to solve problems is a skill that cannot be taught or tested. The imagination makes an intuitive leap that is usually instantaneous and produces a solution that was not logically apparent. Thus, a physician might make a preliminary diagnosis that is systematically confirmed with further questions, examination, or tests. The scientist who discovered how stars age made an intuitive connection between aging stars and humans.

You can learn more about using intuition by reading. Suggested books include: *Drawing on the Right Side of the Brain*, which can help to develop creativity, and *Unicorns are Real: A Right-Brained Approach to Learning*, which describes individual learning styles.

1.5.6 Visual Reasoning

Experimental evidence shows that young infants can reason visually well before they acquire language. The ability to reason visually is the key to solving many science problems.

Visual reasoning skills are directly tied to perceptual abilities, which can be developed both directly and indirectly. Direct observation of mechanisms or processes reinforces mental images of them. Sketching large objects (e.g., bioreactors, houses, trains) develops visual insight and the ability to simplify details. Indirect observation involves imagining mechanisms, molecules, or systems (e.g., drawing a sketch to illustrate words or concepts such as antigen—antibody interactions, pressure, or the path of a bolus of food through the digestive system). Both direct and indirect observation lead to improved perception. The following exercise can help to develop visual reasoning skills.

Exercise 5. Picture a first-floor apartment and a sixth-floor apartment in the same building. Which apartment is likely to have better water pressure in the shower? Why? Which apartment is likely to have better bathtub drainage? Why? How could water pressure or drainage be improved?

Exercise 6. Visualize the Krebs cycle. Explain in one sentence what causes the cycle to work.

Exercise 7. Draw the molecules of epimers and anomers to help you to conceptualize them.

1.5.7 Logical Reasoning

Because it is concerned with proof, logical reasoning is associated with the development of science and scientific methods. Logical reasoning provides a systematic means of testing or proving a hypothesis or conclusion. Conclusions have three degrees of certainty—hypothesis, conclusion suggested, and conclusion confirmed—and may be valid or invalid.

Many books describe the formal rules of logic and provide practice exercises. A recommended text is *With Good Reason: An Introduction to Informal Fallacies.*

1.5.8 Quantitative Reasoning

Quantitative reasoning is the ability to estimate a reasonable answer before calculating it. Unfortunately, many people have have poor skills in this area, partially because of the widespread use of calculators. Students are not permitted to use calculators while taking the VETs, so it is a good idea to practice estimating quantities without using a calculator while preparing for these tests.

A student uses quantitative reasoning when she performs mathematical operations mentally. This type of reasoning is also used to translate words into numbers and numbers into words (e.g., creating a graph showing employment trends in a geographic area).

1.5.9 Proportional Reasoning

Proportional reasoning is used to solve problems in biology and chemistry, such as determining the flow of blood in arteries or veins of varying diameters. This type of reasoning is also used to measure changes in one variable relative to another, for example, in problems applying Boyle's law. Blood pressure and concentration problems often require proportional reasoning. Questions about population tables or charts also may require this type of reasoning.

Proportional reasoning is often aided by visualization, or the ability to picture the elements of a problem (see section 1.5.6). Making a schematic drawing in the margin may be helpful.

1.5.10 Solutions

Exercise 1(A). In Figure 1-6*A*, the outer circle represents daughters because all mothers are daughters, but daughters are not necessarily all mothers. The space between the two circles represents daughters who are not mothers. In Figure 1-6*B*, circles have been added to represent aunts and grandmothers.

Exercise 1(B). Domestic animals may include cats, dogs, or both, as shown in Figure 1-7.

Exercise 2. The Venn diagram is fairly complex, as shown in Figure 1-8.

1.6 ACTIVE PROBLEM-BASED LEARNING

Problem-based learning requires assessment of a situation and identification of the cause of the problem. Examples include a mechanic who is attempting to determine why a car is stalling and a teacher who wonders why a student is having trouble learning algebra.

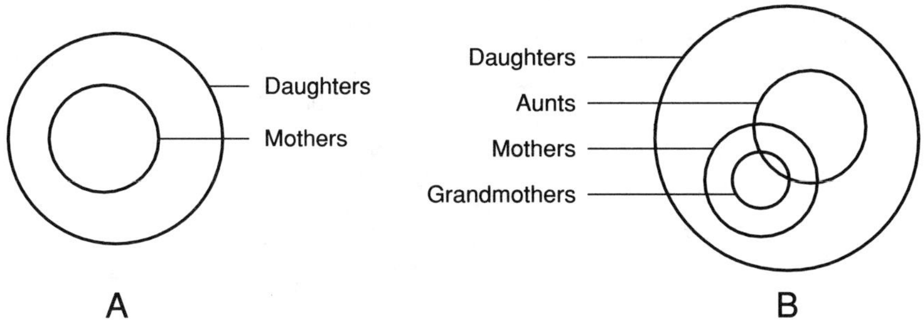

Figure 1-6*A* and *B* Solution to Exercise 1(A).

Figure 1-7 Solution to Exercise 1(B).

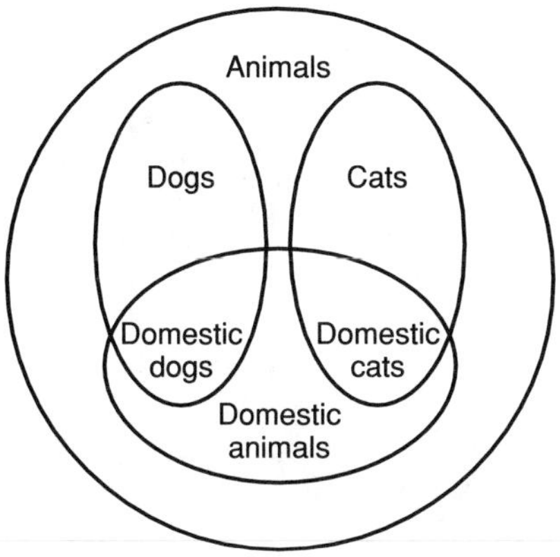

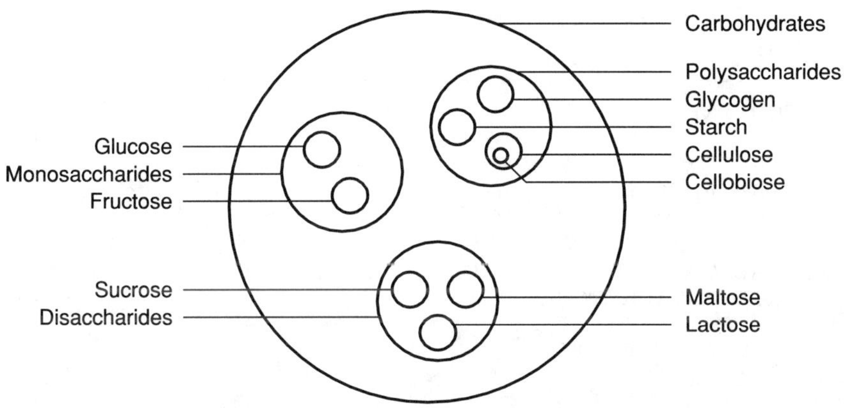

Figure 1-8 Solution to Exercise 2.

Two case studies are presented for analysis. Answering the questions will require reasoning and problem-solving skills. You may want to discuss the answers in a study group session. You can practice analyzing more case histories by visiting animal hospitals, animal shelters, or the zoo, and by watching *National Geographic* on the Discovery Channel.

Case 1. Figure 1-9 shows a receipt for products purchased at a pet shop. Use this receipt to answer the following questions:

1. Name the pet products listed on the attached receipt, and describe one function of each product.
2. Was any discount given on the pet supplies?
3. Who was the UNQ Pig Ear Treat purchased for?

```
# 12113 UNQ PIG EAR TREAT 12 PACK
  1 @      9.99                      9.99T
# 13128 SIERRA HUTCH          LRG
  1 @    169.99                    169.99T
 10.00 PERCENT DISCOUNT            -16.99
# 13134 SIERRA HUTCH PAN KIT  LRG
  1 @     49.99                     49.99T
 10.00 PERCENT DISCOUNT             -4.99
# 12113 UNQ PIG EAR TREAT 12 PACK
- 1 @     -9.99                      9.99T
# 12113 UNQ PIG EAR TREAT 12 PACK
  1 @      9.99                     -9.99T
 10.00 PERCENT DISCOUNT              -.99
#    30 PET SUPPLIES
  1 @      5.00                      5.00T
# 80234 REDI MIN/SALT WHL
  1 @    1.49                        1.49T
 10.00 PERCENT DISCOUNT              -.14
# 80232 REDI SALT WHEEL
  1 @    1.49                        1.49T
 10.00 PERCENT DISCOUNT              -.14
# 80078 FAR RABBIT BOTTLE    32 oz
  1 @      6.99                      6.99T
 10.00 PERCENT DISCOUNT              -.69
----                            ----------
  7                  SUBTOTAL      221.00
                    SALES TAX       18.23
                                ----------
                        TOTAL      239.23
                         CASH      240.00
                                ----------
                       CHANGE         .77

CLERK NUMBER 7
```

Figure 1-9 Receipt for pet supplies.

```
--------------------------------------------------------------------------------
PATIENT ID:  1             SPECIES:  RABBIT      WEIGHT:                SEX:  MALE
PATIENT NAME:  SHADOW      BREED:  RABBIT        BIRTHDAY:  07-94
--------------------------------------------------------------------------------
MAY 15 1995    EXAMINATION - ROUTINE                              $    29.50
               INJECTION                                                19.00
               INJECTION                                                 0.00
               HOSPITALIZATION AVIAN/S EXOTIC                           25.00
               INTENSIVE CARE UNIT (1/2)                                 7.50
               OXYGEN THERAPY                               120         30.00
               DAILY PROFESSIONAL CARE                                   0.00
MAY 16 1995    MEDICATION ADMINISTRATION/DOSE                 2          0.00
               FLUIDS SUBCUTANEOUS/INPATIENT                            16.00
               HOSPITALIZATION AVIAN/S EXOTIC                           25.00
               INTENSIVE CARE UNIT (1/2)                      2         15.00
               OXYGEN THERAPY                               120         30.00
               X-RAY ONE VIEW                                           50.00
               DAILY PROFESSIONAL CARE                                   0.00
MAY 17 1995    MEDICATION ADMINISTRATION/DOSE                 2          0.00
               HOSPITALIZATION AVIAN/S EXOTIC                            0.00
               INTENSIVE CARE UNIT (1/2)                                 7.50
               DAILY PROFESSIONAL CARE                                   0.00
                         ---------------------------------------------------
                         PATIENT SUBTOTAL:                        $   254.50

                                                                  ----------
                         TOTAL INVOICE:                           $   254.50
                         BALANCE DUE:                             $   254.50
                                                                  ==========
```

A

Figure 1-10*A–C*. Invoices for veterinary services.

```
--------------------------------------------------------------------------------
PATIENT ID:  1          SPECIES:  RABBIT           WEIGHT:           SEX:  MALE
PATIENT NAME:  SHADOW  BREED:  LOP, AMERICAN FUZZY BIRTHDAY:  07-94
--------------------------------------------------------------------------------
               BOARDING EXOTIC/SMALL AVIAN                           $      7.50
               MEDICATION ADMINISTRATION/DOSE                 2             4.00
               DAILY PROFESSIONAL CARE                                      0.00
               BAYTRIL ORAL 1/2 OZ                                         11.25
               GENTOCIN OPTHALMIC DROPS                                     9.27
                                  ----------------------------------------------
                                   PATIENT SUBTOTAL:                 $     32.02


                                                                      ----------
                                   TOTAL INVOICE:                    $     32.02
                                   PREVIOUS BALANCE:                 $    254.50
                                                                      ----------
                                   BALANCE DUE:                      $    286.52
                                                                      ==========
```

B

```
--------------------------------------------------------------------------------
PATIENT ID:  1          SPECIES:  RABBIT           WEIGHT:           SEX:  MALE
PATIENT NAME:  SHADOW  BREED:  LOP, AMERICAN FUZZY BIRTHDAY:  07-94
--------------------------------------------------------------------------------
               BOARDING EXOTIC/SMALL AVIAN                           $      7.50
               MEDICATION ADMINISTRATION/DOSE                 3             6.00
               DAILY PROFESSIONAL CARE                                      0.00
                                  ----------------------------------------------
                                   PATIENT SUBTOTAL:                 $     13.50


                                                                      ----------
                                   TOTAL INVOICE:                    $     13.50
                                   PREVIOUS BALANCE:                 $    286.52
                                                                      ----------
                                   BALANCE DUE:                      $    300.02
                                                                      ==========
```

C

Figure 1-10 *(continued)*

Case 2. A man has a pet male rabbit called Shadow. On May 15, 1995, Shadow was taken to the veterinarian for a routine examination. Shadow now seems sick, and the owner brings him to you for an evaluation. He gives you the invoices shown in Figure 1-10*A–C*. You begin your evaluation by identifying all of the treatments and examinations that the rabbit underwent. Answer the following questions:

1. Where was the rabbit kept from May 15, 1995, through May 17, 1995? Why?
2. What tests were performed?
3. Why was the rabbit kept in the intensive care unit?
4. What medications were given to the rabbit?
5. What do you think was wrong with Shadow?

REFERENCES

American Veterinary Medical Association: *Today's Veterinarian*. Schaumburg, IL, AVMA, 1987.

American Veterinary Medical Association: *Your Career in Animal Technology.* Schaumburg, IL, AVMA, 1987.

Atkinson RH, Longman DG: *Reading Enhancement and Development.* St. Paul, MN, West, 1995.

Boyd L (ed): *Zoological Parks and Aquariums in the Americas, 1988-89*. Wheeling, American Association of Zoological Parks and Aquariums.
Duncan JC: *Careers in Veterinary Medicine*. New York, Rosen Group, 1988.
Educational Testing Service: *Directory of Graduate Programs: 1988-89.* Princeton, NJ, ETS.
Educational Testing Service: *Graduate Record Examinations: Annual Descriptions of the Subject Tests.* Princeton, NJ, ETS, 1995.
Educational Testing Service: *Practicing to Take the GRE Subject Tests.* Princeton, NJ, ETS.
Harris AJ, Sipay ER: *How to Increase Reading Ability*. White Plains, NY, Longman, 1985.
Lee MP, Lee R: *Opportunities in Animal and Pet Care Careers.* Lincolnwood, IL, National Textbook, 1984.
Miller LL: *Increasing Reading Efficiency*. Fort Worth, TX, Holt, Rinehart, & Winston, 1984.
Quinn S, Irvings S: *Active Reading in the Arts and Sciences,* 2nd ed. Boston, Allyn and Bacon, 1991.
The Psychological Corporation: *Veterinary College Admission Testing Program* candidate information booklet. San Antonio, TX, The Psychological Corporation, 1995.
Whimbey A, Lochhead J: *Problem Solving and Comprehension.* Hillsdale, NJ, Lawrence Erlbaum Associates, 1994.

2
CHAPTER

Developing Verbal Ability for the VETs

2.0 INTRODUCTION

As discussed in Chapter 1, the skills needed for the VETs are developed over the course of a student's academic career and cannot be learned during a few months of review. However, you can improve your performance on the VETs by following the suggestions offered in this chapter and especially by completing the sample test items.

2.1 WHAT VERBAL ABILITY MEASURES

Verbal skills are essential for professional success. Effective communication requires a good vocabulary and the ability to express ideas clearly and precisely as well as the ability to understand others.

Antonym, synonym, and analogy questions measure vocabulary and the ability to analyze the meanings of words. Answering these questions requires the ability to match similar and opposite concepts, form conclusions about word relations, and categorize ideas, structures, and concepts.

2.1.1 Types of Questions

Antonym questions require you to choose one word, from a list of four choices, with a meaning most nearly opposite that of the given, capitalized word.

Synonym questions require you to chose one word, from a list of four possible answers, with a meaning most nearly the same as the given, capitalized word. To answer these questions, you must know precise definitions and shades of meaning (e.g., *flaming, warm, tepid,* and *hot* are all related terms, but only one is similar in meaning to *cozy*).

Analogies are sets of word pairs that describe a similar, or analogous, relation. Analogy questions require you to choose one word, from a list of four possible answers, that best completes the second word pair by expressing the same relation as the given word pair.

2.1.2 Time Allotment

You have a limited amount of time to complete each section. Because they are more complex, analogy questions generally take longer to answer than antonym or synonym questions. In addition to having a working knowledge of the dictionary definitions of the words, to answer analogy questions, you must extrapolate a relation between the words. Because each question scores the same value, you should spend less time on the relatively easy questions, saving time for the more difficult ones.

Mastering the following strategies can help to increase speed. Building vocabulary is done most effectively in frequent, small increments, perhaps 10 words at a time. It is better to concentrate on expanding your working knowledge of the multiple meanings of words that you know than to memorize lists of unknown words.

2.2 ANTONYMS

2.2.1 Answering Antonym Questions

The correct answer is the word most nearly opposite in meaning to the given word. In most cases, one of the answer choices is a synonym of the given word. If you can identify the synonym, you can eliminate it as a potential answer.

Many words do not have an exact opposite. The correct answer is the word that is most nearly opposite the given word in meaning.

Try to place the capitalized word in context by thinking of a sentence or phrase in which it might be used. Even if you are not sure of its exact definition, you will have a sense of its meaning. If you cannot think of a sentence immediately, try another strategy to determine the meaning of the given word.

English contains many words that differ only slightly in meaning. Context phrases can help you to identify the best use of the given word.

Many words, especially nouns and verbs, have more than one meaning. Some words even have opposite meanings, depending on the context. *Sanguine,* for example, can mean either murderous or optimistic, in addition to red.

If you know the given word, try to identify an antonym before you read the choices. You can then look for the answer that is most similar in meaning to your antonym. If none of the answers provided matches the antonym you selected, think of alternate meanings and contexts suggested by the answer choices.

Identify the prefix, root, and suffix of the given word, especially if it is not familiar. Read each answer carefully, noting its spelling and part of speech. Many words are easily confused (e.g., *ingenuous* and *ingenious*), and one letter sometimes makes a difference.

2.2.2 Unfamiliar Words

Sound out the unfamiliar word. Identify its root and any prefixes or suffixes. Use the clues from these elements to guess the meaning of the word. For example, if the word has a negative prefix (e.g., mal-, dis-, non-), look for a positive element (e.g., bene-, eu-, -ful) in the answer list.

If you can identify the elements of a word, but not their meaning, think of familiar words that contain the same elements.

Sometimes a complicated given word has a simple antonym. Some simple words can be misleading. Read carefully, and consider alternate meanings.

For example:

IRREFRAGABILITY
A. expulsion
B. equivocality
C. incontestability
D. fragrant
ir—re—frag—abil—ity (broken into elements)

Although you may not know this word, you can begin to decode it. The suffixes indicate that it is a noun, having to do with a quality or characteristic. The prefix irr- is negative (e.g., irresponsible, irritating, irresistible). The prefix re- means again. The root, frag, appears in such words as fragment, meaning broken part. You can now approximate the meaning of *irrefragability:* "not-again-break-able-ness," or something similar to permanence, reliability, or decisiveness. Its opposite might be uncertainty or vagueness. "The irrefragability of the research conclusions" and "the irrefragability of the evidence" are possible context phrases.

If a first reading of the answer list does not yield a definite choice, eliminate any choices that do not have clear opposites, such as *fragrant. Fragrant* can also be eliminated because, although it appears to contains the root, frag, it has nothing to do with the meanings of the components. *Incontestability* is similar to the meaning derived from the components of the given word, and can therefore be eliminated because the correct answer must have the opposite meaning. It also has a negative prefix, in-, and is therefore unlikely to be the antonym of a word with a negative prefix. Of the remaining choices, *expulsion* can be eliminated, even if you do not know its meaning, because it has a negative prefix, ex-, and because it is not a noun related to quality, as demanded by the suffixes of *irrefragability.* The only remaining choice is *equivocality,* meaning vagueness, imprecision, or uncertainty. You may, of course, have deduced the meaning of this word by breaking it down into its elements, equi- (same) and vocal (voice).

The best way to achieve a high score on this section of the test is to acquire a broad and varied vocabulary. When a word is unfamiliar, however, following these suggestions aids in solving the puzzles that antonym questions can pose.

2.3 SYNONYMS

2.3.1 Answering Synonym Questions

Synonym questions are often easier to answer than antonym questions because many words do not have clear opposites.

The correct answer is the word or phrase that is closest in meaning to the given word. The answer must be the best available choice. Some questions may seem to have several possible answers, but there is only one whose meaning most closely matches that of the given word.

Often, one answer choice is an antonym of the given word. Identifying and eliminating this word can help you to clarify the meaning of the given word.

Try to place the capitalized word in context by thinking of a sentence or phrase in which it might be used. Even if you are not sure of the exact meaning of the word, you will have a sense of how it is used. If you cannot think of a sentence quickly, try another strategy.

English contains many words that differ only slightly in meaning. Context phrases can help you to identify the best uses of the given word.

Many words, especially nouns and verbs, have more than one meaning. Some words even have opposite meanings, depending on the context.

Identify the prefix, root, and suffix of the given word, especially if it is not familiar. Read each answer carefully, noting its spelling and part of speech. Many words are easily confused, and one letter can make a difference.

2.3.2 Unfamiliar Words

Sound out unfamiliar words. Identify the root, prefixes, and suffixes. The clues from these elements can help you to determine the meaning of the word.

If you can identify the elements of a word, but do not know their meaning, think of words that you know that contain the same elements.

Some complicated words have simple synonyms. Some words are not as simple as they appear. Read all given words and answer choices carefully, and consider alternate meanings.

2.4 ANALOGIES

2.4.1 Types of Analogies

Most analogies are of one of two word types:

NOUN:NOUN pairs, such as LEAF:TREE or ICE:RAIN
or
NOUN:ADJECTIVE pairs, such as SANDPAPER:ROUGH or OVEN:HOT

Occasionally, verbs are included in analogies, such as COW:MOO or BIRD:MOLT

Some analogies are ADJECTIVE:ADJECTIVE pairs, such as HAPPY:SAD or HAIRY:BALD

2.4.2 Common Relations Used in Analogies

Analogies can be classified into several common types. However, other types are possible, and sometimes categories overlap. It is helpful to practice using and recognizing the following types of pairings until you are comfortable with each category.

1. CHARACTERISTIC
   One word describes a characteristic of the other. For example:

diamond:hard	(A diamond is a hard substance.)
owl:wise	(An owl is said to be wise. Note: The characteristic may be fictional.)
sharp:knife	(A knife is usually sharp. Note: The order of the pair may be reversed.)

2. TYPE, OR KIND
   One word is a type of the other. For example:

salmon:fish	(A salmon is a type of fish.)
maze:puzzle	(A maze is a type of puzzle.)
shell:home	(A shell is a type of home or shelter. Note: Some words can be used as either nouns or verbs. Compare the words in the answer choices to determine their usage.)

3. DEGREE
   One word shows a decrease or increase in action or quality. For example:

drizzle:downpour	(A drizzle is a light rain; a downpour is a heavy shower.)
ecstatic:content	(Ecstatic means overjoyed; content is a milder state of pleasure.)
nibble:devour	(To nibble is to eat sparingly; to devour is to consume ravenously.)

4. PART TO WHOLE
   One word is a part, or component, of the other. For example:

sentence:paragraph	(A sentence is a part of a paragraph.)
comb:teeth	(Teeth are part of a comb. Note: The order of the words may be reversed.)
purple:blue	(Blue is a component of the color purple. Note: It is easy to be misled by associations based on similarity. Some relations require more analysis.)

5. PURPOSE, OR FUNCTION
   One word is a function of or has a use for the other. For example:

garage:car	(A garage is a place to store a car.)
pen:write	(A pen is used to write.)
towel:dry	(A towel is used to dry things.)

6. SEQUENCE
   One word is an earlier or later stage of the other. For example:

acorn:oak	(An acorn is the beginning state of an oak tree. Note: Sequence relations can easily be confused with type or degree relations. Read all answer choices to determine the correct relation.)
dusk:dawn	(Dawn is the beginning of the day; dusk is the end.)
crawl:walk	(A baby learns to crawl before he learns to walk.)

7. CAUSE AND EFFECT
One word is either the cause or the effect of the other. For example:

crime:punishment	(A crime leads to punishment.)
height:dizziness	(Height can cause dizziness.)
scar:cut	(A scar is caused by a cut.)

8. TOOL OR INSTRUMENT
One word is a tool for the other. For example:

scalpel:surgeon	(A scalpel is used by a surgeon.)
voice:ventriloquist	(A ventriloquist uses her voice to perform.)
score:musician	(A score is used by a musician.)

9. ANTONYMS
One word is the opposite, or nearly the opposite, of the other. For example:

laugh:cry	(Laughter is associated with happiness; crying is a sign of the opposite emotion, sadness.)
high:low	(High is the opposite of low.)
prefix:suffix	(Prefixes and suffixes are used at opposite ends of a word.)

10. SYNONYMS
The words have similar, or nearly the same, meaning. For example:

stray:wander	(To stray means to wander.)
abundant:plentiful	(Something that is abundant is in large supply, or plentiful.)
forgery:counterfeit	(Both forgery and counterfeit describe something that is faked.)

11. ASSOCIATION
One word is symbolically associated with the other. For example:

red:anger	(The color red is used to represent anger.)
shamrock:luck	(A shamrock is used to symbolize good luck.)
robin:spring	(The arrival of robins is associated with the arrival of spring. Note: Word order may be reversed.)

12. NONSEMANTIC
One word is related to the other by something other than its meaning, such as sound, spelling, or form. For example:

see:sea	(These words are homophones: They are pronounced alike despite different meanings.)
eat:tea	(Eat and tea are anagrams: Their letters are rearranged.)
sit:sat	(Sit is present tense; sat is past tense.)

2.4.3 Answering Analogy Questions

State the relation between the words in the given word pair in a sentence. Recognizing the proper relation depends on the ability to define each word. Consider a variant meaning or context if you cannot construct a simple sentence to illustrate the relation of the pair.

For example:

PHRASE:SENTENCE ::
PARAGRAPH :
A. essay
B. structure
C. theme
D. grammar

Describe the relation between the given words in a short sentence. Visualize how the first word relates to the second word. What does a phrase do in or to a sentence? Which common relation form does this question seem to use? For example, is a *phrase* a degree, cause or effect, or part of a *sentence*? A *phrase* is part of a sentence. Therefore, this analogy is a part-to-whole relation.

Read the third capitalized word, and substitute it and each of the answer choices in turn in the sentence. Which answer choice could a *paragraph* be part of?

A. A *paragraph* is part of an *essay*? Yes, an essay is a short literary composition.
B. A *paragraph* is part of a *structure*? No, a structure is the configuration of a composition of elements.
C. A *paragraph* is part of a *theme*? No, a theme is a topic of discourse or discussion.
D. A *paragraph* is part of a *grammar*? No, grammar is the system of language rules.

Only answer choice A, *essay*, fits this relation sentence. If all of the answers were eliminated by this process, the next step would be to formulate a more specific relation between the given words and then to create a new sentence.

Check the order of relation between the given words. The same order of relation must be used in the given word pair and the answer choice pair. Part-to-whole relations are not the same as whole-to-part relations. Cause and effect relations are not the same as effect and cause relations. This common mistake occurs especially when the analogy question is read quickly.

For example:

MONTH : YEAR ::
MINUTE :
A. second
B. hour
C. season
D. time

This example is a sequence analogy. A *month* is shorter span of time than a *year*. In choice A, a *second* is a shorter span of time than a *minute*, but because the direction of the relation stated in the given word pair is reversed, this answer is not correct. In choice B, an *hour* is a longer amount of time than a *minute*, so this answer is correct. Choices C and D are associated with time as well, but are not specific units of time and thus can be eliminated.

Do not confuse similar relations.

For example:

MILK : YOGURT ::
GRAPES :
A. raisins
B. fruit
C. champagne
D. fermentation

This example is a cause and effect analogy. *Yogurt* is the effect of fermentation on *milk*. The correct answer is choice C, *champagne*. *Champagne* is the effect of fermentation on *grapes*. In choice A, *raisins* are also the product of *grapes*, but the cause and effect relation is different: *Raisins* are the effect of dehydration on grapes. Choice B, *fruit*, would be correct only if this question represented a type analogy. Choice D, *fermentation,* is the process that creates *yogurt* from *milk*, but it does not have the correct relation to *grapes*.

Be aware of multiple meanings.

For example:

BEAR : REJECT ::
SHOULDER :
A. carry
B. shun
C. border
D. bone

In this example, each word has multiple meanings. For example, as a verb, *bear* could mean to support, to produce, to endure, to display, to press, or to turn. Reading the complete analogy shows that *bear* is defined here as a verb meaning to support or maintain. *Reject* is defined as a verb meaning to refuse. Therefore, the given word pair has an antonym relation: To *bear* is the opposite of to *reject*. Likewise, *shoulder* is defined as a verb meaning to assume or undertake. Therefore, the antonym of *shoulder* is choice B, *shun*.

Read all of the choices carefully. Even if you believe that you have identified the correct answer, examine the other answer choices to ensure that you are not overlooking a better choice. Test each answer in the relation sentence to avoid careless mistakes.

For example:

PEANUT:SHELL ::
APPLE:
A. core
B. pare
C. crop
D. plant

Unless you examined each answer carefully, you might miss the correct relation: You *shell* a *peanut* to remove its skin, and you *pare* an *apple* to remove its skin. Choice A, *core,* means to remove the central part. Choice B, *pare,* means to cut away the skin. Choice C, *crop,* can be defined as a verb meaning to reap. Choice D, *plant,* can mean to put into the ground to grow.

2.4.4 Unfamiliar Words

Use the words you know to eliminate clearly incorrect choices. For example, the parts of speech in the answer choice word pair must match those in the given word pair. If some choices are not the correct part of speech, you may be able to eliminate them immediately.

Read each unfamiliar word carefully, and determine as much as you can about its meaning by separating it into its elements (prefix, root, and suffix). Think of contexts suggested by each answer choice. At this point, you may have enough information to make a guess.

For example:

ROCK:IMMUTABLE ::
WATER :
A. stagnant
B. turbulent
C. rapid
D. contaminate

Even if you do not know the word *immutable*, you can immediately eliminate *contaminated,* because it is the wrong part of speech. The other choices are all adverbs, and therefore may be correct. You can describe the relation of the given pair only if you can decode the meaning of the second word. Break it into components: im—mut—able. The prefix im- usually means not, without, or opposing. The suffix -able means something that can be or do. The root, mut, is found in other words that you may know, such as mutant and commute. If you dissect those words as well, you can easily determine the meaning of the root, mut, which is to change or move. You can now construct a relation sentence, such as, "Rocks are unchangeable, or immovable." This analogy shows a characteristic relation.

You also must know the meanings of all of the answer choices, and you can apply the same process to *turbulent* to identify the correct answer. Familiarity with a wide variety of antonyms and synonyms helps in solving analogy problems. Not all antonyms and antonyms are as obvious as *hot* and *cold* or *gentle* and *kind.* If one question is taking too much time, skip it and return to it if you have time later.

2.5 BASIC WORD ELEMENTS

If you know the most common prefixes and suffixes, you can combine them with your knowledge of root words to decipher the meaning of many unfamiliar words. Roots are easier to identify and interpret if you know prefixes and suffixes well.

A number of strategies can help you to remember words and word elements and their meanings. Visualize the meaning of the word or element, and add a symbol or sketch to help you to remember it. For example, use a plus or minus symbol to indicate whether it has positive or negative connotations. This knowledge is especially helpful for answering antonym and synonym questions. Mnemonic and memory aids, such as rhymes, word associations, and visual images, may be helpful. Some students use flash cards. Other students personify adjectives by attributing their characteristics to familiar persons or objects.

2.5.1 Prefixes

A prefix is a word element that is added before the root to modify its meaning. Prefixes are abundant and are often combined with others (e.g., hyperinflation, unrepresented, antidiscrimination). Many prefixes and suffixes come to English from other languages. Prefixes greatly enrich language by denoting specific shades of meaning and allowing vivid expression of concepts. Familiarity with common prefixes is essential to performing well on the verbal portions of the test.

Prefixes pose some special challenges. Some have several, occasionally opposite, meanings. For example, in- sometimes means not (e.g., invalid); it can also mean very (e.g., infuriate) or in or on (e.g., infiltrate). Further, it changes its form to il-, im-, or ir-, depending on the root. Prefixes that look identical can have different meanings, depending on their origin (e.g., a- in apart means away from; a- in amoral means without; a- in atop means on). When prefixes are combined, each element must be decoded and analyzed in terms of the others.

Some resources list prefixes according to their language of origin, noting that Latin prefixes are often attached to Latin roots, Greek prefixes to Greek roots, and so on. Because there are so many exceptions, Table 2-1 lists prefixes according to their function rather than their origin.

2.5.2 Suffixes

A suffix is a part of a word that follows the root. Suffixes indicate conditions, attitudes, objects of a verb, actions, and places. The part of speech is determined by the suffix. When suffixes are used in combination, the part of speech is determined by the final suffix. Some suffixes can form more than one part of speech.

Noun suffixes indicate an act or quality, state or condition, result or product, or rank or status. Verb suffixes indicate action. Adjectival and adverbial suffixes indicate a quality, similarity, or relation. Adverbial suffixes are often used in combination with others: artfully (ful + ly), comically (ic + al + ly).

Table 2-2 lists suffixes by function in determining the part of speech, rather than by etymology. You can add other suffixes as you learn them.

2.5.3 Roots

A root is a core word element accompanied by prefixes, suffixes, or both. Table 2-3 lists common roots and their meanings.

2.6 SUGGESTIONS FOR IMPROVING VOCABULARY

Public and school libraries have a wealth of resources to help you build your word knowledge. Familiarize yourself with the call numbers for books on language (e.g., 378.1 for test preparation materials,

TABLE 2-1. ***Prefixes***

Prefix and Variants	General Meaning	Examples
Positive, adding, or intensifying		
ad, ac, af, ag, al, an, ap, ar, as, at	to, toward, very	admit, accrue, afford, allude, appear, assent, attuned
arch	chief	archbishop, architect
be	around, about, away, very	beset, beloved, bemused
bene	good, well	benefactor, benediction
com, co, col, con, cor	with, together, very	combine, cooperate, collude, convene, corrupt
en, em	in, within, among	enable, empathy
eu	good, well, beautiful	euphemism, eulogy
extra	beyond, outside	extrovert, extracurricular
hyper	excessive, over	hyperactive, hyperbole
in, il, im, ir	very (see negative prefixes)	impress, illuminate, inform, irradiate
over	excessively	overestimate
per	thorough	permeate, pernicious
pro	for, before, favoring	progress, profuse, provide
super, supra	over, above	superimpose, supervise
sur	beyond, above, extra	surfeit, surtax, surtitle
syn, sym, syl, sys	together	synchronize, symbiosis, systematic
ultra	beyond, excessively	ultramodern, ultraviolet
Negative, detracting, or removing		
ad, abs, a	from, off, away	abduct, avert, abstain
an, a	without	anarchy, amoral
anti	against, opposite	antidote, antithesis
apo	from, away	apology
cata	down, away	catalysis, catastrophe
contra, contro, counter	against	contradict, contraceptive, countermand
de	down, away from	devalue, decrease
dis, di, dif	not, apart	discord, divest, diffuse
ex, e, ef	out, off, from	export, elude, efface
for	away, off, from	forego, forbid, forgive
hypo	under, beneath	hypnosis, hypodermic
in, ig, il, im, ir	not, opposing	incorrect, illegal, ignoble, immature, irrational
mal, male	bad, badly	malnutrition, malefactor
mis	wrong, poorly	misfire, misconstrue
non	not	nonsense
ob, oc, of, op	against	object, oppose, offend, occlude
se	apart, away	seclude
sub, suc, suf, sug	under	subsist, succumb, suffice, suggest
un	not	unfit

(continued)

TABLE 2-1. *(continued)*

Prefix and Variants	General Meaning	Examples
Direction, position, location, or order		
ambi	both	ambivalent, ambidextrous
amphi	around, both	amphitheater, amphibian
ana	back, through, against	anagram, anachronism
ante, anti, pre	before, previous	antecedent, anticipate, presuppose
circum, peri	around	circumvent, periphery
dia	through, across	diagnose, diameter
epi	on, over, outside	epicenter, epidermis
fore	before, previous	foreword
inter, intra	between, among	interject, intramural
meta	change of, over	metamorphosis, metaphysics
over	above, beyond	overcast, overnight
para	beside, beyond	paranormal, paramedic, paraphrase
per	through	perforate
peri	around, near	periscope, perimeter
post	after	postpone, postmortem
pre	before	precede
re	back, again	recede, regroup, respond
retro	back, backward	retrospective, retrograde, retroactive
trans	across, beyond, through	translate, transmit, translucent
sub	under	subcutaneous, subbasement
super	above	superscript
Numbers and fractions		
demi, hemi, semi	half	demigod, demitasse, hemisphere, semiconscious, semicircle
poly, multi	many	polygon, polymorphous, multitude
mono, uni	one	monotheism, unity
bi, di	two, twice	bipolar, bisect, diameter
tri	three	triumvirate, tricycle
quadr, tetra	four	quadruped, tetrahedron
quint, quinque, penta	five	quintuplets, pentagram
sex, hexa	six	sextet, hexagon
sept, hepta	seven	September, heptameter
oct, octa, octo	eight	octopus, octagon
nona, nonem, ennea	nine	November, ennead
dec, deca	10	decimate, decalogue, deciliter
duodec, dodeca	12	duodecimo, dodecahedron
cent, hecto	100	century, hectograph
milli	1000	millipede, millennium

TABLE 2-2 ***Suffixes***

Suffix	Meaning	Examples
Noun suffixes		
age	state, place, process	lineage, patronage
al	pertaining to, doing	denial
an, ian	belonging to, concerned with	human, magician
ance, ancy, ence, ency, cy	act, state, condition	dalliance, truancy, emergence, fluency, accuracy, agency
ant, ent	doing, showing	servant, agent, pendant
ar	marked by, pertaining to	regular
ard, art	one doing	braggart, wizard
ary	belonging to, showing	adversary
ate	office or function	magistrate, delegate
ation	act or state of, result	education, maturation
cle, cule, let	little	icicle, molecule, platelet
cy	state	democracy
dom	state, rank, condition	kingdom
er, or	doer, actor, maker	climber, advisor
ery	action, skill, state	surgery, robbery
ese	of, relating to, language	governmentese
ess, ette	feminine	actress, suffragette
et	diminutive	midget
hood	state, condition	womanhood, statehood
ic	caused by, showing	comic
ice	act, state, quality	novice
id	marked by, showing	putrid
ile, il	marked by, showing	juvenile, civil
ine	marked by, dealing with	serpentine, marine
ion	action, state, result	commission, condition
ism	act, manner, state, belief	atheism, purism
ist	practitioner, doer, believer	anarchist, socialist
ite	native, citizen, or member	suburbanite, socialite
ition	action, state, result	abolition
ity, ty	state of being, quality	fluidity, honesty
ive	tending to, belonging	incentive
ment	result, means, action	commencement, adornment
mony	resulting state, condition	acrimony, matrimony
ness	quality, state	loneliness, meekness
oid	something like	anthropoid
ory	a place of, serving for	repository
ry	condition, practice	chivalry
ship	condition, office, skill	friendship, craftsmanship
sion, tion	act or state of	exclusion, fruition
t, th	act, state, quality	height, flight, warmth
tude	that which is, quality	plentitude, fortitude

(continued)

TABLE 2-2 *(continued)*

Suffix	Meaning	Examples
ure	act, result, state, rank	overture, censure
y	result, action, quality	perjury, augury
Verb suffixes		
ate	become, form, make, treat	create, animate
en	become, cause to be	enliven, fasten
esce	grow, continue, become	effervesce, coalesce
fy	make, cause	beautify, solidify
ish	do, make, perform	furnish, embellish
ize	make, cause to be, treat with	familiarize, polarize
Adjectival suffixes		
able, ible	able, fit, likely	doable, edible
acious, aceous	having the quality of	capacious, herbaceous
al	belonging to, characteristic	familial, practical
an	belonging to	human
ant	showing	jubilant
ar	pertaining to	lunar, solar
ary	belonging to, showing	fragmentary
en	made of, like	silken, golden
ent	doing, showing, agent	evident, fluent
escent	beginning, becoming	effervescent
ese	of a place, style, language	Portuguese
esque	like, in the style of	romanesque
fic	making, causing	beatific
ful	full of, marked by	doleful, grateful
ian	pertaining to	mammalian
ic	dealing with, showing	prolific
id	marked by, showing	acrid
ile, il	marked by, showing	fragile
ine	marked by, dealing with	sanguine
ish	rather, suggesting, like	impish, boyish
ist	practicing, characteristic of	feminist
ite	showing, marked by	favorite
ive	tending to, relating to	effective
less	lacking, without	helpless, guileless
ly	like	friendly
ory	pertaining to	compensatory
ose	marked by, given to	comatose
ous, ious	marked by, given to, full of	amorous, sagacious
some	showing, tending to	loathsome
ward	in the direction of	eastward
y	showing, suggesting	throaty
Adverbial suffixes		
ly	in the manner of	quickly, dryly
ward	in the direction of	forward

TABLE 2-3. *Roots*

Root	Meaning	Examples
ag, act	to do	act, agent, inactive
cap, capt, cep, cip	to take	capture, anticipate, perception
cad, cas	to fall	cadence, casual
ced, cess	to yield, to go	proceed, accession
cid, cis	to cut, kill	incisive, homicide
cred, credit	to believe	discredit, credible
curr, curs	to run	cursory, incursion
da, don	to give	data, mandate
dic, dict	to say	indictment, prediction
duc, duct	to lead	abduct, induction
fac, fic, fec, fect	to make or do	infect, factory, fiction, perfection
fer, lat	to bring or carry	translate, infer
graph, gram	writing	telegraph, epigram, grammar
leg, lect	to choose, read	select, eligible
mitt, miss	to send	missile, emissary, admittance
mori, mort	to die	immortal, moribund, mortality
pon, posit	to place	expose, proponent, positive
port, portat	to carry	import, portable, transport
scrib, script	to write	inscribe, circumscript
sequi, secut	to follow	sequel, consecutive
spec, spect	to look at	inspect, spectacular
tang, tact	to touch	contact, tangent
ten, tent	to hold	tenure, tenacious
veni, vent	to come	convene, prevent
anthrop	man, mankind	anthropology
auto	self	automobile, autobiography
bibli	book	Bible, bibliophile
bio	life	biosphere, biology
chrom	color	chromosome, chromatography
chron	time	anachronism
cosm	world	cosmic
crac, crat	power, rule	democracy, autocracy, bureaucracy
cycl	wheel, circle	bicycle, encyclical
dem	people	demographic
dox, doct	belief	orthodox
erg	work, power	energy, ergometric
gen	type, race	genetics
hetero	other, different	heterophile
homo	same	homogenized
metr, meter	measure	thermometer

TABLE 2-4. *Additional Vocabulary Words*

abrogate	deploy	parliament
acclaim	disconsolately	partisan
allege	dominant	phenomenon
anemometer	downturn	precarious
animosity	emblematic	prototype
atrocities	embroil	ramification
augment	expediency	referendum
besieged	extraneous	reignite
bioaccumulate	flagrant	relinquish
boom	founder	retarding
bureaucratic	gouging	shore up
cache	homily	skeptical
cavalierly	hygrometer	slowdown
comprehensive	hyperbole	slump
consolidation	impetuous	solidarity
conspicuous	incursion	sovereignty
augment	index	stopgap
austere	intractable	subsidize
barometer	intransigent	sumptuous
contingent	lionize	surge
counteroffensive	lobby	surrogate
culminate	mandate	thwart
curb	myopia	tribunal
cyclical	nondescript	wake
debenture	obviate	waning
decry	pantheon	yen

428.3 for vocabulary building). Also look in the reference room for books that you can use while at the library.

Look for books that provide clear explanations in a useful format. Check the table of contents for organization. Avoid sources that simply list unusual words and uncommon uses.

Read good books of all kinds; newspapers, especially the *Wall Street Journal* and the *New York Times*; and magazines. When you find an unfamiliar word or a familiar word in an unfamiliar context, look it up in a dictionary. A good thesaurus is a valuable tool for improving vocabulary. A recent Random House edition is organized alphabetically; Roget's editions are organized by topic.

Play with words. Scrabble, crossword puzzles, and other word games can be fun and help to expand your vocabulary. You can also use word games and puzzles for group study. Scrabble, for example, can be played by alternate rules. To increase its usefulness as a learning tool, you can play with all of the tiles exposed. At each turn, all of the players can work together to form the best available word. You might score each word and aim for a high combined total, or you might concentrate on prefixes and award extra points for them. You could ask players to provide synonyms and antonyms for each word formed. The possibilities for enjoyment and learning are endless.

You must know the words used in the questions to analyze and answer verbal questions. Some students believe that they will need these words only for the test, that the words in the sample questions are useless for the future. This type of thinking is a mistake. For example, the words listed in Table 2-4 appeared on 3 consecutive days in either the *Wall Street Journal* or the *New York Times*. Every career requires the ability to communicate clearly, accurately, and effectively.

Most of the words listed in Table 2-4 are probably in your recognition vocabulary. Can you define them without a context to help you? If not, look them up, learn them, and think of current uses and specific contexts for them (e.g., the economy, social sciences, politics).

2.7 SAMPLE TEST ITEMS

2.7.1 Antonyms

1. MILITANT
A. strict
B. passive
C. combative
D. activist

2. AUDACIOUS
A. bold
B. timorous
C. inaudible
D. insolent

3. INDIGENT
A. powerless
B. destitute
C. prosperous
D. calm

4. STRENUOUS
A. effortless
B. passionate
C. strict
D. driven

5. PROCRASTINATE
A. postpone
B. tarry
C. profane
D. accomplish

6. POSTHUMOUS
A. burial
B. postmortem
C. hurry
D. during life

7. ORNATE
A. simple
B. florid
C. flashy
D. ostentatious

8. AGRARIAN
A. urban
B. cultivation
C. sparse
D. unlikable

9. DISCREET
A. judicious
B. diverge
C. obtrusive
D. inconsistent

10. TEMPESTUOUS
A. stormy
B. tumultuous
C. moderate
D. disposition

11. INTRIGUING
A. overt
B. mysterious
C. covert
D. clandestine

12. LEWD
A. licentious
B. vulgar
C. impose
D. refined

13. PRIVATION
A. loss
B. privilege
C. unregulated
D. knowledge

14. SYMMETRICAL
A. unbalanced
B. unsympathetic
C. proportional
D. harmonious

15. STAGNANT
A. motionless
B. polluted
C. sluggish
D. flowing

16. SCOUNDREL
A. villain
B. clean
C. hero
D. recruit

17. COLLEAGUE
A. comrade
B. graduate
C. stranger
D. partner

18. DISCERN
A. confuse
B. detect
C. separate
D. burden

19. EGREGIOUS
A. exit
B. flagrant
C. inconspicuous
D. unreasonable

20. SYCOPHANTIC
A. servile
B. toady
C. obsequious
D. independent

21. SCINTILLATING
A. sparkle
B. copious
C. tedious
D. flashing

22. VIRULENT
A. venomous
B. malignant
C. innocuous
D. unskilled

23. OBESE
A. heavy
B. tractable
C. slender
D. corpulent

24. VIVACIOUS
A. dull
B. lively
C. incandescent
D. sprightly

25. ICONOCLAST
A. revolutionary
B. illustrator
C. conformist
D. cartographer

26. INHERENT
A. acquired
B. empirical
C. given
D. dominant

27. EPHEMERAL
A. peripheral
B. perpetual
C. subliminal
D. etheral

28. INNOCUOUS
A. naive
B. immune
C. vitriolic
D. devious

29. DICHOTOMY
A. cacophony
B. synergy
C. hierarchy
D. union

30. ECLECTIC
A. ordinary
B. catholic
C. exclusive
D. inflexible

31. SAGACIOUS
A. unknowing
B. spicy
C. outrageous
D. serious

32. OBSEQUIOUS
A. edgy
B. nervous
C. truculent
D. sparkling

33. IMMUTABLE
A. unspeakable
B. remarkable
C. stolid
D. tractable

34. SUCCINCT
A. loquacious
B. accomplished
C. reserved
D. moist

35. ABSTRACT
A. diffuse
B. coalescent
C. stylized
D. unrealistic

2.7.2 Answer Key: Antonyms

1. B. passive
2. B. timorous
3. C. prosperous
4. A. effortless
5. D. accomplish
6. D. during life
7. A. simple
8. A. urban
9. C. obtrusive
10. C. moderate
11. A. overt
12. D. refined
13. B. privilege
14. A. unbalanced
15. D. flowing
16. C. hero
17. C. stranger
18. A. confuse
19. C. inconspicuous
20. D. independent
21. C. tedious
22. C. innocuous
23. C. slender
24. A. dull
25. C. conformist
26. A. acquired
27. B. perpetual
28. C. vitriolic
29. D. union
30. C. exclusive
31. A. unknowing
32. C. truculent
33. D. tractable
34. A. loquacious
35. B. coalescent

2.7.3 VCAT Analogies

1. READING:VOCABULARY :: REHEARSAL :
   - A. proficiency
   - B. applause
   - C. iteration
   - D. validity

2. BENEVOLENCE:ALTRUISM :: AVARICE :
   - A. anthropomorphism
   - B. philanthropy
   - C. misanthropy
   - D. amorphousness

3. PRINCIPLE:PROBITY :: DIVINATION :
   - A. sanctity
   - B. scrutiny
   - C. godliness
   - D. augury

4. RANCOROUS:MALICIOUS :: QUIXOTIC :
   - A. utopian
   - B. philistine
   - C. apocryphal
   - D. labyrinthine

5. SOBRIETY:LEVITY :: TEMERITY :
   - A. effrontery
   - B. reticence
   - C. propensity
   - D. duplicity

6. ZEALOUS:LISTLESS :: PUGNACIOUS :
   - A. innocuous
   - B. impious
   - C. ingenious
   - D. insurgent

7. CRYPTIC:ESTOTERIC :: CURSORY :
   - A. didactic
   - B. caustic
   - C. terse
   - D. lackluster

8. IOTA:SCINTILLA :: OMEGA :
   - A. allegorical
   - B. initial
   - C. divine
   - D. ultimate

9. JOCUND:MOOD :: CONVIVIAL :
   - A. party
   - B. ambiance
   - C. perspective
   - D. expression

10. VERBOSE:PROLIX :: RIBALD :
    - A. profane
    - B. glabrous
    - C. hirsute
    - D. scanty

11. INADVERTENT:INCIDENTAL :: INTRACTABLE :
  A. impassive
  B. implausible
  C. implacable
  D. imperturbable

12. PRODIGIOUS:COLLECTION :: SUMPTUOUS :
  A. banquet
  B. propensity
  C. hierarchy
  D. quagmire

13. OBDURATE:ACQUIESCENT :: STRINGENT :
  A. nonchalant
  B. acerbic
  C. miserly
  D. numinous

14. TACITURN:SULLEN :: MEANDERING :
  A. gullible
  B. residual
  C. traipsing
  D. esoteric

15. EVANESCENT:STAGNANT :: UNOBTRUSIVE :
  A. bombastic
  B. ungainly
  C. susceptible
  D. recalcitrant

16. INDIGENT:OPULULENT :: PROFANE :
  A. decorous
  B. pugnacious
  C. innocuous
  D. dissipated

17. MILLIGRAM:DECIGRAM :: DECIGRAM :
  A. decagram
  B. centigram
  C. hectogram
  D. kilogram

18. LICENTIOUS:ASCETIC :: LIBERTINE :
  A. ascendant
  B. lonely
  C. abstemious
  D. political

19. ACRE:ROD :: FATHOM :
  A. link
  B. furlong
  C. yard
  D. league

20. MINUTE:SECOND :: HOUR :
  A. month
  B. week
  C. century
  D. minute

21. BACCHANALIAN:EXCESSIVE :: DRACONIAN :
  A. severe
  B. monstrous
  C. grandiloquent
  D. plaintive

22. INSOMNIAC:FITFUL :: PERFECTIONIST :
  A. deprecatory
  B. altruistic
  C. meticulous
  D. circumspect

23. MISSISSIPPI:TEPEE :: COLORADO :
  A. cabin
  B. lodge
  C. tent
  D. hogan

24. TEEMING:FECUND :: BRISTLING :
  A. discomposed
  B. sardine
  C. penurious
  D. flaccid

25. ROCOCO:ORNATE :: ROMANESQUE :
  A. edacious
  B. unembellished
  C. riparian
  D. ambulatory

26. HOMOPHONE:HOMONYM :: SPOONERISM :
  A. malapropism
  B. oxymoron
  C. paradox
  D. euphemism

27. TORTUROUS:PAINFUL :: TORTUOUS :
  A. doubtful
  B. cursory
  C. meandering
  D. painstaking

28. VIABLE : TROPOSPHERE ::
ABIOTIC :
A. hemisphere
B. spherical
C. biosphere
D. stratosphere

29. PALATABLE : SAVORY ::
PALATIAL :
A. grandiose
B. mitigating
C. paucity
D. superfluous

30. SESSILE : MOTILE ::
RECALCITRANT :
A. circumspect
B. amenable
C. captious
D. ossified

31. EPHEMERAL : SNOWFLAKE ::
BLOSSOM :
A. lily
B. evergreen
C. tuber
D. root

32. FRESCO : PAINTER ::
OPERA :
A. corral
B. symphony
C. composer
D. soloist

33. CARTOGRAPHER : SURVEY ::
SURGEON :
A. prognosis
B. patient
C. scalpel
D. anatomy

34. TOUCH : SENSE ::
SKIN :
A. drum
B. organ
C. shell
D. membrane

35. MYOPIA : EYE ::
TREE :
A. burl
B. crown
C. sap
D. cicada

36. BLUE : SAPPHIRE ::
RED :
A. sanguine
B. garnet
C. crimson
D. chimera

37. METEOR : METEOROLOGIST ::
COSMOS :
A. astronomer
B. astrologer
C. cosmetologist
D. meteorite

38. LUSTER : TARNISH ::
VERTICAL :
A. precipitate
B. perpendicular
C. plumb
D. prone

39. ALTRUISTIC : COMPENSATION ::
FRACTIOUS :
A. union
B. whole
C. harmony
D. sum

40. HIEROGLYPH : WORD ::
DELTA :
A. change
B. coda
C. letter
D. river

2.7.4 GRE Analogies

41. RED : SPECTRUM ::
A. elephant : herd
B. prom : anthology
C. fruit : cornucopia
D. sculpture : museum

42. WINE : GRAPES
A. oven : eat
B. camera : picture
C. soap : lye
D. honey : bee

43. PUGILIST : FIST
A. carpenter : nails
B. diva : voice
C. driver : car
D. actor : script

44. HIEROGLYPHIC:WORD
- **A.** paradigm:puzzle
- **B.** apocryphal:theory
- **C.** omega:infinity
- **D.** fresco:painting

45. LOCKET:VAULT
- **A.** china:closet
- **B.** paste:pearls
- **C.** photo:album
- **D.** box:deadbolt

2.7.5 Answer Key: VCAT Analogies

1. A. proficiency
2. C. misanthrophy
3. D. augury
4. A. utopian
5. B. reticence
6. A. innocuous
7. C. terse
8. D. ultimate
9. B. ambiance
10. A. profane
11. C. implacable
12. A. banquet
13. A. nonchalant
14. C. traipsing
15. A. bombastic
16. A. decorous
17. A. decagram
18. C. abstemious
19. D. league
20. D. minute
21. A. severe
22. C. meticulous
23. D. hogan
24. A. discomposed
25. B. unembellished
26. A. malapropism
27. C. meandering
28. D. stratosphere
29. D. superfluous
30. B. amenable
31. A. lily
32. C. composer
33. D. anatomy
34. B. organ
35. A. burl
36. B. garnet
37. C. cosmetologist
38. D. prone
39. C. harmony
40. A. change

2.7.6 Answer Key: GRE Analogies

41. A. elephant:herd
42. C. soap:lye
43. B. diva:voice
44. C. omega:infinity
45. D. box:deadbolt

REFERENCES

Bader W, et al: *MAT: Miller Analogies Test.* Englewood Cliffs, NJ, Prentice-Hall, 1988.
De Vries MA: *The Complete Word Book.* Englewood Cliffs, NJ, Prentice-Hall, 1991.
Morse-Cluley E, Read R: *Webster's New World Power Vocabulary.* New York, Simon & Schuster, 1988.
Random House Dictionary. New York, Random House, 1987.
Schur NW: *Practical English: 1,000 Most Effective Words.* New York, Ballantine Books, 1983.
The 1,000 Most Challenging Words. New York, Ballantine Books, 1983.
Whimbey A, Lochhead J: *Problem Solving & Comprehension.* Hillsdale, NJ, Lawrence Erlbaum Associates, 1986.

3

CHAPTER

Reading Comprehension Skills for the VETs

3.0 INTRODUCTION

The reading comprehension section of the VETs measures the ability to read, comprehend, organize, and analyze new information in the humanities, social sciences, basic sciences, and veterinary research. Reading comprehension passages are taken from scientific books and journals and are typical of information covered in the first year of veterinary school. The passages are followed by multiple-choice questions.

No knowledge of the topic is required for the reading comprehension test. Table 3-1 summarizes the reading comprehension sections of the Veterinary College Admission Test (VCAT), the Graduate Record Examination (GRE), and the Medical College Admission Test (MCAT). This chapter describes the reading comprehension test and offers strategies for improving your score.

3.1 PREPARATION FOR THE READING COMPREHENSION TESTS

Learning special reading skills may help in preparing for the reading comprehension test. Most students need an average of 1 hour per day to develop these skills.

The reading comprehension section tests the ability to comprehend, analyze, and interpret information.

3.2 COMPREHENSION OF NEW INFORMATION

The VETs test your ability to read and analyze new information. For the purpose of this test, "new" means unseen or unrehearsed, but not necessarily unknown or unfamiliar. In addition to textbooks and lectures, sources of new information include veterinary research reports, magazine articles, and newspapers. These sources are available at most libraries. Recommended newspapers and magazines include: the New York Times, *Scientific American, Discover, American Scientist by Sigma Xi,* and *USA Today.* Recommended medical journals include the *New England Journal of Medicine,* the *Journal of the American Veterinary Medical Association,* and the *Journal of the American Medical Association.*

TABLE 3-1. ***Comparison of the Reading Comprehension Sections of the VCAT, GRE, and MCAT***

VCAT	GRE	MCAT
Usually 5 or 6 long (1300–1500-word) or short (200–300-word) passages containing factual or fictional material drawn from life sciences, physical sciences, social sciences, and humanities.	Usually 2 long passages (followed by 7 or 8 test items) and 2 short passages (followed by 3 or 4 test items) taken from humanities, social sciences, biologic sciences, and physical sciences.	Usually 9 passages, each 500–600 words long, and followed by 6–10 questions. This section is called the verbal reasoning subtest. Passages are drawn from humanities, social sciences, and natural sciences (approximately 26 subject areas).
The questions test: Literal comprehension (based on information in the passage) Inferential comprehension (understanding implied hypotheses and conclusions) Evaluative comprehension (differentiating among opinions, claims, and judgments)	Types of questions: Main idea, or primary purpose of passage Explicit information Information or ideas implied or suggested Application of the author's ideas to other situations Use of logic, reasoning, or persuasive techniques Tone, or the author's attitude revealed through the passage	The questions test major skills and 24 subskills: Comprehension Evaluation Application Incorporation of new information

3.2.1 Reading Ability

Reading ability is a difficult concept to define. It depends on the difficulty of the passage, your concentration level and interest in the subject matter, your speed in reading and understanding the text, and your ability to connect the various parts of the passage. The difficulty of the passage is determined by the vocabulary and the level of detail. You can build your vocabulary by keeping a list of new words that you encounter.

Analytical reasoning (see section 1.5.1 in Chapter 1) consists of breaking a complex passage into short, understandable pieces. Practice using this skill, especially when you read complex and detailed information. Break long sentences into short, understandable phrases.

The reading comprehension test requires a specific approach to reading that includes scanning, correlating, understanding vocabulary, and developing speed and rhythm. To evaluate your skills in these areas, complete Exericse 1, which contains a passage that is similar in format and style to those that appear on the VETs.

Exercise 1. Skim Passage 1 for approximately 30 seconds to determine the main topic. Read the questions, but not the answer choices. Spend 3–5 minutes reading the passage and developing connections among the various parts. Underline or highlight important points as necessary. Answer the questions, consulting the passage as necessary. Check your answers in section 3.5.1.

Passage 1

Connective Tissue:
General Characteristics and Functions
Connective tissue allows movement and provides support. In this tissue, there is an abundance of intercellular material called matrix, which is variable in type and amount and is one of the main sources of difference between the types of connective tissue. It consists of various fibers embedded in a ground substance.

Loose Connective Tissue

The fibers of loose connective tissue are not tightly woven. The tissue, filling spaces between and penetrating into the organs, is of three types: areolar, adipose, and reticular.

Areolar Tissue

The most widely distributed connective tissue is pliable and crossed by many delicate threads; yet, the tissue resists tearing and is somewhat elastic. Areolar tissue contains fibroblasts, histiocytes (macrophages), leukocytes, and mast cells.

Fibroblasts are small, flattened, somewhat irregular cells with large nuclei and reduced cytoplasm. The term fibroblast refers to the ability of a cell to form fibrils. Fibroblasts are active in repair of injury. It is generally believed that suprarenal steroids inhibit and growth hormones stimulate fibroblastic activity. Histiocytes are phagocytic cells similar to leukocytes in blood; however, they perform phagocytic activity outside the vascular system. The histiocyte is irregular in shape and contains cytoplasmic granules. The cell is often stationary (or "fixed"). Mast cells, located adjacent to small blood vessels, are round or polygonal in shape and possess a cytoplasm filled with metachromatic granules. Mast cells function in the manufacture of heparin (an anticoagulant) and histamine (an inflammatory substance responsible for changes in allergic tissue). Depression in mast cell activity results from the administration of cortisol to patients. Areolar tissue is the basic supporting substance around organs, muscles, blood vessels, and nerves forming the delicate membranes around the brain and spinal cord and comprising the superficial fascia, or sheet of connective tissue, found deep in the skin.

Adipose Tissue

Adipose tissue is specialized areolar tissue with fat-containing cells. The fat, or lipid, cell, like other cells, has a nucleus, endoplasmic reticulum, cell membrane, mitochondria, and one or more fat droplets. Adipose tissue acts as a firm, yet resilient, packing around and between organs, bundles of muscle fibers, nerves, and supporting blood vessels. Since fat is a poor conductor of heat, adipose tissue protects the body from excessive heat loss or excessive rises in temperature.

Reticular Tissue

Reticular fibers consist of finely branching fibrils taking a silver stain as observed under the microscope. The primary cell of the reticular fiber is the reticular cell. Reticular fibers form the framework of the liver, lymphoid organs, and bone marrow.

Dense Connective Tissue

Dense connective tissue is composed of closely arranged tough collagenous and elastic fiber. It can be classified according to the arrangement of the fibers and the proportion of elastin and collagen present. Examples of dense connective tissue having a regular arrangement of fibers are tendons, aponeuroses, and ligaments. Examples of dense connective tissue having an irregular arrangement of fibers are fasciae, capsules, and muscle sheaths.

Specialized Connective Tissue

Cartilage

Cartilage has a firm matrix consisting of protein and mucopolysaccharides. Cells of cartilage, called chondrocytes, are large and rounded with spherical nuclei. Collagenous and elastic fibers are embedded in the matrix, increasing the elastic and resistive properties of this tissue. The three types of cartilage are hyaline, fibrous, and elastic.

In utero, hyaline cartilage, the precursor of much of the skeletal system, is translucent with a clear matrix caused by abundant collagenous fibers (not visible as such) and cells scattered throughout the matrix. Hyaline cartilage is gradually replaced by bone in many parts of the body through the process of ossification; however, some remains as a covering on the articular surfaces. The hyaline costal cartilages attach the anterior ends of the upper seven pairs of ribs to the sternum. The trachea and bronchi are kept open by incomplete rings of surrounding hyaline cartilage. This type of cartilage is also found in the nose.

Fibrous cartilage contains dense masses of unbranching, collagenous fibers lying in the matrix. Cells of fibrous cartilage are present in rows between bundles of the matrix. Fibrocartilage is dense and resistant to stretching; it is less flexible and less resilient than hyaline cartilage. Fibrous cartilage, interposed between the vertebrae in the spinal column, is also present in the symphysis pubis, permitting a minimal range of movement.

Elastic cartilage, which is more resilient than either the hyaline or the fibrous type because of a predominance of elastic fibers impregnated in its ground substance, is found in the auricle of the external ear, the auditory tube, the epiglottis, and portions of the larynx.

Bone is a firm tissue formed by impregnation of the intercellular material with inorganic salts. It is living tissue supplied by blood vessels and nerves and is constantly being remodeled. The two common types are compact, forming the dense outer layer, and cancellous, forming the inner, lighter tissue of the shaft of a long bone.

The dentin of teeth is closely related to bone. The crown of the tooth is covered by enamel, the hardest substance in the body. Enamel is secreted onto the dentin by the epithelial cells of the enamel organ before the teeth are extruded through the gums. Dentin resembles bone, but is harder and denser.

Blood and Hematopoietic Tissue

Marrow is the blood-forming (hematopoietic) tissue located in the shafts of bones. The red blood cells (erythrocytes) and most white blood cells (leukocytes) originate in the capillary sinusoids of bone marrow. Some leukocytes are formed in the lymphoid organs. Blood is a fluid tissue circulating through the body, carrying nutrients to cells, and removing waste products.

Lymphoid tissue is found in the lymph nodes, thymus, spleen, tonsils, and adenoids. The germinal centers of lymph tissue produce plasma cells and lymphocytes. Lymphoid tissue functions in antibody production.

Connective tissues perform many functions, including support and nourishment for other tissues, packing material in the spaces between organs, and defense for the body by digestion and absorption of foreign material.

Reticuloendothelial system

Connective tissue cells, carrying on the process of phagocytosis, are frequently referred to as the reticuloendothelial system. The cells ingest solid particles similar to the manner in which an amoeba takes in nourishment. Three types of phagocytic cells belong to this classification: reticuloendothelial cells lining the liver (Kupffer's cells), spleen, and bone marrow; macrophages, termed tissue histiocytes or "resting-wandering" cells; and microglia, located in the central nervous system. The reticuloendothelial system is a strong line of defense against infection.

Synovial Membranes

Synovial membranes line the cavities of the freely moving joints and form tendon sheaths and bursae.

1. Which is NOT a type of areolar connective tissue?
- **A.** Histiocytes
- **B.** Plasma cells
- **C.** Leukocytes
- **D.** Fibroblasts

2. The connective tissue forming the framework for the liver is classified as:
- **A.** loose connective tissue.
- **B.** synovial membranes.
- **C.** fibrous cartilage.
- **D.** areolar tissue.

3. Mast cells function in the production of:
- **A.** histamine.
- **B.** cortisol.
- **C.** A and B only.
- **D.** all of the above.

4. Which is NOT a function of specialized connective tissue?
- **A.** Producing plasma cells and lymphocytes
- **B.** Phagocytosis
- **C.** Protecting the body from an excessive increase or decrease in temperature
- **D.** Producing blood cells

5. Which term does NOT apply to any connective tissue?
- **A.** Squamous
- **B.** Areolar
- **C.** Reticular
- **D.** Lymphoid

6. Which is NOT a characteristic of the reticuloendothelial system?
   A. Microglia cells
   B. Macrophages
   C. Serve as framework for bone marrow and liver
   D. Defense against infection

7. Which type of tissue is largely characterized by the nature of material that lies between the cells?
   A. Connective tissue
   B. Smooth muscle tissue
   C. Nervous tissue
   D. Pseudostratified tissue

8. The most widely distributed connective tissue is:
   A. dense connective tissue.
   B. adipose connective tissue.
   C. areolar connective tissue.
   D. specialized connective tissue.

9. What type of connective tissue acts as a precursor to much of the skeletal system?
   A. Hyaline cartilage
   B. Fibrous cartilage
   C. Elastic cartilage
   D. Synovial membrane

10. Cartilage cells are called:
   A. histiocytes.
   B. erythrocytes.
   C. chondrocytes.
   D. mast cells.

3.2.2 Organizing What You Read

The elements of effective organization include drawing mind maps with the right amount of detail and keeping a vocabulary list or notebook. To help you locate information quickly, you can mark the text with lines, circles, brackets, parentheses, or other marks. Mind maps are charts to record your thoughts as you read.

To evaluate your ability to organize information, answer the following questions about Passage 1.

1. How many words does Passage 1 contain?
2. How much time did you spend reading the passage?
3. What is the main idea conveyed in the passage?
4. Did you mark the passage (e.g., highlight, underline) as you extracted information?
5. Without reading the passage again, can you remember 20 new or difficult vocabulary words?
6. Can you write a short summary of the passage?
7. Which parts of the passage were the most difficult?
8. Did the passage contain any irrelevant information?

If you had trouble answering these questions, you may need more practice in analyzing and organizing text. Marking the text (see section 3.2.3) and creating a mind map (see section 3.2.4) can help you to develop these skills. Some students create a mind map for each article that they read while preparing for the VETs. Practicing these skills allows you to develop a rhythm and increase your speed. To see how effectively you organized the information in Passage 1, see the answers and discussion that follow.

1. To determine the length of a passage, count the average number of words per line and multiply this number by the number of lines in the passage. Passage 1 is approximately one and one-half typed pages, or 500 words, long.

2. Reading this type of passage should take approximately 5 minutes. Students who take the VCAT are given approximately 30 minutes to read a passage and answer 40 questions. Table 3-2 shows the average time taken to read VCAT passages and answer the questions.

   This time distribution assumes that all passages and items are of equal difficulty and length. Most students spend approximately equal amounts of time reading the passages and answering the questions. Marking important terms as you read can save time. It is best to answer answer as many questions as you can, skipping difficult ones. If you have time at the end, you can review the passage and answer the questions that you skipped.

3. A mind map of Passage 1 (see section 3.2.4) shows that the passage describes the structure and function of various types of connective tissue.

TABLE 3-2. ***Average Time to Complete the VCAT Reading Comprehension Test***

Passage	Length	Questions	Time (min)
Model I (5 passages; 40 questions)			
1	Long	10	9
2	Short	4	3
3	Short	4	3
4	Long	10	9
5	Long	12	10
Total (min)			34
Model II (6 passages; 40 questions)			
1	Long	10	9
2	Short	4	3
3	Short	4	3
4	Long	10	9
5	Long	8	7
6	Short	4	3
Total (min)			34

4. Highlighting and using mind maps can help you to locate important information quickly.
5. The mind map can help you to locate vocabulary words. Posssible vocabulary words for Passage 1 include loose tissue, dense tissue, and mast cells.
6. Because it organizes the information according to topic, a mind map can also help you to summarize a passage. In addition, writing a summary helps you to remember the information.
7. Different readers find different material difficult. In this passage, you may have had trouble determining where each type of connective tissue is found because the introduction does not emphasize this point.
8. Textbook or encyclopedia passages usually contain little irrelevant information. Information that is not needed to answer the questions is unused, but not irrelevant.

3.2.3 Marking Text to Improve Comprehension

In Figure 3-1, the important points are indicated by underlines, circles, or other marks. Noting important points in this way helps you to see connections between the ideas. Highlighting important information helps you to answer the test questions more quickly because time is not wasted rereading the passage to search for details.

3.2.4 Mind Mapping

A mind map traces and records your thoughts as you read a passage. Mind maps are used to extract basic information and rearrange it for later use. In a mind map, long arrows, or leaders, are used to connect the ideas or thoughts expressed in the passage. For example, in Figure 3-2, arrows are used to show the relation between "fibroblasts" and "histiocytes." A mind map helps you to organize and understand the details of the passage. With practice, you will be able to draw these maps quickly and accurately. Mind maps can lead you quickly to the right sections when you answer the test questions.

3.2.5 Analyzing Questions and Distractors

Conventional multiple-choice questions are composed of a stem and five answer choices. The format of these questions is similar on tests from the high school-level Scholastic Aptitude Tests (SATs) through the National Veterinary Professional examinations. The choices usually include one correct choice, a few obviously wrong options, and an almost-right answer that is similar to, or easily confused

(1) control passage as it branches from the intro. paragraph → keep looking for differences in structure (S) and function (F)
(2) develop a mental layout of passage as it expands in content

(approx. 500 words)

Connective Tissue: General Characteristics and Functions

Connective tissue allows movement and provides support. In this tissue there is an abundance of intercellular material called matrix, which is variable in type and amount and is one of the main sources of difference between the types of connective tissue. It consists of various fibers embedded in a ground substance.

Loose Connective Tissue

The fibers of loose connective tissue are not tightly woven. The tissue, filling space between and penetrating into the organs, is of three types: areolar, adipose, and reticular.

Areolar Tissue. The most widely distributed connective tissue is pliable and crossed by many delicate threads; yet, the tissue resists tearing and is somewhat elastic. Areolar tissue contains fibroblasts, histiocytes (macrophages), leukocytes, and mast cells.

Fibroblasts are small, flattened, somewhat irregular cells with large nuclei and reduced cytoplasm. The term fibroblast refers to the ability of a cell to form fibrils. Fibroblasts are active in repair of injury. It is generally believed that suprarenal steroids inhibit and growth hormones stimulate fibroblastic activity. **Histiocytes** are phagocytic cells similar to **leukocytes** in blood; however, they perform phagocytic activity outside the vascular system. The histiocyte is irregular in shape and contains cytoplasmic granules. The cell is often stationary (or "fixed"). **Mast cells** located adjacent to small blood vessels are round or polygonal in shape and possess a cytoplasm filled with metachromatic granules. Mast cells function in the manufacture of heparin (an anticoagulant) and histamine (an inflammatory substance responsible for changes in allergic tissue). Depression in mast cell activity results from the administration of cortisol to patients. Areolar tissue is the basic supporting substance around organs, muscles, blood vessels, and nerves forming the delicate membranes around the brain and spinal cord and comprising the superficial fascia, or sheet of connective tissue, found deep in the skin.

Adipose Tissue. Adipose tissue is specialized areolar tissue with fat-containing cells. The fat or lipid cell, like other cells, has a nucleus, endoplasmic reticulum, cell membrane, mitochondria, and one or more fat droplets. Adipose tissue acts as a firm yet resilient packing around and between organs, bundles of muscle fibers, nerves, and supporting blood vessels. Since fat is a poor conductor of heat, adipose tissue protects the body from excessive heat loss or excessive rises in temperature.

Reticular Tissue. Reticular fibers consist of finely branching fibrils taking a silver stain as observed under the microscope. The primary cell of the reticular fiber is the reticular cell. Reticular fibers form the framework of the liver, lymphoid organs, and bone marrow.

Dense Connective Tissue

Dense connective tissue is composed of closely arranged tough collagenous and elastic fiber. It can be classified according to the arrangement of the fibers and the proportion of elastin and collagen present. Examples of dense connective tissue having a regular arrangement of fibers are tendons, aponeuroses, and ligaments. Examples of dense connective tissue having an irregular arrangement of fibers are fasciae, capsules, and muscle sheaths.

Specialized Connective Tissue

Cartilage. Cartilage has a firm matrix consisting of protein and mucopolysaccharides. Cells of cartilage, called **chondrocytes**, are large and rounded with spherical nuclei. Collagenous and elastic fibers are embedded in the matrix, increasing the elastic and resistive properties of this tissue. The three types of cartilage are hyaline, fibrous, and elastic.

In utero, **hyaline cartilage**, the precursor of much of the skeletal system, is translucent with a clear matrix caused by abundant collagenous fibers (not visible as such) and cells scattered throughout the matrix. Hyaline cartilage is gradually replaced by bone in many parts of the body through the process of ossification; however, some remains as a covering on the articular surfaces. The hyaline costal cartilages attach the anterior ends of the upper seven pairs of ribs to the sternum. The trachea and bronchi are kept open by incomplete rings of surrounding hyaline cartilage. This type of cartilage is also found in the nose.

Fibrous cartilage contains dense masses of unbranching, collagenous fibers lying in the matrix. Cells of fibrous cartilage are present in rows between bundles of the matrix. Fibrocartilage is dense and resistant to stretching; it is less flexible and less resilient than hyaline cartilage. Fibrous cartilage, interposed between the vertebrae in the spinal column, is also present in the symphysis pubis, permitting a minimal range of movement.

remember elasticity and springs from Physics (Are density and elasticity related?)

Figure 3-1 Marked-up passage.

Elastic cartilage, which is more resilient than either the hyaline or the fibrous type because of a predominance of elastic fibers impregnated in its ground substance, is found in the auricle of the external ear, the auditory tube, the epiglottis, and portions of the larynx.

Bone is a firm tissue formed by impregnation of the intercellular material with inorganic salts. It is living tissue supplied by blood vessels and nerves and is constantly being remodeled. The two common types are **compact**, forming the dense outer layer, and **cancellous**, forming the inner lighter tissue of the shaft of a long bone.

The dentin of teeth is closely related to bone. The crown of the tooth is covered by enamel, the hardest substance in the body. Enamel is secreted onto the dentin by the epithelial cells of the enamel organ before the teeth are extruded through the gums. Dentin resembles bone but is harder and denser.

Blood and Hematopoietic Tissue. Marrow is the blood-forming (hematopoietic) tissue located in the shafts of the bones. The red blood cells (erythrocytes) and most white blood cells (leukocytes) originate in the capillary sinusoids of bone marrow. Some leukocytes are formed in the lymphoid organs.

Blood is a fluid tissue circulating through the body, carrying nutrients to cells, and removing waste products.

Lymphoid tissue is found in the lymph nodes, thymus, spleen, tonsils, and adenoids. The germinal centers of lymph tissue produce plasma cells and lymphocytes. Lymphoid tissues function in antibody production.

Connective tissues perform many functions, including support and nourishment for other tissues, packing material in the spaces between organs, and defense for the body by digestion and absorption of foreign material.

Reticuloendothelial system. Connective tissue cells, carrying on the process of phagocytosis, are frequently referred to as the reticuloendothelial system. The cells ingest solid particles similar to the manner in which an amoeba takes in nourishment. Three types of phagocytic cells belong to this classification; reticuloendothelial cells lining the liver (Kupffer's cells), spleen, and bone marrow; macrophages, termed tissue histiocytes or "resting-wandering" cells; and microglia, located in the central nervous system. The reticuloendothelial system is a strong line of defense against infection.

Synovial Membranes. Synovial membranes line the cavities of the freely moving joints and form tendon sheaths and bursae.

Figure 3-1 *(continued)*

with, the correct answer. For example, if the stem says, "All of the following are functions of the liver EXCEPT," the exception might be a function of the spleen that students tend to ascribe to the liver.

Because there are normally at least two seemingly correct answers, it is easy to be misled. For example, under the pressure of the test, a student might mark the first answer choice that seems correct. However, this choice may be the almost-right answer, or "the most likely distractor." For this reason, you must read all of the choices before selecting one. Mark choices that are clearly wrong (e.g., with a slash), and reread the remaining choices to select the best one.

The VETs pose many questions on a limited content area. For this reason, taking the VETs is more like a marathon than a sprint. A sprinter simply runs as fast as possible from start to finish. On the other hand, a marathon runner develops an overall plan well in advance, with appropriate strategies for each part of the race. The runner then practices those strategies so that her performance is deliberate, yet automatic. Preparing for and taking the VETs is also aided by an overall plan and well-practiced specific strategies. When you identify an effective strategy for answering multiple-choice questions, for example, it is best to use that strategy consistently.

In many ways, much classroom training runs counter to the strategies suggested for the best performance on multiple-choice items. Many students have learned to compete not only for finding the right answer, but also for identifying it faster. This focus on speed encourages students to rely on rote memory and intuitive leaps rather than deliberation. Many students need to practice deliberate strategies consistently until they become automatic.

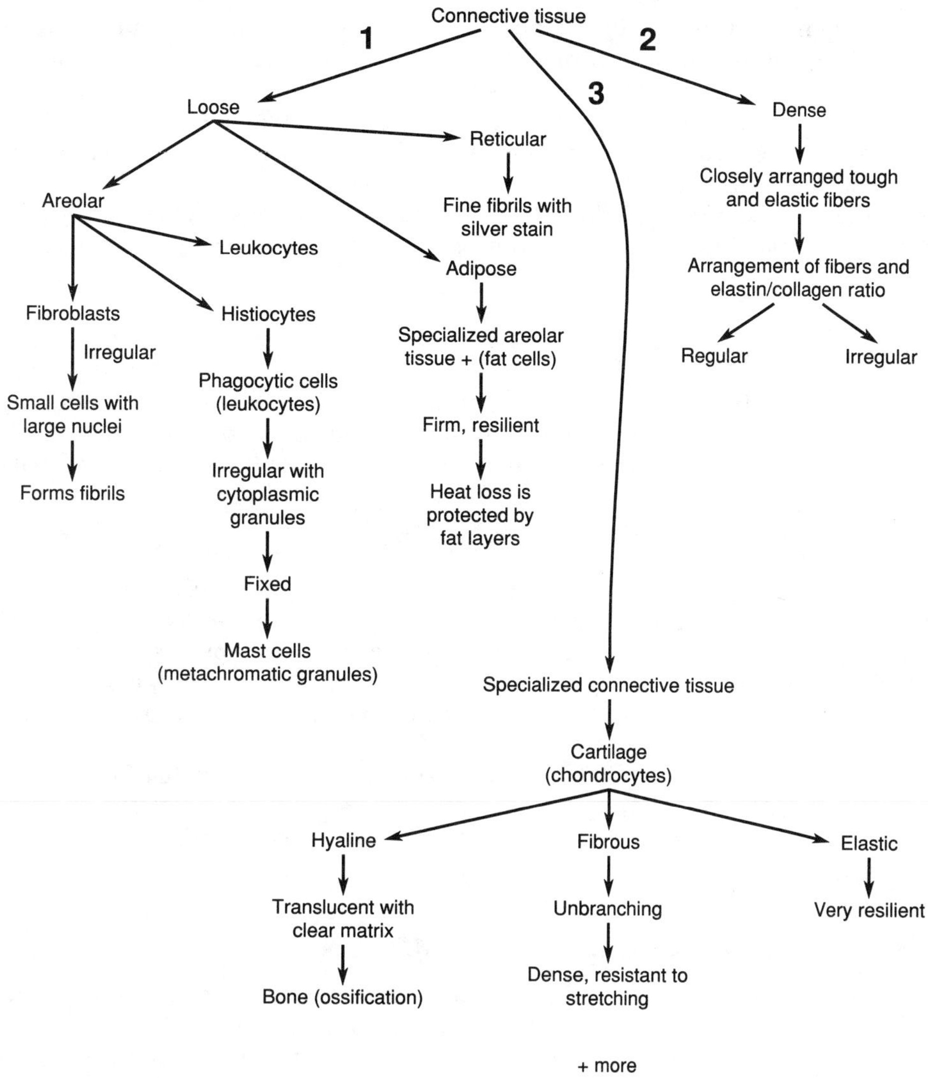

Figure 3-2 Mind map.

3.2.6 Question Analysis Strategy

Most readers cannot identify the best answer on reading subtests based on recall alone. With the strategy of question analyis, the student highlights or marks the text and creates a mind map. Next he reads the question to determine what to look for, and then he searches the passage for the sentence that contains the answer.

The relevent passage typically has a number of important words, primarily significant nouns, in common with the question. For example, if a question asks, "In what historical period was United States population growth the lowest?" the student can scan the passage given for "population growth" and "lowest." The sentence that provides the answer might read: "This was the lowest rate of population growth recorded until the 'Great Depression,' when the net growth rate fell to 7 per 1000 population during the 1930–1935 period." Once you locate the correct sentence in the passage, choosing the right answer depends on a clear understanding of the material. At first, you may find this strategy awkward and time consuming. However, practice increases your accuracy and speed.

With the question analysis strategy, follow these steps:

1. Work with one question at a time. Read the question, and identify the significant words. Try to anticipate the correct and almost-correct answers.

2. Underline the significant words in the question, primarily the nouns and active verbs.
3. Scan the passage, looking for a sentence that contains the same words that you have underlined. These words may appear in a different order.
4. Mark the number of the question in the margin of the test booklet.
5. Slow down and read carefully because you are looking for the difference between the right answer and the almost-right answer.
6. Answer the question carefully, working back and forth between the passage and the question. Pay attention to the remaining words in the sentence, especially the conjunctions, adverbs and adjectives, and restrictive phrases.

3.2.7 Remembering Information

Memorization is linked to diagramming and reasoning skills. Developing your reasoning skills helps to improve your short-term memory. Section 3.2.4 describes the use of mind maps to extract information. Integrating this skill with your reasoning abilities can help you to become a skilled critical reader (see Chapter 2).

To remember important concepts, follow these suggetions:

1. Read with interest. Associate facts and details with your need to achieve a good score on the VETs.
2. To develop good recall, observe and concentrate. People remember best the information that they find interesting, that requires careful examination, and that invokes serious thought.
3. Read with the intention of recalling facts. As you read, decide which facts are important. Not all printed information is worth recalling, and it is impractical to try to recall everything that you read.
4. Develop optimal speed. Speed is tied to your rate of reading. Your rate of reading should never be so high that understanding is affected. Comprehension should never be sacrificed in favor of speed. Excessive speed hurts the performance of a student who has difficulty comprehending ideas and recalling facts.

3.3 COMPREHENSION OF CURRENT INFORMATION

Current information includes lecture and laboratory notes, textbooks and study guides, and information from friends and the news media. To master any type of information, the first step is to understand it and identify the types of reasoning embedded within it. Effective comprehension requires reasoning skills, the ability to identify relations between various types of information, the ability to understand given and implied assumptions, and the ability to derive direct and indirect, or implied, conclusions.

3.3.1 Applying Logic to Comprehension

In standardized tests, form and syntax in written text are governed by the language and rules of logic. Thus, people use logical reasoning both to understand what they read and to determine how they organize their thoughts when they write. Logical reasoning also governs the understanding of test questions.

Logic involves at least three premises. "Premise" is a logician's term. Although each academic discipline is governed by logic, each has a specialized language. In law, for example, the word for premise is "evidence"; in medicine, "symptoms"; and in biology, "data." No matter what the discipline, logic supplies the rules; although the labels might change from discipline to discipline, the rules of academic thinking are the same. Thus, if you recognize a pattern in the data, evidence, or symptoms, you might draw a conclusion. In logic, recognizing a pattern and drawing a conclusion is called "making an inference." Just as each discipline has a word for premise, each has a word for conclusion. In law, this word is "verdict"; in medicine, "diagnosis"; in biology, "results," or "conclusions"; and in an essay, "thesis."

Conclusions have three degrees of certainty (Figure 3-3). A hypothesis is a conclusion that has not yet been tested. A conclusion suggested has been tested somewhat, but not enough to confirm it. The most certain is a conclusion confirmed.

Premises (valid or invalid)			Conclusions (direct or indirect)
Premise 1	→		Hypothesis
Premise 2	→	Inference →	Conclusion suggested

Premise 3	→		Conclusion confirmed
Evidence	→		Verdict
Data	→		Results/conclusion
Facts	→		Conclusion/decision
Symptoms	→		Diagnosis
Supporting sentences	→		Thesis

Figure 3-3 Model of a logical argument.

In Figure 3-3, the broken line between "conclusion suggested" and "conclusion confirmed" represents an important step. For example, the Food and Drug Administration sets the standard that governs when a drug is declared effective and can be sold. That is, if the drug has the desired effect on a certain percentage of patients, the side effects are acceptable, and adequate time has passed to exclude long-term side effects, the drug is approved, or, in the language of the model, the conclusion suggested becomes a conclusion confirmed.

In a text, the syxtax suggests whether a sentence is a conclusion suggested or a conclusion confirmed. For example, if the sentence is a conclusion suggested, it usually contains conditional verbs, such as "may," "seem," or "can" (e.g., "it can be inferred"), or adverbs, such as "primarily," "probably," or "most likely." In logic, these conditional words signify that the conclusion should be judged according to probability. In contrast, a deductively phrased statement should be judged according to logical validity. Logical validity states that if the premises are true, then the conclusion must also be true.

For example, if you ask a friend to dinner and he says that he may come, you must decide whether to expect him on the basis of probability. On the other hand, if your friend says that he will come, you can expect him to be there.

Some students look for the obscure, but possible, answers rather than choosing the probable answer that seems too easy. This tendency can be corrected by understanding the nature of probability and realizing that the syntax of the question stem requires the answer to be selected based on probability only. The answer should not be based on either possibility or certainty.

3.3.2 Interpretation of Scientific Information

The interpretation of scientific reading material is linked to the following reading comprehension skills: identifying the central idea of the passage; identifying cause and effect statements; identifying relations between information (e.g., chronologic relations); comparing and contrasting concepts; identifying and understanding underlying assumptions; and identifying and evaluating conclusions.

Students can sharpen their basic reading skills by reading new and difficult material. National science magazines, such as *Scientific American, Science,* and *Science News;* and the *Encyclopaedia Britannica* are good reading resources for test preparation. They are of approximately the same level of difficulty as the test passages, and they are written for a generally well-educated, but not necessarily scientifically educated, audience. Reading one scientific magazine each week keeps you abreast of current issues in science. A recommended text for improving basic reading skills is *Active Reading in the Arts and Sciences*.

3.3.3 Reading Comprehension Questions

The reading comprehension questions on the VETs measure the ability to read and understand a passage. The test generally has one passage from each of the following categories: in the biologic sciences, medicine, botany, zoology, human biology, and pharmacology; and in the physical sciences, chemistry, astronomy, technology, ecology, and geology.

Reading comprehension questions measure the ability to read with understanding, insight, and discrimination. These questions explore the student's ability to analyze a passage from several perspectives: to recognize explicit statements, underlying assumptions, and the implications of the statements or assumptions. Each passage describes a specific topic and provides a context for analyzing a variety of relations (e.g., the function of a word in two sections of the passage, the connections among several ideas, the relation of the author to the topic or the audience).

There are six types of reading comprehension questions. They focus on:

1. the main idea, or primary purpose, of the passage.
2. explicitly stated information.
3. information or ideas that are implied or suggested.
4. application of the author's ideas to other situations.
5. logic, reasoning, or persuasive techniques.
6. tone of the passage, or the author's attitude as it is revealed through language.

The test usually contains three relatively short (300–400 words) reading comprehension passages, each followed by 10–20 questions. The passages are usually drawn from the biologic or physical sciences.

3.3.4 Strategies for Answering Reading Comprehension Questions

1. Reading passages are drawn from many disciplines and sources. You are not expected to be familiar with the material in all of the passages, and you are not expected to have outside knowledge of the passage topics. In addition, your views or opinions may conflict with the views expressed or the information provided in the passage. Answer the questions on the basis of the information provided in the passage.
2. There are three approaches to answering reading comprehension questions: reading the passage carefully, then answering the questions; scanning the passage before reading the questions; and reading the questions, then reading the passage. You must decide which one works most effectively for you. You may find that one strategy usually works best for you, or you may use different strategies with different passages (e.g., reading the questions first if the material is unfamiliar).
3. Underline or mark key parts of the passage to get a sense of its principal ideas, facts, and organization.
4. Analyze the passage carefully before answering the questions. Look for clues that will help you understand unfamiliar material. Separate the main ideas from supporting ideas, or evidence, and the author's ideas or attitudes from background information. Identify the transitions between ideas, and examine the relations among them. For example, are they contrasting or complementary? Consider the points the author makes, the conclusions she draws, and the relation between them.
5. Read each question carefully, and be certain that you understand exactly what is being asked. Read all of the answer choices before selecting the best answer.
6. The best answer is the one that most accurately and completely answers the question. Do not choose an answer simply because it is a true statement. Do not be misled by answer choices that are only partially true or only partially satisfy the problem posed in the question.
7. In answering questions about the main idea of the passage, do not be distracted by statements that are true according to the passage, but are secondary to the central point.

3.3.5 Common Errors in Reading

Many errors are caused by speed or carelessness. Understanding the common types of errors can help you to avoid them.

1. Problems with Analytical Reading

Analytical reading requires a precise, problem-solving approach. If you have trouble reading the questions precisely enough to identify the correct answer, read *Problem Solving and Comprehension*. Almost any college student can benefit from the exercises in this book.

2. Careless Reading of the Questions

Do you read each question analytically? Do you circle important qualifiers, such as "some"? Do you notice questions that have more than one proposition? If your errors result from reading the question too quickly, slow down until your accuracy improves; then increase your speed gradually.

3. Careless Reading of the Passage

Finding the key sentence in the passage is only one step in answering the question. After you locate the sentence, make sure that you thoroughly understand both the question and the information in the passage.

4. Variations in Degree of Concentration

Most students find some passages more interesting than others. They may spend too much time on an interesting passage and lose concentration while reading an uninteresting passage. It is important to approach each passage and its attendant set of questions as though it were a puzzle.

When you analyze your performance on practice tests, do you notice that your correct answers and wrong answers tend to come in groups? This pattern indicates that you slip in and out of focus. To correct this problem, you need to develop your concentration. See Chapter 1 for suggestions on building your ability to concentrate.

5. Slow Start, Slow Finish

Do you perform better on the second reading passage than on the first? If so, you may improve your performance by working on a practice passage just before the test begins.

If your performance is better at the beginning of the test than at the end, you need to increase your stamina. For many people, 45 minutes is a long time for sustained concentration. As with speed, increase stamina slowly.

6. Early Panic, Late Anxiety

If you look at the first question and your mind goes blank, skip that question and move on until you find a question you can answer confidently. You can answer skipped questions if you have time later. Your anxiety level also may increase if you feel that you are working too slowly and will not have enough time to finish.

It is best to practice pacing yourself before you take the test. Increasing your speed under pressure tends to increase the number of careless errors. Your score on the VETs depends on the number of correct answers, not on the total number of questions that you answer. Unlike the SATs, there is no penalty for wrong answers. Therefore, one approach is to answer all of the questions that you can, and then to return to the skipped questions. Because there is no penalty for incorrect answers, guessing is also a valid approach.

7. Question Type Preference

Many students prefer one type of question to another. If you have trouble with a specific type of question, spend extra time working with it. Many people tend to work hardest on what they do best, so you must practice to overcome that tendency. The best way to improve your performance is to work to overcome your weaknesses.

8. Problems with Multiple-Choice Questions

Multiple-choice questions require more analysis time than open-ended or true and false questions. When answering multiple-choice questions, you normally can eliminate two answer choices immediately. It is best to cross them out so that you do not waste time rereading incorrect choices. Finally, you should carefully consider the remaining two possibilities and select the best one. It is a good idea to practice multiple-choice reading questions because they tend to dominate the reading comprehension portion of the test.

9. Negative Stems or Answer Choices

The use of negative words in a question or answer choice makes the item more difficult. Most people are not accustomed to reading for what is not, or for the exception. Usually, the biolgy subtest contains more negative-stem questions than the chemistry subtest because biology does not offer as many options for definition questions.

When you see a negative-stem question, circle the negative word and slow down. You need a separate strategy for these items. Consider each answer, and decide whether it is true or false, marking "T" or "F" next to each. If you are not sure, mark "?T" or "?F." Force yourself to choose. When you use this approach, the answer should be apparent. However, remember that true answers are often easier to identify than false answers.

Especially time consuming are questions that start, "All of the following are true EXCEPT:" As the test date approaches, if you are still working too slowly in the reading section, consider answering all EXCEPT questions last. Remember, answering the single most difficult or most time-consuming question is not rewarded with extra points. It is a better strategy to spend the same amount of time answering two or three easy questions correctly.

10. Keyed-Choice (I, II, III, IV) Questions

Many students have problems with inductively phrased questions. If you do, compare inductively phrased questions with deductively phrased questions. Inductive phrasing allows for more than one possible answer and is a clue that you should choose the best, or most likely, answer.

If most of your reading has been in textbooks, you may be unfamiliar with inductive reasoning in text. You can familiarize yourself with this type of reasoning by reading research reports and scientific periodicals.

If you need practice with questions that test logical and analytical reasoning, you can find extra practice materials in a Law School Admission Test (LSAT) or GRE guide. An actual test provides the best practice. An excellent book on improving reasoning ability is *With Good Reason: An Introduction to Informal Fallacies.*

11. Verbal Ability

Synonyms cause some students problems. To be synonymous, words must be on the same level of classification. For example, "dog" and "German shepherd" are not synonyms because "German shepherd" is only one type of dog. A discussion of synonyms is actually a discussion about the relation between the two terms under consideration. There are three ways to illustrate this relationship: with outlines (Figure 3-4), Venn diagrams (Figure 3-4; see section 1.4.1 in Chapter 1), and analogical, or associative, reasoning (see section 1.5.3 in Chapter 1) .

I. Canine
   A. Dog
      1. German shepherd
      2. poodle
   B. Wolf
      1. red
      2. gray

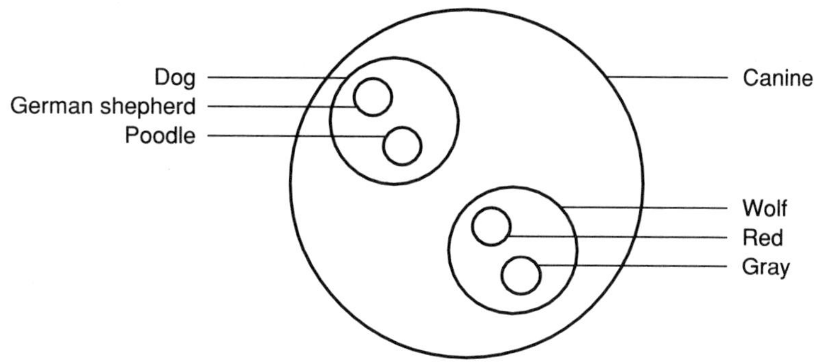

Figure 3-4 Venn diagram.

12. Double Propositions

Many students have trouble with questions that have more than one proposition or answers that have more than one variable. Once again, slow down. Remember that the correct answer must satisfy all of the conditions given.

13. Proportional Reasoning

Students often have trouble with questions that include the words "increase" and "decrease," especially when they require proportional reasoning. Drawing a sketch in the margin of the test booklet and using arrows to help you visualize what is being asked can help with this type of question.

14. Speed, Accuracy, and Concentration

The most common test error is misunderstanding the effects of speed, accuracy, and concentration. Managing time during the test is difficult. Determining how many minutes you have to complete each question or each section does not help because you normally do not spend the same amount of time on each question. Rather, the test contains a mixure of questions of varying degrees of difficulty. You need to develop a sense of timing for working on the questions.

Keep in mind that speed is always a trade-off for accuracy, whether on the VETs or on the highway. Too many students believe that their primary problem on tests is speed, when they really have an accuracy problem. If you build speed before accuracy, you will only select the wrong answer faster.

Negative-stem test questions (i.e., questions that contain FALSE, NOT, or EXCEPT) usually take longer to answer. Negative-stem questions cause difficulty simply because students neither slow down nor change strategy when answering them.

Do not let your unconscious mind determine when you take breaks. Instead, go into the examination with the expectation that after every 30 questions or so, you will sit back, stretch, and roll your head around to ease the strain in your neck and shoulders. Planning your breaks in this way helps you to manage your time more effectively.

15. Learning Error Patterns

Continue to analyze your errors. As you work on reading passages, record your errors and analyze them to identify patterns. An important part of improving your score is developing an awareness of your performance (see section 3.3.4).

You should spend about two-thirds of your study time working to correct your errors and one-third of your time reviewing what you already know or do well. Unless you schedule time in this way, you may work longest on what you already know.

3.4 PRACTICE PASSAGES AND QUESTIONS

Exercise 2. Exercise 2 contains advanced level, logical reading questions that have appeared in some versions of the VETs. Read the passages, and answer the accompanying questions. Each question consists of a given logical statement. Classify each statement according to one of the keyed choices (I, II, III, or IV). The answers are shown in section 3.5.2.

I. Explicitly supported

II. Implicitly supported

III. Contradicted

IV. Neither supported nor contradicted

Passage 2

From the earliest medical records to the present, physicians and laymen have postulated an association between diet and the development of cancer. This has proved a fertile area for a wide range of speculation extending from food faddists to epidemiologists. An objective approach views diet composition and practices in food preparation as possible environmental factors which may influence tumor development.

There are large demographic differences in the prevalence of gastric cancer. Japan, Chile, Austria, Finland, and Iceland have rates (predominantly in men) four or more times those of white men in the United States. In the United States and Europe, higher rates are noted for gastric as well as esophageal cancer among low-income groups.

Certain ethnic groups in the United States appear to have increased risk. Studies of dietary practices in patients with gastric cancer have yielded few or no significant differences from control groups. An association with alcohol intake has been suggested and denied. The increased use of laxatives or mineral oil in affected individuals has been noted. It has been suggested, but remains unproved, that the high incidence of this tumor in Iceland is related to the large intake of smoked food in association with a low intake of vitamin C. It has been pointed out that Japanese prefer talc-dusted rice and that the talc may contain asbestos. The latter is implicated in the development of gastrointestinal cancer, especially gastric cancer. It is postulated that the asbestos-contaminated talc on rice is the carcinogen or cocarcinogen responsible for the high incidence of stomach cancer in Japan.

Death rates for carcinoma of the large bowel (colon cancer) have a strong negative correlation with those of gastric cancer, the one being common where the other is rare. In the United States and England, colon cancer is second only to lung cancer in numbers of deaths. It has been suggested that cancer of the colon in residents of New York is associated with a high fat intake. In Japan, where colon cancer is uncommon, fat intake is about 12% of calories and mostly of the unsaturated type compared with the 40% to 44% figure in the United States.

Japanese immigrants, and especially their children born in the United States, have a much higher incidence of this disease than those in Japan. The same has been noted for Puerto Ricans living in Puerto Rico and on the mainland of the United States.

Japanese people with colon cancer have a higher socioeconomic status than those with rectal cancer and tend to eat diets with more calories in the form of fats and fresh fruit. Czechs have approximately twice the United States rate of intestinal cancer. Their dietary intake is appreciably lower in animal-derived protein and fat and in vitamins. Although their caloric intake is the same, it is derived more from vegetable sources than is the American diet. Contrary to the observations with carcinoma of the esophagus and stomach, the incidence of colon cancer in the United States does not vary appreciably with race or socioeconomic status.

Possible keyed choices:

I. Explicitly supported

II. Implicitly supported

III. Contradicted

IV. Neither supported nor contradicted

1. Environmental factors, such as cooking methods (e.g., frying, steaming) may mitigate the effects of cocarcinogens, such as the talc used on Japanese rice.
2. The incidence of colon cancer is likely to be related to the amount of unsaturated fat present in the diet, regardless of ethnic origin.
3. Scientists have not yet determined which factors in socioeconomic status, diet, and other environmental conditions are most pertinent in determining the risk of cancer, but certain patterns in isolated ethnic groups are at least partially useful as predictors of the risk of specific cancers.
4. A diet high in vegetables, but low in fat, is a reliable prophylaxis for intestinal carcinomas.

Passage 3

Proton magnetic resonance testing enables researchers to distinguish magnetically different protons present in a molecule by counting the signal emitted. Each magnetically different proton sends a separate signal.

There are two means by which protons can be considered "identical"—by symmetry or by being geminal (twins on the same carbon atom). The four protons of methane are all geminal and so only one signal is observed. Similarly, all six protons of ethane are identical by symmetry. But the two methyl groups of methyl ethanoate (methyl acetate) are not identical. One methyl group is attached to a carbonyl carbon, whereas the other is attached to an oxygen. Each methyl group is then in a different magnetic environment. Propane is symmetrical about carbon-2 and so has two magnetically different types of protons. Propane offers the chance to make a careless error in selecting the number of magnetically different protons present. There are four.

Protons (c) and (d) are not identical. Proton (c) is cis to a methyl group, while proton (d) is trans to the methyl group. Again, this gives a different magnetic environment to these protons. In an analogous fashion, protons (c) and (d) of 1,2-dimethyl-cyclopropane are not identical. Here, (d) is cis to two methyl groups, whereas (c) is cis to two protons. With different magnetic environments, (S)-2-bromobutane is a more difficult case. Protons (c) and (d) here are again superficially the same, but in fact they are not. They are "diastereotopic" protons. Replacing each of these protons with some other group will give diastereomers—easily distinguished by chemical and physical properties. Proton (d) will "feel" the effects of the bromine atom of carbon-2 more than will proton (c) in the configuration shown. Each is in a magnetically different environment. If replacement of each of two suspected identical protons with another group yields enantiomers, the protons are called "enantiotopic" and are magnetically indistinguishable.

5. The author advocates the use of diastereomers to distinguish geminally identical proton nuclei in methane.
6. Diastereotopic protons are either geminal or symmetrical.
7. If apparently identical protons yield enantiomers when another group is substituted for each member of the original pair, then the original proton pair may be considered identical.
8. Propane offers a good example of diastereotopic protons.

Exercise 3. The following passages and questions are similar to the VETs reading comprehension section. Read the passages, and answer the questions. The answers are shown in section 3.5.3.

Passage 4

Growth and Formation of Bones

The "cartilage" skeleton is completely formed at the end of 3 months of pregnancy. During subsequent months of gestation, ossification and growth occur.

Longitudinal growth of bones continues in a definite sequence until approximately 15 years of age in girls and 16 in boys. Longitudinal growth should not be confused with bone maturation and remodeling, which are processes continuing until the age of 21 in both men and women. This pattern of maturation is so regular that an individual's age can be determined with amazing accuracy from radiologic examination of his or her bones.

It is sometimes stated that bone is preformed in the cartilage, since the majority of embryonic bones do resemble the future skeleton in shape and composition; however, it is incorrect to state that cartilage actually turns into bone. Cartilage merely represents the environment in which the bone develops.

Formation

Chemical Composition

The strong protein matrix of bone is responsible for its resilience when tension is applied, whereas the salts deposited in this matrix prevent crushing when pressure is applied. A substance known as hydroxyapatite $[Ca_3(PO_4)_2]_3 \cdot Ca(OH)_2$ makes up the major portion of salts present in bone. Small amounts of calcium carbonate ($CaCO_3$) are also present.

Deposition of Bone

Bone develops from spindle-shaped cells called osteoblasts, which are found beneath the periosteum (the fibrovascular membrane covering the bone) and in the endosteum, which lines the marrow cavity. The first function of the osteoblasts is that of secreting a protein substance that polymerizes to form the tough, leather-like matrix. Calcium salts are then precipitated within the matrix, giving the bone its characteristic quality of hardness. For these salts to be deposited, it is necessary that calcium first combine with phosphate, producing calciumphosphate ($CaH\ PO_4$); this substance is slowly converted over a period of several weeks into hydroxyapatite.

Regulation of Deposition

Deposition of bone is regulated partially by the amount of strain on the bone—the more strain, the greater the deposition. Bones in casts, therefore, will waste away, whereas continued and excessive strain will cause the bone to grow thick and strong. In addition, a break in the bone will stimulate injured osteocytes to proliferate, secreting large quantities of matrix for the deposition of new bone.

Reabsorption of Bone

Large cells called osteoclasts are present in almost all cavities of bone, and function to cause reabsorption of bone. It is thought that this is brought about by the secretion of enzymes that digest the protein portion of bone and split the salts. These phosphate and calcium salts are then absorbed into the surrounding extracellular fluid.

The strength and, in some instances, the size of the skeletal bone will depend on the comparative activity of the bone. For example, it is obvious that during the growth period, deposition is more active than reabsorption. The role of the osteoclast has not been definitely established, but it is known to be associated with the removal of dead bone from the inner side during remodeling. As a result, the medullary cavity enlarges, and the bone itself is prevented from becoming overly thick and heavy. Osteoblastic deposition continues to counteract the never-ending process of reabsorption, even when the bones are no longer capable of growth.

It is possible for crooked bones to become straight due to this continual process. A broken bone that has healed crooked in a child will straighten in a matter of a few years.

During the 4-day flight of Gemini IV in 1965, one of the astronauts lost between 1% and 12% of his bone mass, as measured by x-ray of his hands and feet. The flight of Gemini V, which lasted 8 days, caused losses of more than 20%. As a result of these findings, exercises in flight were prescribed that were found to reduce this loss.

Intramembranous Ossification

There are two types of ossification. The first of these is intramembranous ossification, a process in which dense connective membranes are replaced by deposits of inorganic calcium salts, thus forming bone. The membrane itself becomes the periosteum (around bone), whereas immediately within the periosteum can be found compact bone with an inner core of spongy, or cancellous, bone.

Endochondral Ossification

Most bones form by the process of endochondral ossification, the replacement of cartilaginous structures with bone. Growth in length of a bone occurs at the growth plate, which consists of a number of layers of cartilage cells lying between the epiphysis (knoblike extremity of a bone) and the diaphysis (the shaft, or central portion, of a bone). The basal layer of cells is abundantly supplied with blood, and this layer proliferates, producing more cartilage cells and adding to the length of the bone. The upper layers of cells are thus lifted away from the source of blood and nutrients and are subsequently ossified.

As a long bone increases in length, there is a proportional increase in its diameter, owing to periosteal deposition of layers of compact tissue. These layers are thickest in the middle of the shaft and taper toward the epiphysis, which remains essentially cancellous. Simultaneously, the cancellous interior of the diaphysis is destroyed, leading to the formation of the marrow canal. The spongy bone of the epiphysis is left intact.

Ossification of the epiphysis follows a generally predictable pattern. The age of the skeleton can be determined by the presence and size of various mesossification centers. For instance, the physician can determine if a baby is at term by ascertaining whether the distal femoral epiphysis is ossified.

Longitudinal growth is dependent, then, on the growth plate at the junction of the diaphysis and epiphysis. Growth in the diameter of bone occurs primarily by the deposit of bony tissue beneath the periosteum. In a short time, only two thin strips of tissue, the growth plates, remain between the epiphysis and the diaphysis. When these two final sites have filled with osseous tissue, longitudinal growth is complete and growth is no longer possible. The initial shape assumed by a bone during its formation is genetically determined. Extrinsic factors, such as muscle strength, mechanical stress, and biochemical environment, assume a function in determining the shape of a bone. Wolff's law reflects the role of mechanical forces acting on bone and, briefly stated, suggests that the structure of a bone is dependent on its function.

1. Which of the following is NOT a function of the skeletal system?
   A. Support tissues
   B. Protect vital organs and other tissues
   C. Hematopoiesis
   D. Filtration of blood
2. The skeletal system is composed of ____ bones?
   A. 1206
   B. 601
   C. 2010
   D. 206
3. Which of the following is NOT a part of the appendicular skeletal system?
   A. Shoulders
   B. Vertebrae
   C. Pelvic girdle
   D. Arms
4. Ossification of the skeletal system begins:
   A. in utero.
   B. during puberty.
   C. during the first 3 months of pregnancy.
   D. after the first 3 months of pregnancy.
5. The major portion of salts found in bone is represented by:
   A. hydroxyapatite.
   B. calcium carbonate.
   C. calcium chloride.
   D. sodium chloride.
6. Bone develops from cells responsible for secreting a protein matrix, in which salts are precipitated. These cells are called:
   A. fibroblast.
   B. ameloblast.
   C. osteocytes.
   D. osteoblast.
7. Bone deposition is regulated primarily by:
   A. genetic coding.
   B. stress.
   C. age.
   D. cartilage.
8. Before hydroxyapatite can be formed, calcium must combine with:
   A. phosphate.
   B. protein.
   C. oxygen.
   D. carbon.
9. Phosphate and calcium salts freed as a result of bone reabsorption are absorbed into the:
   A. small intestine.
   B. lymphatic system.
   C. extracellular fluids.
   D. bone matrix.
10. Bones of the face and skull are formed by the process of:
    A. endochondral ossification.
    B. osteoclastic activity.
    C. intramembranous ossification.
    D. Wolff's law.
11. Longitudinal growth of bones continues until:
    A. age 25 in men and 24 in women.
    B. age 16 in boys and 15 in girls.
    C. age 19 in men and 18 in women.
    D. puberty in boys and girls.
12. The bone found immediately beneath the periosteum is called:
    A. spongy bone.
    B. compact bone.

C. cancellous bone.
D. long bone.

13. Growth in bone length occurs:
A. in the shaft.
B. at the sutures.
C. at the epiphysis.
D. in the growth plate.

14. Which statement is INCORRECT?
A. Longitudinal growth of bone is complete when the growth plates are completely ossified.
B. Cartilage skeleton will turn to bony skeleton.
C. Strain and injury will cause bone to grow thick and strong.
D. Osteoclast is associated with bone reabsorption.

15. The fibrovascular membrane covering bone is called the:
A. peritoneum.
B. osseous membrane.
C. endosteum.
D. periosteum.

16. All of the following statements are correct EXCEPT:
A. Reabsorption is less active than deposition in the growth period of the bone.
B. Some bones form by the process of mitrochondrial ossification.
C. In a long bone, the periosteal deposition of layers makes the bone taper toward the cancellous epiphysis.
D. The age of the skeleton can be determined by the location and size of mesossification centers.

Passage 5

Mitosis and Meiosis

All organisms that reproduce sexually develop from a single cell, the zygote, produced by the union of two cells, the germ cells or gametes (a spermatozoon from the male and an ovum from the female). The union of an egg and a spermatozoon is called fertilization. The zygote produced by fertilization develops into a new individual of the same species as the parents. Every cell of the individual, with the exception of gametes, contains the same number of chromosomes. In the somatic cells of a plant or an animal, chromosomes are paired, one member of each pair originally derived from one parent, the other member from the other parent. A member of a pair of chromosomes is called a homologue, and commonly we speak of pairs of chromosomes (or of homologues) when we refer to the chromosome number of a species. Humans have forty-six chromosomes, or twenty-three pairs, an onion has eight pairs, a toad has eleven pairs, a mosquito has three pairs, and so on. Homologues of each pair are alike, but the pairs are generally different. The original chromosome number of each cell (diploid number) is preserved during successive nuclear divisions involved in the growth and development of a multicellular organism.

Mitosis

The continuity of the chromosomal set is maintained by cell division, which is called mitosis. At the time of cell division, the nucleus becomes completely reorganized. Mitosis takes place in a series of consecutive stages known as prophase, anaphase, and telophase. In a somatic cell, the nucleus divides by mitosis in such a fashion that each of the two daughter cells receives exactly the same number and kind of chromosomes as the parent cell.

Each chromosome duplicates some time during interphase, before the visible mitotic process begins. At this stage and at early prophase, chromosomes appear as extended and slender threads. At late prophase, chromosomes become short, compact rods by a process of spiral packing. A spindle arises between the two centrioles, and the chromosomes line up across the equatorial plane of the spindle at the metaphase plate. At anaphase, each chromosome separates, forming two daughter chromosomes, which go to opposite poles of the cell. Finally, at telophase, the daughter chromosomes at each pole resolve themselves into a reticulum, and two daughter nuclei are formed.

In mitosis, the original chromosome number is preserved during the successive nuclear division. Since the somatic cells are derived from the zygote by mitosis, they all contain the normal double set, or diploid number (2^n), of chromosomes.

Meiosis

If the gametes (ovum and spermatozoon) were diploid, the resulting zygote would have twice the diploid chromosome number. To avoid this, each gamete undergoes a special type of cell division called meiosis, which reduces the normal diploid set of chromosomes to a single (haploid) set (n). Thus, when the ovum and spermatozoon unite in fertilization, the resulting zygote is diploid. The meiotic process is characteristic of all plants and animals that reproduce sexually, and it takes place in the course of gametogenesis.

Meiosis is the reduction of the chromosome number by means of two nuclear divisions, the first and second meiotic divisions, that involve only a single division of the chromosomes.

The essentials of the process are simple. The homologous chromosomes, distinguished by their identical morphologic characteristics, pair longitudinally; they lie in close contact, forming a bivalent. Each chromosome is composed of two spiral filaments called the chromatids. The bivalent thus contains four chromatids and is also called a tetrad. In the tetrad, each chromatid of the homologue has a single pairing partner. Portions of these paired chromatids may be exchanged from one homologue to the other, giving rise to cross-shaped figures, which are called chiasmata. Chiasma is a cytologic manifestation of an underlying genetic phenomenon called crossing over.

At metaphase I, the bivalents arrange themselves on the spindle, and at anaphase I, the homologous chromosomes and their two associated chromatids migrate to opposite poles. Thus, in the first meiotic division, the monologous pairs of chromosomes are segregated. After a short interphase, the two chromatids of each homologue separate in the second meiotic division, so that the original four chromatids are distributed into each of the four gametes. The result is four nuclei with only a single set of chromosomes.

In the male, all four cells develop into spermatozoa. In the female, one cell develops into an ovum, and the other three become small polar bodies. The formation of germ cells in plants is complicated because before fertilization, the haploid products of meiosis undergo two or more mitotic divisions. However, the essential features of the meiotic process are similar in all sexually reproducing plants and animals.

17. All organisms that reproduce sexually develop from the:
- **A.** gamete.
- **B.** zygote.
- **C.** ovum.
- **D.** homologue.

18. The chromosomes duplicate during:
- **A.** anaphase.
- **B.** telophase.
- **C.** interphase.
- **D.** prophase.

19. The zygote contains the ____ number of chromosomes.
- **A.** haploid
- **B.** tetraploid
- **C.** quadroploid
- **D.** diploid

20. Which statement is NOT true of mitosis?
- **A.** It is a process of cell division.
- **B.** The original chromosome number is preserved.
- **C.** The daughter cells will have the haploid number of chromosomes.
- **D.** The nucleus is completely reorganized.

21. The process of gametogenesis occurs during:
- **A.** mitosis.
- **B.** fertilization.
- **C.** implantation.
- **D.** meiosis.

22. Meiosis is the process by which:
- **A.** the zygote is formed.
- **B.** the diploid number of chromosomes is preserved.
- **C.** continuity of the chromosomal set is maintained.
- **D.** nuclear division occurs, with a reduction in the chromosomes to the haploid number.

23. The bivalent contains four chromatids. It is also called:
- **A.** tetrad.
- **B.** polar bodies.
- **C.** homologues.
- **D.** gametes.

24. During meiosis, the homologous chromosomes and their chromatids migrate to opposite poles during:
- **A.** the second meiotic division.
- **B.** metaphase I.
- **C.** the first meiotic division.
- **D.** anaphase II.

25. In mitosis, the chromosomes line up across the equatorial plate during:
A. anaphase.
B. metaphase.
C. prophase.
D. interphase.

26. During the first meiotic division, the major accomplishment is when:
A. tetrads are formed.
B. gametes are formed.
C. chromosomes come together to form the bivalent.
D. the homologous chromosomes are segregated.

27. A member of a pair of chromosomes is called a:
A. polar body.
B. ovum.
C. sperm cell.
D. homologue.

28. The chromosomes become coiled and visible, and the nuclear membrane disintegrates during what phase of mitosis?
A. Interphase
B. Prophase
C. Metaphase
D. Telophase

29. The correct sequence of steps in mitosis is:
A. Prophase, metaphase, interphase, anaphase, telophase
B. Interphase, anaphase, metaphase, prophase, telophase
C. Interphase, prophase, metaphase, anaphase, telophase
D. Anaphase, prophase, interphase, metaphase, telophase

30. The number of mature gametes resulting from meiosis in the male is:
A. 1.
B. 2.
C. 3.
D. 4.

31. The key difference between anaphase I of meiosis and anaphase of mitosis is:
A. crossing over occurs in anaphase I of meiosis.
B. centromeres divide in anaphase I of meiosis.
C. homologous chromosomes move to opposite poles in anaphase I of meiosis.
D. anaphase in mitosis creates polar bodies.

32. A key difference in the mechanism of mitosis and meiosis is:
A. mitosis has crossing over of homologous chromosomes during prophase.
B. meiosis has a second duplication of DNA during interphase I.
C. meiosis has alignment of homologous chromosomes in metaphase I and separation of homologous chromosomes in anaphase I.
D. mitosis has a reductional division.

33. The main difference in the outcome of mitosis versus meiosis is:
A. meiosis produces identical daughter cells, and mitosis produces different daughter cells.
B. mitosis occurs only in vertebrates.
C. meiosis produces somatic cells.
D. meiosis results in haploid cells, and mitosis results in diploid cells when the parent cells are diploid.

Passage 6

Viruses and Bacteria (Procaryotes)

Procaryotes (bacteria and blue-green algae) differ from eucaryotes by the latter having (1) genetic material in a nucleus and DNA conjugated with proteins; (2) organelles bound within membranes; (3) subcellular structural units to carry out specific functions (e.g., ATP production, photosynthesis); and (4) presence of cell walls made of cellulose or chitin versus murein (amino sugars and amino acids), as in procaryotes. The DNA of procaryotes is found in a nonmembrane region called the nucleoid; enzymes for metabolism and energy production are either free in the cytoplasm or bound to the cell membrane, and the ribosomes are smaller than in eucaryotes. Viruses are not procaryotes or eucaryotes, but constitute their own group.

Viruses

Viruses are usually called "nonliving" and differ from bacteria and other "living" organisms because they (1) do not contain both DNA and RNA; (2) have no metabolic machinery for energy production or protein synthesis; (3) do not arise directly from other viruses, but depend on the host's metabolic machinery to synthesize them; and (4) have no membranes to regulate exit and entry. Structurally, most viruses consist of a protein coat surrounding a core (center) of either DNA or RNA.

The many variations of the basic life cycle of a virus are given below. A cell may have a special receptor or region that is recognized by the virus. The virus attaches and may enter via a process similar to phagocytosis. In the cell, the central core of DNA or RNA and occasionally special enzymes or proteins take over the host's metabolic machinery to produce new coat proteins and new viral DNA or RNA. This may occur in the nucleus, the cytoplasm, or both. The viral coat and viral core (DNA or RNA) then combine to form complete viral particles. At a certain point, the host cell lyses (bursts) and releases the new viral particles as well as uncombined viral coats and viral cores. Sometimes the viral particles exit by a process similar to reverse phagocytosis and incorporate part of the host's cell membrane onto their protein coat in doing so. The above is typical of a virus that attacks an animal or plant cell.

Viruses that attack bacteria are called bacteriophages. Bacteriophages in general consist of a head made of a protein coat and a core as before, and they also contain a tail made of protein that is specialized for attaching to bacteria. A bacteriophage attaches to the surface of bacteria, the core of RNA or DNA is injected into the bacteria, and the protein coat remains on the surface. Then the cycle may proceed as described above for viruses and is called lytic or virulent. However, the bacteriophage nucleic acid may become combined with the bacterial nucleic acid and remain as such for long periods before new bacteriophages are produced and cell rupture occurs. In this case, the bacteriophage is called lysogenic or temperate. The nucleic acid from the bacteriophage is called a prophage. Newly released bacteriophages may contain some of the bacteria's nucleic acid that may be passed onto other bacteria when they are attacked by these bacteriophages. This is the mechanism of transduction.

Bacteria

The general characteristics of bacterial structure are discussed above under procaryotes. More specifically, from inside out, bacteria may have a capsule that is usually made of a polysaccharide mucoid-like material and protects the bacteria from phagocytosis. Inside the capsule is the cell wall, and this prevents the hyperosmotic bacteria from bursting. Inside the cell wall is the cell membrane that may contain invaginations called mesosomes, where localization of enzymes concerned with similar functions may be found. The cytoplasm and nucleoid are as described above. The DNA is circular and is haploid. Some bacteria contain flagella or cilia for locomotion—these are structurally different than their eucaryotic counterparts.

Bacteria have three common shapes: cocci (spherical or ovoid), bacilli (cylindrical or rod-like), and spirillia (helically coiled). The cocci are often found in clusters: diplococci (two bacteria together), streptococci (linear chains of cocci), or staphylococci (grape-like clusters of cocci). All of these are made up of individual bacteria with distinct cell walls.

Metabolically, bacteria may be aerobic or anaerobic. Anaerobic bacteria may use fermentation (where an organic molecule, such as pyruvate lactate, is the final electron acceptor) or inorganic substances as final electron receptors (such as S—H_2S). An obligate anaerobe is one that is killed if exposed to oxygen. This is usually because they cannot handle the peroxides (very toxic) produced in oxidative metabolism. A facultative anaerobe can metabolize in the presence or absence of oxygen. Bacteria may use a great variety of molecules as nutrients. Some are photosynthetic, others are heterotrophic (using organic molecules made by other organisms), and others are chemosynthetic (making organic molecules and energy from inorganic precursors). The last group are important in fixation of nitrogen for use by all organisms. The variety of metabolic nutrients required and products produced are extremely important in studying basic questions of genetics as well as biochemistry, and also in differentiating between the different types of bacteria.

Most bacteria reproduce asexually by the process of binary fission that produces two identical haploid daughter cells by the simple process of mitosis. Genetic recombination (e.g., transfer and rearrangement of genetic information) may occur by three distinct means: transformation, transduction, and conjugation. Transformation involves a bacterium picking up free DNA from a medium, the free DNA being from a different bacterium. Transduction is the transfer of parts of DNA between bacteria by bacteriophages. In conjugation, there is pairing of "male" and "female" forms. DNA is passed sequentially between them via structures called pili. All or a fraction of the DNA may be passed in this way.

The above three genetic mechanisms allow extraordinary adaptability and variability of bacterium. Since bacteria can reproduce in a span as short as 20 minutes, a new trait, such as drug resistance, can spread rapidly in a given population.

34. Bacteriophages:
A. cause disease in humans.
B. are viruses.
C. are bacteria.
D. can reproduce by binary fission.

35. Which substance is NOT ordinarily found in viruses?
A. Carbohydrates
B. Proteins
C. RNA
D. DNA

36. Viruses:
A. are considered living organisms.
B. consist of protein, lipids, and carbohydrates only.
C. do not arise from other viruses directly.
D. have an incomplete metabolic machinery for energy production.

37. Eucaryotes are characterized by all of the following EXCEPT:
A. genetic material in a nucleus.
B. organelles bound within membranes.
C. the presence of cell walls made of murein.
D. subcellular structural units to carry out specific functions.

38. "Contains DNA or RNA, no means of energy production, cannot reproduce self directly" would be a description of :
A. an animal cell.
B. a plant cell.
C. a bacterium
D. a virus.

39. In the replication of a virus in a host cell:
A. the virus directs the metabolic machinery of the host.
B. the host directs synthesis of new viral particles.
C. viral particles are made as a single unit (i.e., coat and core).
D. coat and core structures are released from the host and then combined.

40. Structurally, bacteriophages differ from the usual virus by:
A. having a protein coat.
B. having a core of DNA or RNA.
C. being able to replicate independent of a host cell.
D. having a tail region made of protein for attaching to cells.

41. The part of the cycle of a bacteriophage that may be different from that of a typical virus is:
A. taking over of the host cell's metabolic machinery.
B. incorporation of its nucleic acid into the host cell's.
C. lysis of the host cell.
D. synthesis by the host cell of coat and core separately, followed by combination to form a complete particle.

42. Which structure may protect bacteria from phagocytosis by white blood cells?
A. Mesosome
B. Capsule
C. Nucleoid
D. Cell wall

43. Which association is NOT correct?
A. Cocci—spherical
B. Bacilli—rod-like
C. Diplococci—two cocci
D. Staphylococci—linear combinations of cocci

44. The process whereby a bacterium picks up DNA from a medium and incorporates it into its own DNA is called:
A. binary fission.
B. conjugation.
C. transformation.
D. transduction.

45. Bacteria transfer (exchange) genetic information between themselves by all of the following EXCEPT:
A. transformation.
B. transduction.
C. budding.
D. conjugation.

46. Methods used to distinguish between bacteria may include all of the following EXCEPT:
A. shape.
B. nutrient requirements.
C. products of metabolism.
D. none of the above.

47. A form of hepatitis (inflammation of the liver) is caused by a virus. The serum of patients with hepatitis may contain antigens from the virus hepatitis B surface antigen (HB_sAg) and hepatitis B core antigen

(HB_cAg). An antigen is a substance foreign to the body and capable of eliciting an immune response. Which statement is correct?

A. This information is inconsistent with what is known about modes of viral replication.
B. HB_cAg is probably a lipid.
C. HB_sAg is probably a protein.
D. Enzymes found in liver cells probably do not increase in the serum during the acute disease.

48. Assume that all of these agents can affect only the host cell and its contents. Which of the following would interfere most with the replication of a virus?

A. An agent that blocks synthesis of lipids
B. An agent that blocks synthesis of carbohydrates
C. An agent that blocks synthesis of proteins
D. An agent that blocks synthesis of lysogenic enzymes

49. In the treatment of viral infections, a drug is discovered that directly blocks the synthesis of the viral protein coat. This drug:

A. probably adversely affects protein synthesis by the host cell and hence may cause side effects in the host.
B. probably does not affect host protein synthesis.
C. probably destroys final electron receptors.
D. probably makes the viral protein coat thicker to penetrate.

50. Given a bacterial population without resistance to a certain drug, all of the following may cause introduction of bacterial resistance EXCEPT:

A. transformation.
B. binary fission.
C. transduction.
D. conjugation.

3.5 ANSWER KEY

3.5.1 Exercise 1

1. B	**6. C**
2. A	**7. A**
3. C	**8. C**
4. C	**9. A**
5. A	**10. C**

3.5.2 Exercise 2

1. [IV] Cooking is only mentioned as food preparation in paragraph 1; no relation between cooking and talc or cooking and cancer is made, and no mention of ameliorating any environmental factors is introduced as a remedy or preventive action.
2. [II] See paragraphs 4 and 5.
3. [II] This sentence is a fair statement of the key idea of the passage, and is therefore implicitly supported.
4. [III] See paragraph 6 description of the Czech diet.
5. [IV] This statement is primarily nonsense and depends on a misreading of the entire passage. The clue is that the author advocates nothing.
6. [III] See definition in lines 8–10.
7. [I] See lines 35–39.
8. [II] See lines 19 and 31.

3.5.3 Exercise 3

1. D	**4. D**	**7. B**	**10. C**	**13. D**
2. D	**5. A**	**8. A**	**11. B**	**14. B**
3. B	**6. D**	**9. C**	**12. B**	**15. D**

16. B	**23. A**	**30. D**	**37. C**	**44. C**
17. B	**24. C**	**31. C**	**38. D**	**45. C**
18. C	**25. B**	**32. C**	**39. A**	**46. D**
19. D	**26. D**	**33. D**	**40. D**	**47. C**
20. C	**27. D**	**34. B**	**41. B**	**48. C**
21. D	**28. B**	**35. A**	**42. B**	**49. A**
22. D	**29. C**	**36. C**	**43. D**	**50. B**

REFERENCES

Atkinson RH, Longman DG: *Reading Enhancement and Development,* 4th ed. St. Paul, MN, West, 1992.

Finegold, Baron: *Diagnostic Microbiology*, 7th ed. St. Louis, Mosby-Year Book, 1986.

Flesch RF: *The Art of Clear Thinking*. San Francisco, Harper & Row, 1973.

Giroux JA, Williston GR: *Comprehension Skills, Isolating Details to Recalling Specific Facts, Advanced Level.* Providence, Jamestown, 1974.

Quinn S, Irvings S: *Active Reading in the Arts and Sciences*, 2nd ed. Boston, Allyn and Bacon, 1991.

4

CHAPTER

Preparing for the VETs Biology Test

4.0 INTRODUCTION

The biology section of the VETs includes the Medical College Admission Test (MCAT) Biological Sciences Test, the Graduate Record Examination (GRE) Biology Test, and the Veterinary College Admission Test (VCAT) Biology Section. These examinations measure knowledge of elementary biology. The VCAT Biology Section is the most direct and basic test, the GRE Biology Test is slightly more difficult, and the MCAT Biological Sciences Test is the most difficult, especially for students with no clinical background. This chapter describes the topics covered, the level of subject matter, and the types of questions on the VETs. However, it does not provide a formal review of biology. While preparing for the VETs, review college textbooks on biology, general chemistry, and organic chemistry. A detailed subject outline is shown in section 4.1.

A useful book for measuring competency is *A Complete Preparation for the MCAT.* The GRE biology and chemistry books are useful for testing aptitude. Biology review software is also available.

4.1 BIOLOGY TOPICS FOR THE VETs

This chapter provides an overview of the biology topics covered on the VETs. A biology review test is included (see section 4.9) to illustrate the difficulty of test questions. Use these questions to evaluate your understanding of biology and to identify topics that require more independent study. Students who are preparing for the VETs should be familiar with the following topics:

I. Cell biology and bioenergetics
   A. Origin of life
   B. Cell metabolism
      1. Cellular respiration
         a. Aerobic respiration
         b. Anaerobic respiration
      2. Photosynthesis
         a. Autotrophs

b. Heterotrophs
c. Equation
3. Respiration versus photosynthesis
C. Enzymology
1. Function and example
2. Coenzymes
3. Specificity of an enzyme
4. Enzyme and substrate (lock and key) model
5. Feedback inhibition
a. Enzyme reaction kinetics
b. Chart of digestive enzymes
D. Thermodynamics and cellular bioenergetics
1. Definitions
a. Heat and internal energy
b. Thermal equilibrium and temperature
2. Scales for temperature measurement
a. Thermometer
(1) Freezing point
(2) Boiling point
b. Four temperature scales
(1) Celsius
(2) Fahrenheit
(3) Rankine
(4) Absolute
3. Heat capacity
a. Specific heat capacity
b. Equation
c. Calorie and joule
4. Thermodynamics
a. First law of thermodynamics
(1) Entropy
(2) Enthalpy
b. Second law of thermodynamics
5. Bioenergetics
a. Definitions
b. Energy production
(1) Glycolysis
(2) Citric acid cycle
(3) Electron transport system
(4) Oxidative phosphorylation
E. Organelles
1. Structure and function
2. Definition of cell and organelle
a. Eukaryotic cell
b. Prokaryotic cell
3. Parts of a eukaryotic cell
a. Cell membrane and transport
(1) Phospholipids
(2) Unit membrane model
(3) Fluid mosaic model
(4) Diffusion
(5) Osmosis
(6) Tonicity
(7) Facilitated diffusion
(8) Active transport

(9) Phagocytosis
(10) Pinocytosis
b. Cytoplasm and cytoplasm organelles
(1) Location of organelles
(2) Function of organelles
c. Nucleus and cell mitosis
(1) Chromatin
(2) Chromosomes
(3) Cell division
(4) Cell cycle
(a) Interphase
(b) Prophase
(c) Metaphase
(d) Telophase
(e) Centrioles
3. Example of a eukaryotic cell
a. Fungi
(1) Characteristics
(2) Life cycle and reproduction
b. Protista
II. Microbiology of bacteria and fungi
A. Bacteria and viruses
1. Structure, shape, metabolism, and life cycle
2. Life history of human immunodeficiency virus and acquired immune deficiency syndrome
3. Viral and rickettsial diseases
B. Characteristics of bacteriophages and rickettsiae
C. Schizomycetes class of bacteria
1. Order Eubacteriales
a. Suborder Eubacteriineae
b. Suborder Caulobacteriineae
c. Suborder Rhodobacteriineae
2. Order Actinomycetales
3. Order Chlamydobacteriales
4. Order Myxobacteriales
5. Order Spirochaetales
6. Order Beggiatoales
D. Nutritional grouping of bacteria
1. Autotrophic bacteria
2. Saprophytic bacteria
3. Parasitic bacteria
E. Bacteria and enzymes
1. Hydrolytic enzymes
a. Amylolytic enzymes
(1) Diastase
(2) Cellulase
(3) Disaccharidases
b. Lipolytic enzymes
c. Proteolytic enzymes
2. Oxidizing enzymes
a. Alcoholnidase
b. Zymase
F. Bacterial respiration
G. Mechanisms of infection
1. Pathogenic bacteria
a. Virulence
b. Specificity

2. Sources of infection
    a. Outside the host
    b. Within the host
    c. Transmission of disease-producing organisms

III. Plant biology
  A. Cellular anatomy and physiology
    1. Adenosine triphosphate and energy-producing pathways
      a. Respiration
      b. Fermentation
      c. Photosynthesis
      d. Experimental biosynthesis
      e. Guttation
    2. Extracellular matrix
      a. Plant cell walls
      b. Collagen
  B. Plant structure and function (morphology)
    1. Roots, stems, leaves, and their tissues
    2. Meristems
    3. Water relations
      a. Absorption
      b. Transport
      c. Transpiration
    4. Mineral nutrition
    5. Translocation and storage
    6. Control mechanisms
      a. Hormones
      b. Photoperiods
      c. Tropisms
  C. Plant reproduction and development
    1. Sex and alternation of generations
    2. Flowers, fruits, and seeds
    3. Mendelian genetics
  D. Histology (laboratory techniques)
  E. Mycology
  F. Phycology
  G. Paleobotany
  H. Taxonomy
  I. Pathology

IV. Animal biology
  A. Integumentary system
    1. Skin and thermodynamics
    2. Layers of skin
    3. Functions of skin
    4. Thermoregulation
      a. Mechanisms of heat conservation
      b. Mechanisms of heat loss
  B. Skeletal system
    1. Structure of bones
      a. Spongy bone
      b. Compact bone
      c. Human bone
        (1) Flat bone
        (2) Long bone
    2. Human skeleton

C. Muscular system
   1. Types of muscles
      a. Smooth
      b. Striated
      c. Cardiac
   2. Attachment and structure of muscles
      a. Antagonistic muscle
      b. Synergistic muscle
      c. Muscle groups
         (1) Flexor and extensor
         (2) Abductor and adductor
      d. Functional units of muscle
         (1) Myofibril
            (a) Sarcomeres
            (b) Myosin
            (c) Actin complex
         (2) Sarcoplasmic reticulum
   3. Oxygen debt and voluntary muscle control
      a. Oxidative metabolism
      b. Endurance and cramps

D. Circulatory system
   1. Heart
      a. Structure
      b. Heartbeat
         (1) Systole
         (2) Diastole
   2. Circulatory blood vessels
      a. Arteries
      b. Veins
      c. Arterioles
      d. Capillaries
   3. Blood
      a. Red blood cells
      b. White blood cells
      c. Platelets
      d. Lymphocytes
   4. Blood circulation
      a. Resistance
      b. Ejection fraction
      c. Critical velocity
      d. Cardiac output

E. Immunologic system
   1. Types of immunity
      a. Natural
         (1) Racial
         (2) Individual
      b. Acquired
         (1) Active
         (2) Passive
   2. Mechanisms of immunity
      a. Opsonins
      b. Bacteriolysins
      c. Agglutinins
      d. Precipitins
      e. Antitoxins

f. Hypersensitivity
   (1) Anaphylaxis
   (2) Allergy

F. Digestive system
   1. Structure and functional relations
   2. Digestive functions of key nutrients
   3. Origins and functions of digestive enzymes
G. Respiratory system
   1. Structure and function
   2. Effects of smoking
H. Renal fluid composition
   1. Body fluid composition
      a. Extracellular
      b. Intracellular
      c. Acidity of plasma
   2. Excretory system
      a. Structure
      b. Function
   3. Homeostasis of body fluids
   4. Buffers in the renal system
I. Nervous system
   1. Central and peripheral systems
      a. Neurons
         (1) Sensory neurons
         (2) Motor neurons
         (3) Associate neurons
      b. Neurotransmitters and impulse transmission
   2. Autonomic system
      a. Sympathetic system
      b. Parasympathetic system
   3. Hindbrain
      a. Structure
      b. Function
   4. Spinal cord
   5. Types of nerves
      a. Cranial nerves
      b. Spinal nerves
J. Endocrine system
   1. Anatomy and function of endocrine glands
   2. Hormones
K. Reproductive system
   1. Female and male anatomy
   2. Gametogenesis
      a. Females
      b. Males
   3. Meiosis
   4. Menstrual period
L. Effects of disease on animal body systems
   1. Mechanisms of disease
   2. Diseases of the circulatory system
   3. Diseases of the digestive system
   4. Diseases of the respiratory system
   5. Diseases of the excretory system
   6. Diseases of the nervous system

M. Evolution and adaptation
   1. Mechanisms of evolution
      a. Mutation
      b. Hardy-Weinberg law
   2. Consequences of evolution
      a. Speciation
         (1) Reproductive isolation
         (2) Geographic isolation
      b. Patterns of evolution
         (1) Convergent
         (2) Divergent
         (3) Parallel
   3. Population growth
      a. Growth curves
      b. Parallel growth
N. Social behavior
   1. Basic behavioral responses
   2. Effect of evolution of neurologic structures on behavior
   3. Behavioral modes in populations
      a. Social factors
      b. Interspecific interactions
   4. Communication between individuals
O. Respiratory systems
   1. Animals without specialized respiratory organs
      a. Harvey's luminescent organism equation
      b. Nonspherical organisms
   2. Animals with respiratory organs
      a. Fish gill ventilation
      b. Animals with lungs
         (1) Ventilation lungs
         (2) Diffusion lungs
         (3) Mammalian lungs
         (4) Avian air sacs
      c. Insect tracheae
   3. Comparison of air and aquatic respiration
P. Vertebrate circulation
   1. Total body water distribution
      a. Extracellular
      b. Intracellular
   2. Vertebrate heart size
      a. Heartbeat related to size
      b. Colloidal osmotic pressure
Q. Digestive systems
   1. Food size related to feeding method
      a. Using mucus traps (e.g., trinicates)
      b. Using tentacles (e.g., sea cucumbers)
      c. Using setae (e.g., flamingos)
      d. Using cilia (e.g., sponges)
      e. Ingesting inactive masses (e.g., earthworms)
      f. Chewing (e.g., insects, snails)
      g. Swallowing prey (e.g., snakes)
      h. Sucking nectar (e.g., bees)
      i. Ingesting blood (e.g., leeches)
      j. External digestion (e.g., spiders)

2. Energy metabolism
    a. Oxygen storage
    b. Metabolic rate and body size
    c. Oxygen consumption
        (1) Swimming
        (2) Flying

R. Biophysical parameters
1. Temperature
    a. Antifreeze glycoproteins in fish
    b. Nonshivering thermogenesis
    c. Body size related to evaporation rate
2. Osmotic regulation
    a. Osmoconformers (e.g., aquatic invertebrates)
    b. Ionic concentrations in body fluids
    c. Osmoregulation
    d. Aquatic vertebrates
        (1) Eslasmobranchs
        (2) Cyclostomes
        (3) Teleosts
        (4) Amphibians
    e. Air-breathing vertebrates
3. Biomechanics and locomotion
    a. Movement by cilia and flagella
    b. Jumping mechanics
    c. Channels and gates
        (1) Nerve cell potentials
        (2) Nerve impulses

V. Population biology and genetics

A. Biologic organization and relation of major taxa
1. Linnaeus's classification chart
2. Five-kingdom classification chart
    a. Characteristics of kingdoms
    b. Examples of kingdoms
        (1) Kingdom Protista
        (2) Kingdom Fungi
        (3) Kingdom Monera
        (4) Kingdom Plantae
            (a) Prokaryota
            (b) Eukaryota
        (5) Kingdom Animalia: phylum Chordata
            (a) Subphylum Invertebrates
            (b) Subphylum Vertebrates
                (i) Class Amphibia
                (ii) Class Reptilia
                (iii) Class Aves (birds)
                (iv) Class Mammalia
                (v) Class Osteichthyes (bony fish)

B. Fertilization, descriptive embryology, and developmental mechanics
1. Fertilization
2. Developmental mechanics of embryos
3. Descriptive embryology
    a. Differentiation
    b. Determination
    c. Induction

C. Chromosomal, molecular, and human genetics
   1. Nucleic acids
      a. Nucleotides
      b. Nucleosides
      c. Nucleic acids
   2. RNA structure
      a. Types of RNA
      b. Differences between DNA and RNA
   3. Biosynthesis and molecular genetics
      a. Genetic code
      b. Duplication and transcription of DNA
      c. Translation of RNA
      d. Activation of amino acids by activating enzymes
      e. Protein synthesis
         (1) Base-pairing rule
         (2) Chart of amino acids and DNA codons

D. Mendelian genetics
   1. Alleles
      a. Homozygous
      b. Heterozygous
   2. Mendelian inheritance
      a. First law of segregation
      b. Second law of independent assortment
   3. Chromosomal mutations
   4. Pedigree charts and Punnett squares
   5. Hardy-Weinberg principle

4.2 CELL BIOLOGY AND BIOENERGETICS

The earth is approximately 4.5 billion years old, and life on earth started 3 billion years ago. Most scientists believe that chemical events that occurred over a period of hundreds of millions of years resulted in the formation of bioorganic cells.

For thousands of years, people believed in spontaneous generation, or the routine appearance of living organisms from nonliving matter. Francesco Redi, an Italian scientist, disproved spontaneous generation in 1668 by laboratory experiments on maggots. The theory of spontaneous generation was disproved in 1850 by Louis Pasteur in France.

4.2.1 Origin of Life

The origin of life is rooted in four basic requirements: the presence of certain chemicals, the absence of oxygen, an energy source, and millions of years.

These requirements were tested in 1936 in a laboratory apparatus based on ideas proposed by Russian scientist Alexander Oparin and again in 1953 by American scientist Stanley Miller. The laboratory equipment was rich in hydrogen, ammonia, and methane, and was used to produce proteinoids, or chains of amino acids. Adding water to proteinoids formed microspheres that were similar to living cells.

4.2.2 Prokaryotic and Eukaryotic Cells

Table 4-1 compares prokaryotic cells with eukaryotic cells. Learn the structures, life history, and sources of disease for bacteria, bacteriophages, viruses, and fungi. Learn the detailed structure and functions of eukaryotic cells. Study both generalized eukaryotic cells and specialized eukaryotic cells, such as neural cells, or neurons; muscle cells; epithelial cells; and connective cells. Evaluate the physical and chemical aspects of cell membrane transport models, ion channels, chromosome movement mechanics, cellular adhesion, and membrane receptors. Section 4.3 discusses bacteriology and viral diseases.

TABLE 4-1. ***Comparison of Prokaryotic and Eukaryotic Cells***

		Eukaryote	
Cell Structure	**Prokaryote**	**Animal Cell**	**Plant Cell**
Cell membrane	Present	Present	Present
Cell wall	Present	Absent	Present
Nucleus	Absent	Present	Present
Chromosomes	Single DNA molecule	Multiple DNA and protein	Multiple DNA and protein
Endoplasmic reticulum	Absent	Usually present	Usually present
Mitochondrium	Absent	Present	Present
Ribosomes	Present	Present	Present
Golgi bodies	Absent	Present	Present
Lysosomes	Absent	Often present	Similar structures
Vacuoles	Absent	Small or absent	Present
9 + 2 cilia/flagella	Absent	Often present	Present
Centrioles	Absent	Present	Absent

4.2.3 Bioorganic Molecules

Proteins, amino acids, phospholipids, and carbohydrates have complex classification techniques and experimental analysis techniques. Learn the types and configurations of biologically significant molecules. Memorize the 22 α-amino acids and their structures, along with the RNA genetic code showing the base sequence. Distinguish between epimers and anomers with respect to carbohydrates. Know the basic molecular structures of phospholipids and sphingolipids. Understand the classification and experimentation techniques for bioorganic molecules (e.g., How are steroids classified? How are steroids tested in the laboratory to determine pK_{a1}, pK_{a2}, and isoelectric points?)

4.2.4 Enzymology

Enzymes are chiral molecules and behave as stereospecific or geometry-specific biochemicals. Focus on the molecular structure and functions of enzymes for the animal body. Remember the classification of enzymes as isomerases, ligases, oxidoreductases, transferases, hydrolases, and lysases. Review the molecular structure and special functions of elastase, plasmin, trypsin, urease, α-amylase, enterokinase, and bovine pancreatic ribonuclease. Recognize allosteric effectors and the role they play in enzymology. Identify important coenzymes, such as biotin, nicotinamide, and lipoic acid. Learn how to graph enzyme reactions and the feedback inhibition characteristics of enzymes.

4.2.5 Protein Synthesis

Protein synthesis, or biosynthesis, has two subprocesses: translation and transcription. Each subprocess consists of three major steps: initiation, elongation, and termination, or release of the biochain. Link the structure and chemistry of biologic molecules to the mechanics of translation and transcription. Understand Crick's law of molecular biology: DNA information is passed onto the RNA, which in turn transfers it to the proteins. Focus on how information is passed from DNA to RNA, how information is passed from RNA to proteins, and how research is performed to prove the law.

4.2.6 Cellular Metabolism

Cellular metabolism consists of a series of complex biochemical reactions. These reactions are of four types: carbon bond reactions (i.e., making and breaking of C bonds); isomerization, substitution, and reorganization reactions; oxidation and reduction reactions; and electrophilic group-transfer reactions (i.e., nucleophile to nucleophile).

Apply these types of reactions to the four major biochemical processes of glycolysis, the citric acid cycle, the electron transport chain, and oxidative phosphorylation. Understand the mechanisms that determine and control the biochemical synthesis of lipids, fatty acids, lipoproteins, amino acids, and urea. Relate biochemical synthesis to basal metabolic rate. Relate Gibbs' free energy theory to cellular metabolism. Compare and contrast exergonic and endergonic reactions related to $\Delta G = \Delta G° + RT (\ln[P_1][P_2]/[R_1][R_2])$. P_1, P_2 are the biochemical products, and R_1, R_2 are the biochemical reactants. Understand Lipmann's law as it applies to eukaryotes and prokaryotes: The ADP–ATP coupling is the receptor and distributor of biochemical energy in all living organisms or more complex systems.

4.2.7 Cell Metabolism

Metabolism is the total of all chemical reactions in a cell, including anabolism, catabolism, respiration, and photosynthesis. ATP, which is produced as a result of cellular respiration, is the source of energy for most endothermic reactions in cells. Cellular respiration is divided into two types:

1. Aerobic respiration (i.e., with oxygen):

   $C_6H_{12}O_6 + 6O_2 \rightarrow 6CO_2 + 6H_2O + 38ATP$
   (glucose) 2ATP

   Net ATP gained = 36

2. Anaerobic respiration (i.e., without oxygen):

   $C_6H_{12}O_6 \rightarrow 2C_2H_5OH + 2CO_2 + 4ATP$
   2ATP (ethyl alcohol)

   Net ATP gained = 2

Autotrophs are organisms that make food (i.e., organic molecules) from inorganic molecules. In contrast, heterotrophs are organisms that take in preformed food. Plants, algae, and some bacteria are autotrophs; animals, fungi, and many unicellular organisms are heterotrophs. These organisms are further classified as chemoautotrophs, photoautotrophs, chemoheterotrophs, and photoheterotrophs.

Photosynthesis (Figure 4-1) is a complex set of reactions by which autotrophic organisms make food. Chlorophyll is the green pigment found in plants and leaves. The equation for photosynthesis is the opposite of that for aerobic respiration. Respiration is exergonic, whereas photosynthesis is endergonic. Sunlight is converted into ATP during photosynthesis. Glucose is the most important molecule for any form of life.

4.2.8 Formation and Properties of Enzymes

Enzymes are secretion products formed within the cells by the living protoplasm. Some of them, known as intracellular enzymes, or endoenzymes, remain within the cell during its lifetime. Others, known as extracellular enzymes, or exoenzymes, diffuse through the cell membranes and into the surrounding medium. In some cases, the secretion from the cell is not the true enzyme, but a proenzyme or zymogen that is converted into the true enzyme after it leaves the cell. Some types of enzymes, such as oxidases, are produced by all species and aid in respiration. Others are produced only by certain species.

The best known enzymatic changes are catabolic. These changes result in products that are chemically simpler than the substance that is destroyed. Others, however, are synthetic and aid in the creation of more complex substances, even protoplasm. When the first few enzymes were discovered, no naming scheme was followed, but the suffix -ase is now generally added to the name of the material affected (e.g., maltase, gelatinase, urease). This method of naming is complicated by the fact that different types of enzymes may act on the same substance and form a different product. For example, alcohol,

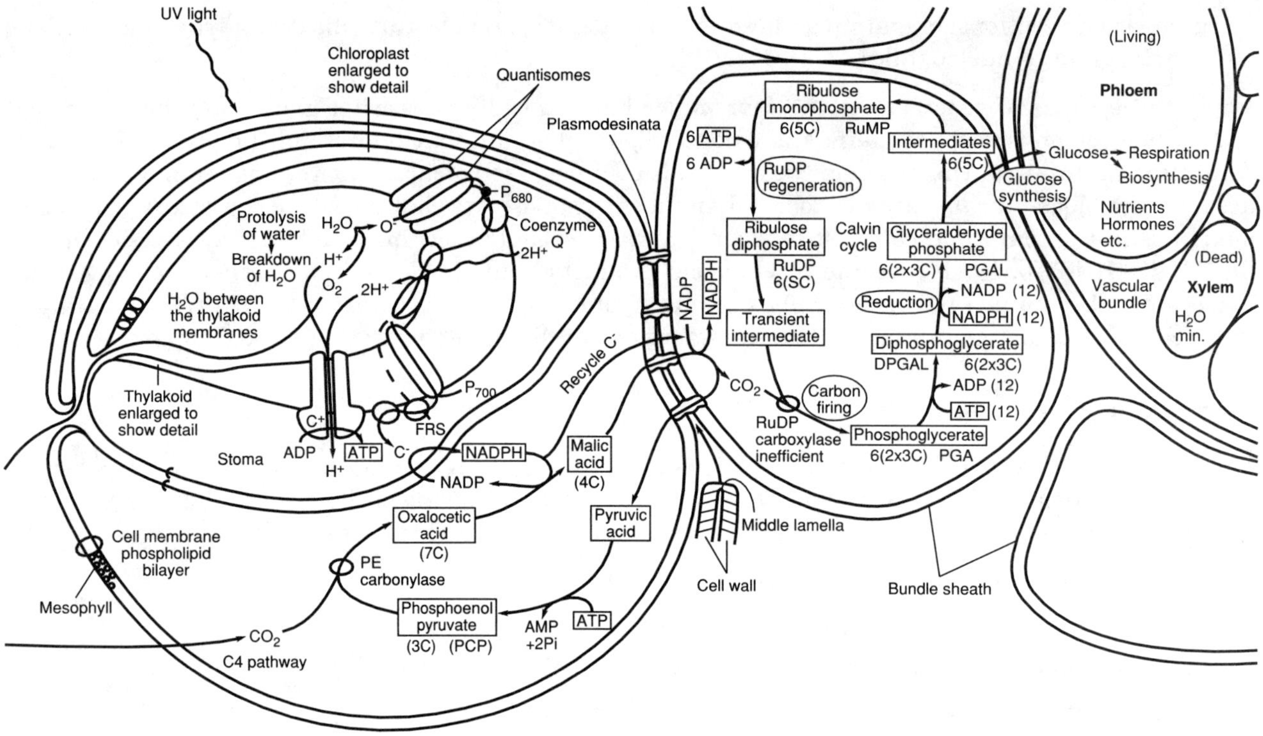

Figure 4-1. Photosynthesis.

glycerol, lactic acid, or oxalic acid may be formed from glucose. Enzymes cannot be classified by their appearance because most have not been seen in their pure state; neither can they be classified by their chemical composition until it is determined. Two methods of classifying enzymes are in common use. One is based on the type of substrate affected by the enzyme (e.g., carbohydrates, fats, proteins). The other is based on the reaction that the enzyme catalyzes (e.g., hydrolysis, oxidation, reduction).

On the basis of the chemical change produced by the enzyme, two classes are distinguished: hydrolases, which promote hydrolysis; and oxidases, including reductases, which promote oxidation and reduction.

4.2.9 Partial Classification of Enzymes

The hydrolytic group includes enzymes that cause one or more molecules of water to combine with each molecule of substance, such as starch, and form a new substance. Because most amylolytic and proteolytic enzymes produce changes through hydrolysis, this group is large.

The amylolytic group, known as carbohydrases, consists of enzymes that hydrolyze complex carbohydrates into simpler carbohydrates. Diastase (e.g., amylase, ptyalin) which varies slightly, depending on the source, hydrolyzes starch to maltose. Cellulase converts cellulose into the sugar cellobiose. This reaction is similar to the destruction of starch because cellulose has the same empirical formulas as starch. Cellulase is produced by many fungi, but by only a few types of bacteria, chiefly some *Bacterium* species and some *Clostridium* species. Both diastase and cellulase are exoenzymes. Disaccharidases change disaccharides into monosaccharides. The action of maltase, for example, is shown in the following formula:

$$\underset{\text{Maltose}}{C_{12}H_{22}O_{11}} + H_2O \rightarrow \underset{\text{Glucose}}{2C_6H_{12}O_6}$$

Similarly, invertase converts sucrose into glucose and fructose, and lactase converts lactose into glucose and galactose. Disaccharidases are produced by many species of fungi, yeasts, and bacteria. They are exoenzymes.

The lipolytic, or streatolytic, group includes approximately a dozen exoenzymes that hydrolyze fats and esters. Lipases hydrolyze fats into fatty acids and glycerol. Few types of bacteria produce lipase, but when sufficient water is present in fats and oils to support bacterial life, fats are hydrolyzed by certain species of bacteria. The storage capacity of fats is largely a result of their dryness.

The proteolytic group includes extracellular enzymes that hydrolyze proteins and related substances. The best known of these are pepsin and trypsin, which are important in animal digestion. No bacteria are known to produce pepsin. The proteases produced by many types of bacteria and fungi are similar in action to trypsin. Gelatinase, which hydrolyzes and liquefies gelatin when it is mixed with water to form a gel, is produced by many bacteria and fungi. Rennin hydrolyzes the casein of milk, forming paracasein, which combines with calcium to form a precipitate. The enzyme is produced abundantly by the stomachs of young mammals, such as pigs, sheep, and calves, as well as by some types of bacteria.

The oxidizing group includes enzymes that promote the addition of oxygen to other substances. These enzymes play a part in the respiration of all living things. The action of oxidizing enzymes is easily demonstrated by cutting open an apple and noting the browning that occurs as a result of oxidation when the cut surface is exposed to air. Dehydrogenases are oxidizing enzymes in the sense that they remove hydrogen from water with aerobic bacteria. Alcoholoxidase oxidizes the alcohol produced by yeasts to the acetic acid of vinegar. It is produced chiefly by bacteria of the genus *Acetobacter*. Alcoholoxidase may be a group of enzymes rather than a single enzyme. Zymases are endoenzymes that convert glucose and other monosaccharides into ethyl alcohol and carbon dioxide.

4.2.10 The Structure of DNA and RNA

DNA and RNA are complex biomolecules. The Watson-Crick model that was traditionally proposed as a right-handed double helix for DNA was challenged, and a new Z-DNA model uses a left-handed double helix.

Compare the old and new DNA models. Focus on stated and implied assumptions,molecular biology applications, and current research trends. Understand target and vehicle DNA, plasmids, genomes, modern DNA cloning techniques, and genetic repair. Link the specific roles of mRNA, tRNA, and rRNA to translation and transcription mechanisms.

4.2.11 Cell Division

Cell division, the process by which cellular material is divided between two new daughter cells, increases the number of individuals in the population of one-celled organisms. It is the means by which an organism grows and, in multicelled organisms, the means by which injured tissues are replaced and repaired. The new cells are structurally and functionally similar to the parent cell and to one another. Each new cell inherits an exact replica of the hereditary information of the parent cell.

In prokaryotic cell division, two daughter chromosomes are attached to different sites on the interior of the cell membrane. As the membrane elongates, the chromosomes are separated. The cell membrane then pinches inward, and a new cell wall forms to complete the division of the daughter cells.

The animal and plant cell cycle consists of five major phases: gap $(G)_1$, synthesis (S), G_2, mitosis or meiosis, and cytokinesis. The G_1, S, and G_2 steps are collectively known as interphase.

During the G_1 step of interphase, the cell doubles in size. Its enzymes, ribosomes, mitochondria, and other cytoplasmic molecules and structures approximately double in number. Membranous structures derived from the endoplasmic reticulum are renewed and enlarged by the addition of phospholipid and protein molecules. These strucutres include the nuclear envelope, Golgi bodies, lysosomes, vacuoles, and vesicles. Mitochondria and chloroplasts are produced from previously existing mitochondria and chloroplasts. During the S step of interphase, DNA is synthesized. During the G_2 step of interphase, the cell assembles the special structures required for the separation of chromosomes during mitosis and the separation of the two daughter cells during cytogenesis.

During mitosis, the chromatid slowly coils and condenses into chromosomes, which consist of two replicas. The point of attachment is the centromere, which contains disk-like structures known as kinetochores. The function of mitosis is to maneuver the replicated chromosomes so that each new cell receives a full complement of chromosomes, one of each. Mitosis occurs in four stages: prophase, metaphase, anaphase, and telophase.

During prophase, the chromosomes condense and move toward the equator of the spindle. The centriole pairs move apart to form a spindle of fibers made of microtubules. As these fibers separate, the nuclear envelope degrades.

During metaphase, the chromatid pairs move back and forth within the spindle, tugged first toward one pole and then toward the other. They finally become arranged precisely at the midplane, or equator, of the cell.

During anaphase, the centromeres in all of the chromatid pairs separate simultaneously. The chromatids of each pair move apart, and each becomes a separate chromosome. The centromeres move first, and the arms of the chromosomes drag behind.

During telophase, the chromosomes reach the opposite poles, the spindle disperses, and nuclear envelopes form around the two sets of chromosomes. In the nucleus, the nucleoli reappear, and four new centrioles begin to form adjacent to the previous ones.

During cytokinesis, the cytoplasm divides into two nearly equal parts. The cleavage always occurs at the midline of the spindle. This step usually accompanies mitosis.

Meiosis consists of two consecutive nuclear divisions. During meiosis I, the homologues separate in four stages: interphase I, prophase I, anaphase I, and telophase I. During meiosis II, the chromatids also separate in four stages: interphase II, prophase II, anaphase II, and telophase II.

In addition to the types and phases of cell division, learn when cells divide through mitosis and when they divide through meiosis. Figure 4-2 shows the stages of human sexual reproduction.

4.3 BACTERIA AND VIRUSES

Bacteria are one class of the lowest division of the plant kingdom. Viruses are minute disease-producing agents.

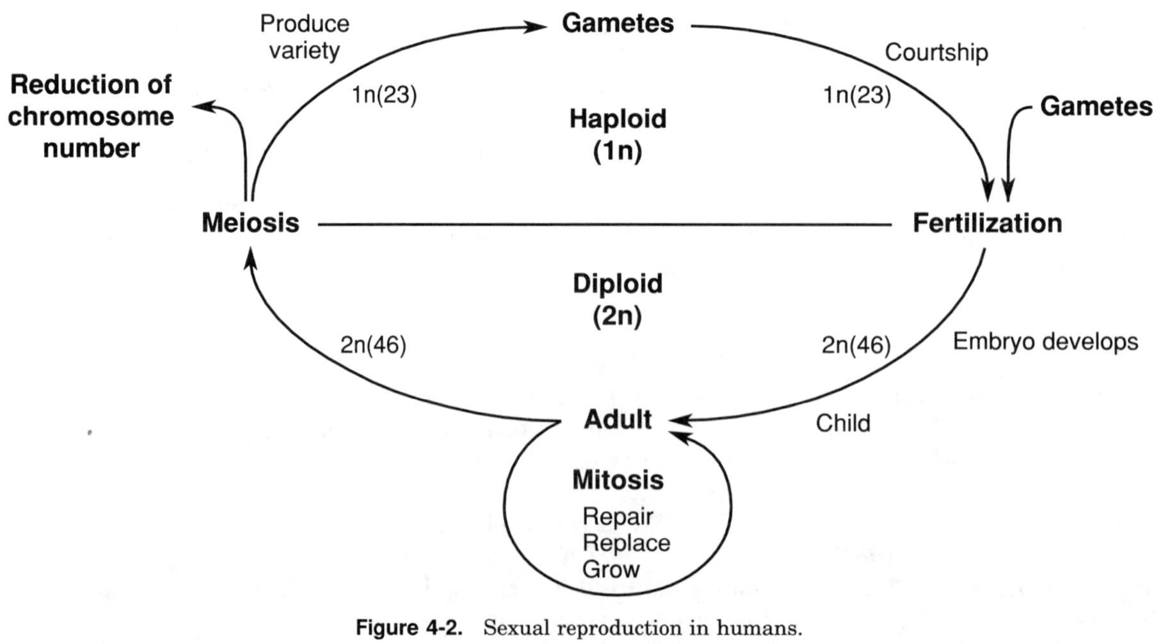

Figure 4-2. Sexual reproduction in humans.

4.3.1 Classification of Bacteria

Because of the chaotic condition of bacterial classification at the time, the Society of American Bacteriologists attempted to establish a more useful system. At its annual meeting in Urbana, Illinois, in 1915, the society assigned to the Committee on Classification the task of formulating a new system of classification.

Five orders of bacteria are known. Some of the orders are divided into suborders, and all are subdivided into families, families into tribes, tribes into genera, and genera into species.

4.3.2 The Class Schizomycetes

Organisms of the class Schizomycetes are mostly unicellular plants. Individual cells may be spherical, curved, or spiral rods. Some species produce pigments. The sulfur purple and green bacteria possess pigments that are similar to the true chlorophylls of higher plants and have photosynthetic properties. The phycocyanin found in blue-green algae is not found in Schizomycetes.

Multiplication typically occurs through cell division. Endospores are formed by some species in the order Eubacteriales. Sporocysts are found in some species in the order Myxobacteriales. Ultramicroscopic reproductive bodies are found in species in the order Borrelomycetaceae. These organisms cause diseases of either plants or animals. Five orders are recognized: Eubacteriales, Actinomycetales, Chlamydobacteriales, Myxobacteriales, and Spirochaetales.

4.3.3 The Order Eubacteriales

The order Eubacteriales contains spherical or rod-shaped organisms composed of simple, undifferentiated rigid cells. The organisms are short or long, and straight, curved, or spiral. Some organisms are nonmotile, and others move by means of flagella. Elongated cells divide by transverse fission and may remain attached to each other in chains. Spherical organisms divide either by parallel fission, producing chains, or by fission, alternating in two or three planes, producing either tetrads or cubes of eight and multiples of eight cells. Many spherical cells form irregular masses in which the plane of division cannot be determined. Endospores occur in some species. Some species are chromogenic, and in a few (e.g., bacteriopurpurin and chlorophyll), the pigment is photosynthetic.

4.3.4 The Suborder Eubacteriineae

Organisms of the suborder Eubacteriineae are true bacteria in the narrow sense of the word. The cells are rigid and free. Branching occurs only under abnormal conditions. The cells are not attached by holdfasts or stalks, and they do not form sheaths. One-third of the species form pigments, but they have no photosynthetic properties. Endospores are found in the family Bacillaceae, but rarely in other families.

This suborder includes most common bacteria studied in the laboratory, both saprophytes and parasites, and some autotrophic species. The suborder Eubacteriineae contains many more species than the other orders combined.

4.3.5 Families in Eubacteriineae

The suborder Eubacteriineae has 13 families. Most bacteria that cause diseases of plants are classified into two genera in this suborder: *Xanthomonas,* rods that usually have monotrichic flagella and are related to *Pseudomonas;* and *Erwinia,* rods that have peritrichic flagella, and some species of which are probably related to *Aerobacter* or *Escherichia.*

The family Nitrobacteriaceae contains mostly gram-negative, non–spore-forming rods that are autotrophic. They obtain energy through the oxidation of hydrogen, methane, carbon dioxide, ammonia, nitrites, sulfur, or thiosulfates. They are nonparasitic and are mostly inhabitants of soil and water.

This relatively small family, with only nine genera and approximately twenty-two species, is of tremendous economic importance to humans. It contains the nitrifying organisms that, living in enormous numbers in nearly all well-aerated soils, convert the ammonia of decaying organic matter to the nitrates that are essential for soil fertility. The benefits obtained from the action of these bacteria more than offset the harm done by all disease-producing species combined.

The family Pseudomonadaceae contains gram-negative, non–spore-forming rods that are usually motile by polar flagella that occur singly or in tufts. Some are straight, and others are spirally curved, but rigid and dividing transversely. Many are saprophytes in soil or water, and others are parasitic on plants or animals. This large, important family contains 12 genera and approximately 250 species, including *Vibrio comma,* the cause of Asiatic cholera, and other *Vibrio* species that cause less important diseases. *Pseudomonas* species from soil, water, and diseased plants sometimes produce green, fluorescent, water-soluble pigments that diffuse into the surrounding medium, forming colored halos around the colonies. *Xanthomonas* is a large genus of plant pathogens that cause many important diseases, including blights of bean, walnut, and cotton. *Acetobacter* is a genus of pleomorphic organisms that are important in completing the carbon cycle and producing vinegar and commercial acetic acid through the oxidation of alcohol.

The family Azotobacteriaceae contains pleomorphic organisms with both motile and nonmotile forms and large cocci. These organisms are strongly aerobic, oxidize carbohydrates for energy, and fix atmospheric nitrogen when they grow in media or soils that are deficient in nitrogen compounds. This family has one genus, and the type species is *Azotobacter chroococcum.* These organisms are widely distributed in the soil, where they perform nonsymbiotic nitrogen fixation. They and the species of the genus *Rhizobium* of the family Rhizobiaceae are the chief agents in the recovery of nitrogen from the atmosphere. The family Rhizobiaceae contains straight, non–spore-forming, mostly gram-negative rods.

Micrococcaceae is a family with three genera of mostly gram-negative, nonmotile cocci that divide in two or three planes and form sheets, tetrads, packets, or irregular masses. Many species are pigmented, usually yellow, orange, pink, or red. In the most important genus, *Micrococcus*, the cells are arranged in plates or irregular masses because the successive planes of division are oblique to each other and perhaps because of reorientation after division. Some species cause boils, abscesses, or infection of wounds. *Sarcina* contains species of saprophytes and facultative parasites. These mostly gram-positive organisms are pigmented orange or yellow. By division in three planes, they form definite packets. They are common in air, water, soil, and milk.

The family Neisseriaceae contains gram-negative cocci that form pairs or masses. They grow best at 37°C, but most of them require special media containing blood, serum, or ascitic fluid. This family has two genera and thirteen species.

Neisseria is a genus of nearly strict mammalian parasites. These organisms grow best on blood media, and some grow poorly even on such media. By division in two planes, they form pairs or small irregular masses. One species, *Neisseria gonorrhoeae* causes a serious widespread venereal disease; another, *Neisseria meningitis,* causes a common form of meningitis.

The family Lactobacteriaceae includes two tribes: Streptococceae, composed of spheres or short rods in chains, and Lactacilleae, composed of longer rods. These mostly nonmotile, gram-positive organisms ferment carbohydrates and form lactic acid and other products.

The family Lactobacteriaceae has seven genera and sixty-two species. It contains both saprophytic and pathogenic species. *Streptococcus lactis* and some species of *Lactobacillus* are responsible for the souring of milk. Several species of *Streptococcus* are pathogenic, causing scarlet fever, septicemia, puerperal fever, and other infections. *Diplococcus pneumoniae* is responsible for the most common types of pneumonia in humans and animals. Members of this family are used extensively in the microbiologic assay of vitamins and amino acids.

Corynebacteriaceae is a new family of three genera and twenty-nine species. These usually gram-positive, slender, straight to slightly curved rods have irregularly stained segments or granules. These organisms are usually nonmotile and may show positive reactions in various physiologic tests. One species, *Corynebacterium diphtheria,* produces a powerful exotoxin that causes diphtheria in humans.

Achromobacteriaceae is a new family composed of three genera and forty-five species. These gram-negative to gram-variable, small to medium rods are usually uniform in shape. If motile, cells have peritrichic flagella. Growth on agar slants is nonchromogenic to gray-yellow in milk. Many organisms of this family are found in water and soil. None are active in the fermentation of sugars, especially lactose.

The family Enterobacteriaceae consists of non–spore-forming, gram-negative rods, most of which have peritrichic flagella. These organisms ferment carbohydrates and reduce nitrates to nitrites.

This large family contains eight genera and one-hundred ninety-eight species. Many species are harmless saprophytes that are widely distributed in nature, and others inhabit the alimentary tract of humans and other mammals, either as part of the normal flora or as causative organisms of specific diseases. *Shigella dysenteriae* causes bacillary dysentery, *Salmonella typhi* causes typhoid fever, and *Salmonella pullorum* causes white diarrhea of chicks. In the genus *Salmonella,* serologic relations are the chief means of identifying new strains, known as serotypes rather than species. Approximately 150 serotypes have been identified.

One genus, *Erwinia*, contains species of plant pathogens, including *Erwinia amylovora,* the cause of fire blight of apples and pears.

The family Parvobacteriaceae contains gram-negative rods that are mostly parasitic and grow poorly on artificial media, except those that contain body fluids. They do not form gas in the fermentation of carbohydrates.

This family of 10 genera and 56 species is important in medical bacteriology. In the genus *Pasteurella, Pasteurella multocida* is the type species and includes hemorrhagic septicemic bacteria. *Pasteurella* species are found in fowl, swine plague, and bubonic plague of humans and rodents. *Pasteurella tularensis* causes tularemia in humans and animals. *Malleomyces mallei* causes glanders in horses and other animals, including humans; and *Brucella melintensis, Brucella abortus,* and *Brucella suis* cause brucellosis in humans and domestic animals. In humans, *Haemophilus pertussis* is the probable cause of whooping cough, and *Noguchia granulosis* is the probable cause of trachoma.

The family Bacteriaceae contains non–spore-forming rods. The relation of this heterogeneous collection of species to one another and to other groups of bacteria has not been determined. This family contains one genus and fifty-six species. Most of them are harmless saprophytes, but a few cause minor diseases. One species, *Bacterium bibula,* digests the cellulose of plant refuse in the soil.

The family Bacillaceae contains the only organisms that produce endospores, which are more resistant than vegetative cells to unfavorable environmental conditions. This family of rod-shaped, mostly gram-positive bacteria contains only two genera: *Bacillus,* with thirty-three species of aerobes, and *Clostridium,* with sixty-one species of anaerobes or microaerophiles.

Because they decompose proteins, the members of this family are valuable scavengers. Most species of *Bacillus* are saprophytic; however, *Bacillus anthracis* causes anthrax. Although most species of *Clostridium* are nonpathogenic, *Clostridium perfringens* and related species cause the fatal gas gangrene of wounds, and *Clostridium botulinim,* growing saprophytically in the absence of air, produces the deadly toxin of botulism.

4.3.6 The Suborder Caulobacteriineae (Stalked Bacteria)

The suborder Caulobacteriineae contains four families of organisms that constitute another group of iron bacteria, which store ferric hydroxide, not in a sheath, as do the organisms in the order Chlamydobacteriales, but in a stalk by which the cells are attached to a solid support.

These kidney-shaped or spherical cells occur singly. The stalk is secreted from the concave surface of the cell. Cell division is transverse in most genera, but longitudinal in the family Pasteuriaceae. As the cell divides, the tip of the stalk at the point of attachment also divides, producing branched colonies. In most genera, reproduction is by fission only, but in the family Pasteuriaceae, budding occurs as well.

The characteristic stalks of this suborder vary from slender, threadlike structures many times the length of the cell at its tip to short, broad, disk-like holdfasts.

Most species are harmless saprophytes or autophytes of minor economic importance. One species, *Pasteuria ramosa,* is parasitic in the body cavities of the crustaceans *Daphnia pulex* and *Daphnia magna.*

4.3.7 The Suborder Rhodobacteriineae (Purple and Green Bacteria)

The suborder Rhodobacteriineae has three families, twenty-one genera, and forty-eight species of organisms that possess photosynthetic purple or green pigments. Some purple cells contain free sulfur. In certain genera, the cells are spherical or ellipsoidal and divide in two or three planes within a gelatinous matrix that holds them together temporarily in groups or a mass. Later, they escape, and in some species, achieve motility.

Two types of chemical reactions are believed to occur in the photosynthetic process of different members of the suborder Rhodobacteriineae:

1. $CO_2 + 2H_2S \rightarrow HCOH + H_2O + 2S$
2. $3CO_2 + 2S + 8H_2O \rightarrow 3HCOH + 3H_2O + 2H_2SO_4$

In the first reaction, hydrogen sulfide replaces the water used in photosynthesis by the typical green plant; in the second reaction, both water and sulfur are used. Both reactions occur anaerobically, and oxygen is not an end product.

The family Thiorhodaceae contains 13 genera and 34 species. The cells of these organisms contain bacteriopurpurin, with or without sulfur granules. Most of these organisms are found in soil and water.

The family Athiorhodaceae contains two genera of rod-shaped or spiral, generally motile organisms with polar flagella. These organisms contain bacteriopurpurin, which gives them a red, purple, or violet hue. When seen in masses, they are strikingly beautiful. This family is interesting because its members perform photosynthesis. Bacteriopurpurin is a complex of two or more pigments. One of these, bacteriochlorophyll, is green and appears to play an active part in using the energy of light for photosynthesis. The function of the red pigment is uncertain. In this process, carbon from carbon dioxide is used to form organic compounds, perhaps carbohydrates, which are used for growth. Red and infrared light rays are more effective in supplying energy for this process than are those with shorter wavelengths.

Unlike most bacteria, those of the family Athiorhodaceae grow better in light than in darkness. They lose their red color in the dark and regain it in the light. In an unevenly lighted field or one in which the rays of light are separated by passage through a prism, motile forms swim about until they find a region of the right intensity or color of light, where they rest.

Chlorobacteriodaceae is a new family that includes green bacteria that do not contain sulfur. This family has six genera and eight species.

4.3.8 The Order Actinomycetales (Fungus Bacteria)

Compared with the great order Eubacteriales, the order Actinomycetales is small, with only three families, five genera, and approximately one-hundred twenty-five species.

The cells of these mostly aerobic, gram-positive organisms are cylindrical, and in certain genera, notably *Actinomyces,* they are firmly united to form filaments that resemble the mycelium of a true fungus, but much more slender. True branching is fairly common. True endospores are not produced. In general, the members of this order are less aquatic than those of the order Eubacteriales, as shown by their lack of motility and their absence from natural waters.

In the family Mycobacteriaceae, as in the suborder Eubacteriineae, the cells occur singly or in short chains. In addition, there is no differentiation into vegetative and reproductive parts. Branching is rare. The one genus, *Mycobacterium*, is highly significant in medical bacteriology. This genus includes

12 species, about half of which are pathogenic, causing leprosy in humans and different types of tuberculosis in humans and other vertebrates. These organisms have slender, nonmotile, acid-fast rods. Most species grow poorly or not at all on common laboratory culture media.

The family Actinomycetaceae contains organisms that tend to form filaments. Several genera show no differentiation into vegetative and reproductive portions. The species of one genus, *Nocardia*, can use paraffin, phenol, and m-cresol for energy.

The morphologic characteristics of organisms of the genus *Actinomyces* are so radically different from those of other bacteria that some regard them as true fungi of the group Fungi Imperfecti. These organisms are filamentous and are sometimes called the "ray fungus." The filaments are slender, approximately 1 μm in diameter, and without cross walls. This much-branched, mycelium-like structure forms a definite vegetative body that may fragment into elements of various sizes, but does not produce conidia.

Several species are pathogenic to animals. *Actinomyces bovis* causes actinomycosis, or lumpy jaw, in cattle, *Actinomyces israelii* causes actinomycosis in humans, and *Norcardia madurae* causes Madura foot in humans.

The family Crenothrichaceae includes the species *Crenothrix polyspora*, the filaments of which are not branched, but are attached at the base to a rock or another submerged object. The sheath of young filaments is composed of organic material. With age, the sheath, especially the basal portion, becomes encrusted with ferric hydroxide. As the filament matures, its terminal portion expands and opens, forming a trumpet shape.

Reproduction occurs through the formation of nonmotile conidia. These ovoid structures are formed by three-plane division of the cells at the tip of the filament. They escape through the open end of the sheath, become attached, and form new filaments through growth and transverse division.

This species often grows luxuriantly in water supplies, where it causes no harm, although it imparts a disagreeable odor and flavor to the water when masses of these organisms die and decay.

The family Beggiatoaceae contains organisms that form filaments, the tips of which usually have an oscillating motion similar to that of the blue-green algae of the *Oscillatoria* group. Some move by a gliding motion. No conidia are formed. The cells reproduce by constriction, and the filaments reproduce by fragmentation. Sulfur granules are formed, but no bacteriopurpurin is produced. This family contains four genera and eighteen species.

The best known species of this family is *Beggiatoa alba,* which forms gray, slimy masses on the vegetation of swamps, sulfur springs, and sewage-polluted streams. This species is highly pleomorphic, and the cells of the thick filament, located within a delicate sheath, separate into free-swimming cells that grow into few filaments. Many species, known as sulfur bacteria, oxidize hydrogen sulfide as a source of energy.

4.3.9 The Order Chlamydobacteriales (Sheathed Bacteria)

The small order Chlamydobacteriales has three families, eight genera, and twenty-seven species. The normal habitat for these organisms is water. For this reason and also because of their structure, they are known as alga-like bacteria. They form long, slender filaments, mostly 1–2 μm in diameter. In some genera, these filaments are attached at the base to some object; in others, they float freely.

4.3.10 The Order Myxobacteriales (Slime Bacteria)

The order Myxobacteriales is characterized by the production of a mass of slime that enables these bacteria to carry on a remarkable communal life that is not found elsewhere in the bacterial world.

During the vegetative, or swarm, stage, the bacterial cells live and multiply within a slimy matrix that forms a flat, irregularly shaped pseudoplasmodium. The cells are slender, flexible rods. They have no flagella, but show slow motility both individually and in masses. As the cells grow and multiply, they secrete more slime. The pseudoplasmodium enlarges and moves along slowly, carrying the bacteria in its terminal portion. The movement is probably the result of asymmetrical slime production that increases in the back portion of the mass and crowds the colony along. The individual movement of cells probably aids in the process. The mechanics of this process are perplexing and not well understood. The gliding motion of individual cells is similar to that of the *Oscillatoria* group and certain diatoms.

When the pseudoplasmodium reaches a certain degree of maturity, a striking change occurs. The cells collect in a compact on a gelatinous base, and a fruiting body, or cyst, is formed. This cyst may be simple and round or variously lobed. The size, shape, and color are characteristic of the species. In most species, the cysts have stalks that are composed of slime and are devoid of bacteria because the bacteria have collected in the sellings at the top. The fruiting bodies, which are rarely more than 1 mm high, are usually yellow, orange, or red. In some species (e.g., *Chondromyces crocatus*), they are exquisite in appearance, although a hand lens is needed for detailed observation.

As the cysts mature, the cells become shorter and thicker, and in some species, nearly spherical. Their activity ceases temporarily, and the slime dries below and around the cells.

After a short resting period, the cells, singly or in tiny masses bound together by the dried slime, escape from the cysts, largely through the action of wind and air. Under favorable conditions, they form new swarms and excrete slime as before.

This order contains five families, thirteen genera, and seventy-one species. They are mostly saprophytes, absorbing food from their substratum, which at best is decaying wood, fleshy fungi, or animal dung. One species, *Polyangium parasiticum*, is parasitic on the green alga of *Cladophora*. Another, *Podangium lichenicolum*, is parasitic on lichens.

4.3.11 The Order Spirochaetales (Flexuose Spiral Bacteria)

The organisms in the small order Spirochaetales are flexuose spiral rods. In some species, the pointed ends of the rods taper into a slender thread that probably is not a true flagellum. Some species have an axial filament that consists of a relatively straight, cylindrical, protoplasmic core about which the spiral ridges of the cell are wound. Movement in these organisms occurs through the contraction of the protoplasm, which gives the flexible cell an undulating motion that propels it through the water. In some cases, this motion is wriggling; in others, the cell revolves screw-like on its major axis.

Most members of the order are not readily stained by methods that are generally successful with other types of bacteria. Special stains have been devised for some, and dark-field illumination is used extensively to supplement stained preparations.

Because the flexible body, type of movement, and axial filament of these bacteria are strongly suggestive of certain protozoa, some members of the order Spirochaetales may be transferred to that group. However, their apparent lack of nuclei, lack of sexuality, and transverse division justify classifying them as bacteria.

This order contains two families. Spirochaetaceae, with three genera and eleven species, contains some harmless saprophytes found in water, especially water polluted with sewage, and some parasites found in the intestinal tract of bivalve mollusks. The family Treponemataceae consists of three genera and twenty-six species, many of which are parasitic on vertebrates and some of which are pathogenic. Some species of *Borrelia* cause relapsing fever, which is often transmitted by insects, and *Treponema pallidum* causes syphilis.

4.3.12 Class Schizomycetes Bacteria

Order I: Eubacteriales
- Suborder I: Eubacteriineae (true bacteria)
  - Family I: Nitrobacteriaceae
    - 3 tribes, 9 genera, 22 species
      - Example: *Nitrobacter winogradsky*

Family II: Pseudomonadaceae
2 tribes, 12 genera, 250 species
Example: *Pseudomonas aeruginosa*
Family III: Azotobacteriaceae
1 genus, 3 species
Example: *Azotobacter chroococcum*
Family IV: Rhizobiaceae
3 genera, 13 species
Example: *Rhizobium leguminosarum*
Family V: Micrococcaceae
3 genera, 33 species
Example: *Micrococcus luteus*
Family VI: Neisseriaceae
2 genera, 13 species
Example: *Neisseria gonorrhoeae*
Family VII: Lactobacteriaceae
2 tribes, 7 genera, 62 species
Example: *Lactobacillus acidophilus*
Family VIII: Corynebacteriaceae
3 genera, 29 species
Example: *Corynebacterium diphtheriae*
Family IX: Achromobacteriaceae
3 genera, 45 species
Example: *Alcaligenes faecalis*
Family X: Enterobacteriaceae
5 tribes, 8 genera, 198 species
Example: *Escherichia coli*
Family XI: Parvobacteriaceae
4 tribes, 10 genera, 56 species
Example: *Brucella abortus*
Family XII: Bacteriaceae
1 genus, 56 species
Example: *Bacterium triloculare*
Family XIII: Bacillaceae
2 genera, 94 species
Example: *Bacillus subtilis*
Suborder II: Caulobacteriineae (stalked bacteria)
Family I: Nevskiaceae
1 genus, 2 species
Example: *Nevskia ramosa*
Family II: Gallionellaceae
1 genus, 4 species
Example: *Gallionella ferruginea*
Family III: Caulobacteriaceae
1 genus, 1 species
Example: *Caulobacter vibrioides*
Family IV: Siderocapsaceae
2 genera, 3 species
Example: *Siderocapsa treubii*
Suborder III: Rhodobacteriineae (purple and green bacteria)
Family I: Thiorhodaceae
13 genera, 31 species
Example: *Thiosarcina rosea*
Family II: Athiorhodaceae
2 genera, 6 species

Example: *Rhodopseudomonas palustris*
Family III: Chlorobacteriaceae
6 genera, 8 species
Example: *Chlorobium limicola*

Order II: Actinomycetales (fungus-like bacteria)
Family I: Mycobacteriaceae
1 genus, 12 species
Example: *Mycobacterium tuberculosis*
Family II: Actinomycetaceae
2 genera, 35 species
Example: *Actinomyces bovis*
Family III: Streptomycetaceae
2 genera, 78 species
Example: *Streptomyces albus*

Order III: Chlamydobacteriales (alga-like bacteria)
Family I: Chlamydobacteriaceae
3 genera, 12 species
Example: *Leptothrix ochracea*
Family II: Crenotrichaceae
1 genus, 1 species
Example: *Crenothrix polyspora*
Family III: Beggiatoaceae
4 genera, 18 species
Example: *Beggiatoa alba*

Order IV: Myxobacteriales (slime bacteria)
Family I: Cytophagaceae
1 genus, 9 species
Example: *Cytophaga hutchinsonii*
Family II: Archangiaceae
2 genera, 6 species
Example: *Archangium gephyra*
Family III: Sorangiaceae
1 genus, 8 species
Example: *Sorangium schroeter*
Family IV: Polyangiaceae
5 genera, 30 species
Example: *Chondromyces aurantiacus*
Family V: Myxococcaceae
4 genera, 18 species
Example: *Myxococcus fulvus*

Order V: Spirochaetales (flexuose spiral bacteria)
Family I: Spirochaetaceae
3 genera, 11 species
Example: *Spirochaeta plicatilis*
Family II: Treponemataceae
3 genera, 26 species
Example: *Treponema pallidum*
Supplement I: Order Rickettsiales
10 genera, 35 species
Example: *Rickettsia prowazekii*
Supplement II: Order Virales
242 species described

Supplement III: Family Borrelomycetaceae
1 genus, 7 species
Example: *Asterococcus mycoides*

4.3.13 Nutritional Grouping of Bacteria

The types of bacteria that now live on the earth have different food requirements, especially the sources of carbon and nitrogen and the substances that they can oxidize to release energy. One convenient way to group bacteria is into autotrophic, saprophytic, and parasitic species.

Millions of years ago, the first primitive bacteria appeared on the earth. Because few other forms of life were present, little organic matter was available for food. Therefore, this first living substance had to obtain its energy from inorganic food. Forms of life with this ability are known as autotrophic. The inorganic substances that various types of bacteria oxidize include ammonia, nitrites, hydrogen, sulfide, sulfur, and ferrous compounds. A few species oxidize hydrogen, and a few others, carbon monoxide. Most of these substances apparently were dissolved in the sea water from which primitive bacteria originated. Carbon dioxide and carbon monoxide were probably the source of carbon.

Based on the source of the energy used to synthesize simple compounds or elements into more complex ones, plants are classified as either photosynthetic or chemosynthetic.

Photosynthetic plants include most seed plants as well as ferns, mosses, and algae. In the process of photosynthesis, these plants, with the aid of chlorophyll, use the energy of light to combine carbon dioxide and water into some form of carbohydrate. A few of the Rhodobacteriineae species also use a green pigment, bacteriochlorophyll, which is a constituent of bacteriopurpin and performs a function similar to that of chlorophyll. The most primitive bacteria probably could not perform photosynthesis because both chlorophyll and bacteriochlorophyll apparently are products of evolution. However, a simple form of photosynthesis that does not require these pigments may have occurred in the earliest forms of life.

Chemosynthetic plants, most of which are bacteria, appear to be the most primitive now in existence. These plants obtain energy by oxidizing simple inorganic compounds. They degrade carbon dioxide and combine its components with other simple inorganic compounds to produce the constituents of protoplasm.

Most autotrophic bacterial species obtain most of their food from nonliving organic material (e.g., plant and animal bodies and their secretions and excretions). In addition, most of these species use some inorganic compounds, such as ammonia, nitrates, and sulfates.

Organic compounds (i.e., carbohydrates, fats, proteins), supplemented by a few inorganic salts, are easily used by saprophytes to supply the materials for growth and the energy required to synthesize substances in the cell. Some of this material, such as glucose, is ready for use without preliminary treatment. Other types, such as starches and fats, must be digested. Nearly all culture media consist of combinations of organic and inorganic foods for saprophytes and facultative parasites, or organisms that can grow either saprophytically or parasitically.

Some bacteria have evolved into parasites, or organisms that live intimately associated with the living cells of an organism of a different species, usually a higher animal or plant, and obtain nourishment from the host. These bacteria commonly cause disease; when they do, they are known as pathogenic.

Strict parasites can multiply only within the cells or fluids of a living host. They do not grow in a culture medium unless it contains living tissue. With the exception of the rickettsiae, viruses, and the species that causes leprosy, few true bacteria are strict parasites. Facultative parasites multiply either within the cells or fluids of a suitable host or in nonliving substances, such as culture medium.

Although bacterial parasitism was once believed to be restricted to humans and higher animals, more than 100 species of plant parasites have been identified, some of which cause destructive diseases, such as fire blight of apple and pear trees.

Some authorities describe bacteria that can live without organic food (e.g., autotrophic species) as "prototrophic." For some of these bacteria, the presence of organic matter, such as sugars and gelatin, is unfavorable. In the same grouping, saprophytic bacteria are known as metatrophic, and parasitic bacteria are known as paratrophic. These three groups have considerable overlap because most bacteria can obtain their food in more than one way; however, these terms are convenient and widely used when sharp distinctions are not needed.

For convenience, it is often desirable to group living things in ways that do not describe their relations. Thus, "carnivorous" animals may be mammals, birds, fish, or insects; "parasitic" plants may be flowering plants, fungi, or bacteria; and "aquatic" plants include members of all four plant divisions. This grouping does not correspond to the phylogenetic relations of these organims. Some autotrophic bacteria are primitive in the sense that they have changed relatively little from the ancestral condition, whereas others have descended from saprophytic ancestors. Some are included in the order Eubacteriales and some, in the order Chlamydobacteriales.

Because little organic food was available, early bacteria must have been autotrophic. As time passed, other types of plants and animals emerged and died, leaving a supply of organic matter. Some bacteria could not adapt to the use of this organic food and remained autophytes. Others, however, acquired the ability to produce digestive enzymes, underwent other less obvious changes, and became saprophytes, although they still used some inorganic salts.

At some point, both autophytes and saprophytes existed without parasites. Parasitism undoubtedly evolved from saprophytism. These changes probably occurred repeatedly and were separated by long intervals. The steps in this evolution are not known, but they probably included the following events.

In the parasitism of plants, certain saprophytic bacteria were introduced into wounds, water pores, and other openings. These bacteria survived, and evolutionary changes enabled them to live and multiply in their new environment and penetrate deeper into their hosts. In this way, they became plant pathogens.

In animals, parasitism probably originated by at least three mechanisms: (1) saprophytes were accidentally introduced into wounds and evolved into wound parasites; (2) saprophytes of the intestinal contents evolved into parasites, such as those that cause typhoid fever, dysentery, and Asiatic cholera; and (3) saprophytes were drawn into the respiratory tract and evolved into parasites, such as those that cause pneumonia and perhaps tuberculosis.

In the most highly developed form of parasitism, such as that of the protozoan *Gregarena melanopli* in grasshoppers or *Trypanosoma lewisi* in rats, the parasite obtains the full benefit of parasitic life without seriously damaging the host, leaving it alive to support thc parasitc.

4.3.14 Bacteria and Enzymes

Bacteria produce enzymes that correspond closely to those produced by other plants and animals, including humans. These enzymes are necessary for the life of these organisms.

4.3.15 Classification Based on Bacterial Respiration

All living things require oxygen. Some of the oxygen enters into the composition of protoplasm and other constituents of the body, and some combines with carbon, hydrogen and other elements or compounds, with the release of chemical energy. This union usually produces carbon dioxide and water.

In 1861, Pasteur discovered that certain bacteria could perform butyric fermentation in the absence of free oxygen. Since Pasteur's time, knowledge of this phenomenon of anaerobiosis has been greatly extended. As a result of this knowledge, bacteria are grouped, on the basis of their oxygen requirements, into aerobes, anaerobes, facultative anaerobes, and microaerophiles.

Aerobes require oxygen in the free state. Anaerobes require oxygen in a combined form (e.g, a sugar). Free oxygen inhibits the growth of obligate anaerobes. Three theories have been suggested to explain this phenomenon: (1) oxygen is toxic to the cell; (2) hydrogen peroxide is produced by the cells, and because the organisms do not secrete the enzyme catalase to break it down to water and oxygen, the hydrogen peroxide is toxic to the anaerobes; and (3) the growth of obligate anaerobes is dependent on a low oxidation-reduction potential, which is not possible in the presence of free oxygen. None of these theories is adequate to explain why obligate anaerobes do not grow in the presence of free oxygen, but the last theory seems the most satisfactory.

Facultative anaerobes can use free oxygen if it is available, or they can use combined oxygen, as do strict anaerobes. Microaerophiles use free oxygen, although their growth is inhibited by the full oxygen content of the atmosphere. In a stab culture made in nutrient agar, they grow best at some distance below the surface, where the oxygen tension is low.

4.3.16 Types of Respiration

Aerobic respiration occurs in most animals and plants. Anaerobic respiration occurs in two ways, intermolecularly and intramolecularly. Intermolecular respiration occurs when oxygen is removed from one compound, an oxygen donator, and added to another, an oxygen receptor (e.g., a nitrate is reduced to a nitrite, and the oxygen that is released is combined with sulfur and water or thiosulfate to form sulfuric acid). In other words, an oxygen donator is oxidized by the removal of hydrogen, and another compound acts as a hydrogen acceptor and is reduced. Reduction of the hydrogen acceptor may involve the loss of oxygen and the formation of water.

Intramolecular anaerobic respiration occurs when an organic compound is broken down, with partial release of energy and the formation of one or more new compounds that may be oxidized further. The formation of ethyl alcohol from glucose is an example.

The complex series of reactions in the anaerobic decomposition of carbohydrates includes both intermolecular and intramolecular anaerobic respiration. The oxidation of unstable inorganic compounds is performed by autotrophic bacteria.

Some members of the family Nitrobacteriaceae oxidize hydrogen to water, carbon monoxide to carbon dioxide, and hydrogen sulfide to sulfuric acid. Other members of this family oxidize ammonia to nitrites and nitrites to nitrates.

4.3.17 Fermentation

Fermentation has so much in common with respiration that the two are easily confused. The term "fermentation" was first applied to the evolution of bubbles of carbon dioxide in fermenting wine. It was considered a type of cold boiling. The term is still applied to decomposition processes in which gases are evolved in liquids. It is now used, however, to include the formation by microorganisms of organic acids, alcohol, and other substances by oxidative decomposition of carbohydrates and their derivatives.

Putrefaction is the chemical decomposition of proteins and other nitrogenous substances, with the production of disagreeable odors. This process is usually anaerobic. The term "decay" is used to describe any aerobic decomposition of organic matter. In a broad sense, it includes putrefaction. All of these processes are caused by enzymatic action and are similar to digestion.

4.3.18 Nitrogen Metabolism of Bacteria

Nitrogen, in some form, is needed for the production of protoplasm. Most species of bacteria, like other forms of life, cannot use free nitrogen, but must be supplied with some nitrogenous compound.

Recent work shows that bacteria require a supply of the amino acid tryptophan. Some manufacture it from ammonium salts or other amino compounds, but others must have it supplied to them. This need is a basic principle in the nitrogen metabolism of bacteria.

Proteins are widely distributed in plant and animal tissues, both living and nonliving. For saprophytic and parasitic bacteria, proteins are valuable sources of nitrogen. Most bacteria secrete proteases that digest proteins. Proteins are first broken down by the enzymes into proteoses, peptones, and amino acids. Amino acids are then synthesized into protoplasm or broken down into a variety of end products.

Amino acids that have been formed by some digestive process before they reach the bacteria are ready for use in the synthetic metabolism that occurs within the bacterial cell. Commercial peptone, which is used extensively in artificial culture media for both saprophytic and parasitic species, contains amino acids as well as more complex substances that require digestion. Peptone is not useful to most autotrophic bacteria and is harmful to many of them.

Many types of bacteria use ammonium compounds. The ability to use these compounds is primitive. This ability was acquired by autotrophic bacteria and was passed down to the others. Except in autotrophic species, an ammonium compound can be used only in the presence of a carbohydrate or a similar source of energy. Ammonium compounds are especially valuable as foods for many fungi.

The antiseptic properties of nitrites make them injurious to most types of bacteria. However, the members of the genus *Nitrobacter,* of the tribe Nitrobacterieae, oxidize them to nitrates. Some species of *Actinomyces* use nitrites in dilute solution, and some bacteria reduce nitrites to ammonia and obtain oxygen.

Many bacterial species synthesize nitrates into their own proteins, and some use them as a source of oxygen in intermolecular respiration. Nitrates are valuable to higher plants.

A few species of bacteria fix the free nitrogen in the atmosphere into nitrogen compounds. The six species of *Rhizobium* perform this function in symbiosis with the roots of the leguminous plants in which they live, and the two species of *Azotobacter* and at least one species of *Clostridium, Clostridium butyricum,* perform it nonsymbiotically.

4.3.19 Mechanisms of Infection

Pathogenicity is the ability of an organism to cause disease. Virulence is the degree of pathogenicity of an organism as indicated by case fatality rates or the ability to invade host tissues.

Virulence is variable. Some strains of a pathogenic species cause severe forms of a disease, and other strains cause mild forms. In a specific species or strain, however, virulence may be fairly constant (e.g., *Malleomyces mallei,* the cause of glanders in horses, humans, and other animals) or may vary. For example, *Salmonella typhi* freshly removed from a patient is highly virulent, but its virulence is decreased by continuous growth on artificial media. In some cases, virulence is restored by inoculation into a susceptible animal.

Susceptibility of the host to disease is also variable, ranging from little resistance to complete resistance to a specific disease. Under favorable conditions, disease occurs when the virulence of the organism is great enough to overcome the resistance of the host.

The idea of specificity was introduced by Von Plenciz in 1762, after it had been suspected, but not proved, that some types of disease are produced by bacteria. Organisms with complete specificity attach to only one type of host and produce only one type of disease. *Salmonella typhi,* which causes typhoid fever in humans, is a good example. Specificity is rarely so perfect. Most pathogens attack several species of host that may or may not be closely related. The finding that monkeys, rabbits, guinea pigs, and mice may be infected artificially with some human diseases is of great value in experimental medicine.

No pathogen is known to attack both plants and animals, and few attack both birds and mammals, or both warm-blooded and cold-blooded animals. An important step in studying any infectious disease is determining the range of susceptible hosts.

4.3.20 Sources of Infection

An important consideration in infectious disease is the source of the responsible organisms. Few species of pathogenic bacteria normally multiply outside the body of the host. Even though they grow in specially prepared culture media, most pathogenic bacteria cannot grow in other substances, such as water, soil, or manure. If they are found in these materials, it is because they happened to be cast there, and in these locations, their numbers are diminishing rather than increasing. However, milk and some cooked foods offer suitable media for bacterial growth.

Most pathogens reproduce within the body of the host. During the early stages of disease, their numbers increase dramatically, and organisms leave the host through excretion. As the host recovers, the number of organisms usually decreases, and the organisms eventually disappear. However, in a few diseases, the organisms continue to inhabit the body. People and animals harboring these pathogens are known as carriers. The role of carriers is particularly important in diphtheria, typhoid fever, Asiatic cholera, scarlet fever, cerebrospinal meningitis, and pneumonia. Avoiding contact with symptomatic people or animals is much easier than avoiding contact with asymptomatic carriers. Human diseases are contracted from people more often than from objects or materials.

4.3.21 Transmission of Disease-Producing Organisms

Bacteria do not pass from the diseased to the well population by their own locomotion. Most bacteria that are cast off by a patient or a carrier die without reaching a susceptible host, but a small proportion are more fortunate.

For many communicable diseases, direct contact is the most common method of transmission. With some, such as venereal diseases, it is the exclusive method. Through direct contact, an infected person touches another person, and through indirect contact, a person infects an object that is later touched by another person. If the infected object is not touched by another person for some time (i.e., weeks or months), the object is known as a fomite. This method of transmission is important only for diseases caused by resistant organisms (e.g., *Clostridium tetani* and *Bacillus anthracis,* which are spore formers; *Mycobacterium tuberculosis;* the virus that causes smallpox).

Transmission through the air occurs when water or food becomes contaminated and is later swallowed by people or animals. This mode of transmission is important for *Salmonella* species and a wide range of diseases.

Disease vectors are usually insects, but may be other animals. Vectors are the exclusive method of transmission of such important diseases as malaria, Rocky Mountain spotted fever, and African sleeping sickness.

4.3.22 Viruses, Rickettsiae, and the Pleuropneumonia Group

Some disease-producing agents are too small to be seen, even light microscopically. Because many of them readily pass through filters that trap bacteria, they have been called “filterable viruses,” but the term “virus” is now preferred. Viral diseases include influenza, smallpox, measles, infantile paralysis, yellow fever, rabies, foot and mouth disease of cattle, dog distemper, and mosaic diseases of plants, peach yellows, and the curly tops of sugar beets.

Several animal diseases, notably hog cholera, parrot fever, and dog distemper, were once believed to be of bacterial origin because cultures thought to be pure caused these diseases when inoculated into susceptible hosts. Later studies showed that these diseases were caused by a virus that contaminated the cultures.

Viruses share several characteristics. In nature, viruses are always associated with diseased plants or animals. Because no saprophytic viruses are known, they are all classified as strict parasites. If a small amount of virus is inoculated into a susceptible host, the number of organisms increases dramatically. There is no evidence of the spontaneous generation that has been described at various times for animals, bacteria, and viruses.

Viruses are specific, with each type attacking only one or a limited number of host species and causing a definite disease with characteristic symptoms. Most viruses are antigenic, causing animal hosts to produce antibodies that aid in recovery and protect against later attacks. Viruses are also particulate. In other words, as extracted for study, viruses consist of a liquid in which ultramicroscopic particles are suspended. These particles range in size from 10 millimicrons to approximately 300 millimicrons. Most viruses that cause animal infections are spherical. Viruses are more resistant to injurious conditions, such as heat, dryness, and disinfectants, than are the vegetative cells of bacteria, but they are less resistant than bacterial spores.

Some viruses show a special affinity for certain tissues of the body. For example, in smallpox and measles, the skin and mucous membranes are affected, and in rabies and infantile paralysis, the central nervous system is most affected and contains the greatest quantity of virus.

The most widely accepted view of the origin of viruses was presented by Green and Laidlaw. They reported that viruses are degenerate descendants of larger pathogenic microorganisms. The most convincing argument for this origin is the almost continuous range of forms between typical bacterial pathogens and the smallest viruses.

The rickettsiae have the appearance and staining characteristics of small bacteria, but like viruses, must be cultivated in a living medium. Some viruses, such as the psittacosis group, which cause parrot fever, are large. Their staining characteristics are similar to those of bacteria, and their behavior is more similar to that of pathogenic bacteria than to that of typical viruses. However, they are strict parasites. Vaccinia, which causes cowpox, is a complex, medium-sized virus that may be a descendant of bacteria. The smaller viruses also may be derived from protozoa, spirochaetes, or higher fungi because they have so few features in common with bacteria. Burnet proposed the belief that as viruses evolved, their structure became simpler and their dependence on their host for their metabolic needs increased. Eventually, small viruses contained neither enzymes nor organs, nothing but a self-residuum of genetic mechanism. Although the agent that causes one viral disease may differ from the agent that causes another, they may have much in common.

In many viral diseases of humans and animals, visible bodies, known as inclusion bodies, are found in diseased cells, but not in corresponding healthy cells. In some diseases, these bodies are associated with the nucleus; in others, they are associated with the cytoplasm. Their nature is not well understood. Some believe that an inclusion body is a single parasite; others believe that it is a visible collection of ultramicroscopic particles of the virus. However, more consider inclusion bodies degeneration products of diseased host cells.

In both the plant and animal kingdoms, viral diseases are comparable in importance to bacterial diseases. Plants have more viral diseases than do humans and animals; More than 200 have been identified, and others are constantly being added to the list. Some of the most serious human and animal diseases are viral.

Bacterial diseases may have carriers, based on the finding of organisms in healthy people, either by culture or microscopic examination. This type of evidence cannot be obtained for viral diseases because the causative agent is invisible and does not grow on culture media. However, epidemiologic evidence suggests the role of carriers in some viral diseases, such as influenza and infantile paralysis, which often appear in specific localities. There appears to be no alternative to the view that many disease-producing viruses survive between epidermic periods in the tissues of human carriers.

The uniform behavior of viral diseases from year to year, with periods of high or low virulence, has been attributed to the evolution of their genetic mechanism of reproduction. The virus is continuously affected by the law of survival of the fittest. When a virulent form develops, it may disappear rapidly if all the of hosts are killed and no particles of virus remain.

Because most viral diseases of humans and animals confer a high degree of immunity, successful vaccines are possible. Two of the earliest vaccines were for protection against the viral diseases smallpox and rabies. These vaccines contain virus that has been attenuated, or weakened, so that it is safe to use, although still antigenic. Rabies virus is attenuated by drying, and smallpox virus is attenuated by growing in a bovine animal.

The virus of yellow fever is attenuated by passage through the brains of mice and then cultivated in chick embryos. Fertilized eggs with live embryos 7 days old are used for this purpose. The shell of the egg is disinfected, a small hole is drilled in the end, and the embryo is inoculated with the attenuated virus with a syringe and needle. The hole is then sealed, and the eggs are incubated at 37° C for 3–4 days, after which they are aseptically opened and the embryos removed. The embryos are pooled, weighed, and ground up in a saline–serum mixture. After centrifuging and filtering are performed, the fluid portion is placed in vials and desiccated. Several sterility and potency tests are performed before the vaccine is released for use.

Two types of epidemic influenza virus are established: type A and type B strains. Each type produces a specific infection. Influenza virus vaccine is prepared by inoculating diluted influenza virus particles into the embryonic fluid of 10-day-old incubated fertile hen eggs. After 48 hours of incubation, the egg is opened aseptically and the membranes surrounding the embryos, together with the larger blood vessels, are ruptured. The virus is absorbed on the red blood cells. This mixture is removed, and by a process of refrigeration and centrifugation, the virus is obtained in a saline solution free of the red blood cells. The purified and concentrated virus is then inactivated with formalin, and a preservative is added. Type A and type B vaccine lots are pooled in equal amounts, and immunization and sterility tests are performed before the vaccine is administered.

4.3.23 Bacteriophages

A bacteriophage is a type of virus that is parasitic on specific bacteria. Literally translated, the name means "eater of bacteria." Twort, and later d'Herelle, first observed the lysis of bacteria. This action is known as the Twort-d'Herelle phenomenon. These bacterial viruses are specific and are commonly present in sewage and feces. If these materials are passed through a bacteriologic filter, the filtrate contains material that, on inoculation, soon clarifies a heavily clouded broth culture of bacteria. Similarly, the agent can be added to an active culture. After a few minutes, this material can be streaked on a Petri dish. After incubation, clear spots, or plaques, are seen in the streaked areas because some of the cells in that area are killed by a specific bacteriophage.

With the advent of electron microscopy, two strains of coliphage were identified. These strains, designated alpha and gamma, were cultured on the same strain of *Escherichia coli.* These sperm-shaped bodies appear to have heads and tails of different sizes. Particles of a micrococcal bacteriophage appear similar, but are larger.

Lysis of bacteria by bacteriophages is a rapid process in which the bacterium is the host and the virus particle is the parasite. Delbrueck and Luria reported that the first step is the adsorption of the virus on the cell. The next step is the penetration and multiplication of the bacteriophage within the cell. Only one particle appears to enter the cell. After 21–25 minutes, approximately 135 particles are released as the cell is lysed. These particles may enter other cells, and lysis continues. Additional study is needed to identify the mechanism of multiplication of bacterial viruses and the method of bacterial lysis.

4.3.24 The Rickettsia Group

The rickettsiae are small, often pleomorphic, gram-negative bacteria that live and multiply in arthropod tissues. They behave as obligate intracellular parasites and stain lightly with aniline dyes. These organisms are considered intermediate between true bacteria and viruses. They resemble bacteria in size, shape, staining characteristics, and nonfilterability. Their obligate intracellular parasitism is similar to that of viruses. However, viruses multiply only when the cells in a tissue culture are active, whereas rickettsial multiplication occurs and is often maximal when the tissue cells are metabolizing slowly or are no longer viable.

The 10 genera in the order Rickettsias are pathogenic. *Rickettsia prowazekii* is the cause of louse- and flea-borne typhus fever, a disease that may reach epidemic proportions when a population becomes infected with lice, generally during war or famine. Rocky Mountain spotted fever and other diseases of this group are caused by *Rickettsia ricketsii*. All diseases of this group are spread by various species of ticks, in which the pathogens have been found in nearly every type of cell and in every organ. The rickettsiae that cause Rocky Mountain spotted fever multiply well in the cytoplasm and in the nuclei of cells in tissue cultures. Those of the typhus group multiply exclusively in the cytoplasm and are never seen in the nuclei.

Other important rickettsial diseases include Q fever and tsutsugamushi disease, which affects humans, and heartwater, a fatal and economically important disease in goats, cattle, and sheep. In most cases, human symptoms of the rickettsial diseases are similar, characterized by fever, rashes caused by lesions of the blood vessels, and involvement of the brain. The lesions of Rocky Mountain spotted fever first appear on the hands and feet. In typhus fever, lesions first appear on the abdomen and back.

In typhus fever and Rocky Mountain spotted fever, recovery is accompanied by a high degree of long-term active immunity. Vaccines for these diseases have been prepared by a number of methods. Some methods are no longer used because they require living cultures. One current method involves the cultivation of these strict parasites in the bodies of vectors. Either the entire vector or certain heavily invaded tissues are ground up, centrifuged, and filtered. The concentrated rickettsiae are then treated with phenol to disinfect the preparation and inactivate the organisms.

The yolk sac method developed by Cox, which is similar to the methods described for the cultivation of viruses, is the most common method for preparing vaccines for rickettsial diseases. The organisms are inactivated by a chemical, such as phenol, and formalin is added as a preservative. Because the active immunity developed for Rocky Mountain spotted fever is of short duration, the vaccine must be administered annually. One inoculation of the typhus fever vaccine confers long-term active immunity. Passive immunity against these diseases has not been established.

4.4 ANIMAL BIOLOGY

Approximately 1.5 million species of animals have been identified. The life cycle of these multicellular, motile heterotrophs includes a period of embryonic development. Comparing the body plans of existing animal groups and integrating this information with the fossil record shows major trends in animal evolution. The most important elements of the animal body plan are the symmetry of the gut and the body wall; the presence of a distinct head end; and segmentation. Table 4-2 shows that sponges have no body symmetry and no tissue organization, whereas Cnidarians have radial symmetry and some tissue organization.

In terms of their numbers and distribution, insects and other arthropods are the most successful invertebrates. Their hardened exoskeleton, specialized segments, joined appendages, specialized respiratory and nervous systems, and division of labor in the life cycle contribute to their success.

Several evolutionary trends can be followed without considering all 30 animal phyla. Animals are multicellular organisms, and except for sponges, their cells form tissues. The tissues usually are arranged into organs and organ systems. Animals are heterotrophs; they cannot produce their own food. They eat other organisms or absorb nutrients produced by them.

Animals are diploid organisms that reproduce sexually and, in many cases, asexually. Cell division transforms the zygote into a ball-shaped, multicelled embryo. Cells are arranged in germ tissue layers (i.e., ectoderm, endoderm and, in most species, mesoderm). These layers form all tissues and organs of the adult. Most animals are motile, at least during part of the life cycle.

4.4.1 Invertebrate Nonchordates

Invertebrates include a tremendous array of diverse types of animals with many specializations. Common themes are seen in various groups. Structurally, the cells of protozoa, especially ciliates, have the most highly evolved forms departing from the typical cell. Unusual features often provide a focus for studying various phyla (e.g., sponge choanocytes, coelenterate nematocysts, flatworm rhabdites). Remarkable similarities exist between chordates and various invertebrate phyla. The absence of distinctive cytologic characteristics among complex individuals of advanced phyla shows a recent common origin or an older origin that is so successfully integrated that little variation occurs.

Almost any natural organic material can be used as food for some invertebrates. Intracellular or extracellular processes may be involved in digestion. Food in solution can be used by many protozoans and parasites. Particulate food is used by most animals. Small particles of food are most commonly acquired by pseudopodial, ciliary, tentacular, mucoid, or setose mechanisms.

In addition to simple ingestion of mud or other material by relatively unspecialized mouth parts, many feeding specializations have developed. The mandibles of many crustaceans and insects, the radula of mollusks, Aritsotle's lantern of arbacia, the valves of teredo, chelicerae, and the gnathobases of arachnids are used to fragment solid foods. Starfish perform external digestion by inversion of the

TABLE 4-2. *Characteristics of the Major Animal Phyla*

Phylum	Environment	Lifestyle of Adult	Nervous System	Digestive System	Respiratory System	Circulatory System	Reproduction
Porifera Sponges	Most marine, some freshwater	Attached filter feeders	None	No gut	None	None	Sexual, usually hermaphroditic, some asexual
Cnidaria Hydras, anemones, corals, jellyfish	Most marine, some freshwater	Attached, creeping, swimming, floating, carnivores	Nerve net	Saclike gut	None	None	Sexual
Ctenophora Comb jellies	Marine	Mostly planktonic	Nerve net	Branched saclike	None	None	Sexual
Platyhelhelminthes Flatworms, flukes, tapeworms	Marine, freshwater, terrestrial, parasitic	Herbivores carnivores, scavengers	Brain, nerve cords	Saclike gut (some branched)	None	None	Sexual, usually hermaphroditic, some asexual
Nemertea Ribbon worms	Marine, freshwater	Carnivores	Brain, nerve cords	Complete gut	None	None	Sexual
Nematoda Roundworms	Marine terrestrial	Scavengers, carnivores, parasites	Nerve ring, nerve cords	Complete gut	None	Pseudocoele	Sexual
Rotifera Rotifers	Marine, freshwater, wet terrestrial	Filter feeders	Brain, nerve cords	Usually complete gut	None	Pseudocoele	Mostly parthenogenetic
Mollusca Snails, slugs, clams, squids, octopuses	Marine freshwater, terrestrial	Herbivores, carnivores, scavengers, filter feeders	Brain, nerve cords, major ganglia	Complete gut	Ctenidia, other gills	Usually open	Sexual
Annelida Earthworms, leeches, polychaetes	Marine, freshwater, wet terrestrial	Herbivores, carnivores, scavengers, filter feeders	Brain double ventral nerve cord	Complete gut	Gas exchange	Usually closed	Sexual
Arthropoda Crustaceans, spiders, insects	Marine, freshwater, terrestrial	Herbivores, carnivores, filter feeders, parasites	Brain, double ventral nerve cord	Complete gut	Gills, tracheal tubes, book lungs	Open system	Sexual
Echinodermata Starfish, sea urchins	Marine	Carnivores, some herbivores	Radially arranged nervous system	Usually complete gut	Gas exchange	Coelom around viscera	Sexual, some asexual
Chordata Fish, birds, reptiles, mammals	Marine, freshwater, terrestrial	Herbivores, carnivores, omnivores, scavengers	Well-developed brain	Complete gut	Lungs in most gills in fish, perforated pharynx	Closed in most, many lymphatic systems	Sexual, few asexual

stomach. Worms use sucking mouth parts, or piercing and sucking mouth parts, often accompanied by a muscular pharynx, to ingest liquids and soft tissues. Among these worms are many leeches, nematodes, suctorians, lepidopterans, and other arthropods. Internal structural modifications of the digestive tract include the mastax and the gastric mill for grinding as well as various filtering and digestive surfaces for storage. Secretions of salivary and other glands include anticoagulants, poisons, and enzymes.

On the cellular level, circulation occurs by diffusion and protoplasmic movements. The circulatory systems of larger organisms range from vessels with peristaltic contractions to well-developed, chambered hearts with valves and complex vessel systems. Open systems have a heart and arteries, with blood returning through sinuses or hemocoelic spaces. Closed systems have a heart, arteries, capillaries, and veins that return blood to the heart. Heart muscles usually have some spontaneous rhythm of contraction. The intercalated disks of some invertebrate heart muscles increase the evidence of close vertebrate–invertebrate relation. Blood often contains amebocytic cells, proteins, and respiratory pigments as well as food, wastes, antibodies, and hormones. Body fluid is important as a hydrostatic skeleton and in the locomotion of some groups.

Respiratory surfaces are typically moist, thin-walled, and often highly vascularized tissues. The four general types are the general body surface or the surface of appendages, gills, lungs, and tracheae. Organisms of the order Oligochaeta are an example of the body surface type. Many mollusks and crustaceans have gills. Pulmonate snails have a lung-like mantle cavity, spiders have a lamellated type of lung, and holothurians have a water-lung known as a respiratory tree. The tracheae of insects and some other anthropods differ from lungs in the extent of the penetration of body parts: the tracheal type is less dependent on transport by circulating fluids. Some invertebrates perform anaerobic respiration for short periods. Species that commonly depend on anaerobic processes, such as many intestinal parasites, live in organically rich environments.

The end products of metabolism are eliminated by a variety of organs. In aquatic species, carbon dioxide and other solid waste products are partially eliminated by diffusion from respiratory and other surfaces. Water produced by metabolism or taken in by other means is the typical medium of transport for nitrogenous and other waste products. Specialized structures for these purposes include contractile vacuoles (e.g., protozoa), flame cells (e.g., flatworms), nephridia (e.g., annelids), maxillary glands (e.g., crustacea), and coxal glands (e.g., arachnids). The malpighian tubules of insects and some other terrestrial arthropds eliminate uric acid, which is excreted with little water loss. Ammonia is the principal nitrogenous waste product of most aquatic species. Some species store waste products.

Most nervous systems are polarized and synaptic. The system is diffuse in coelenterates, flatworms, and echinoderms. However, in arthropods and higher mollusks, nerve cell bodies are not distributed along the bundles of the processes that form the nerves. Even in some species without an obvious head, cephalization of the nervous system and cerebral ganglion development are found.

Asexual reproductive phenomena include fission, budding, and regeneration of fragments. Sponge gemmules and bryozoan statoblasts are types of internal buds. Reproduction from eggs occurs parthenogentically in some groups. Fertilized sexual eggs are produced by both hermaphroditic and dioecious species. The mechanism of male production varies. Some species produce males from unfertilized eggs and females from fertilized eggs. In many species, sex is determined by chromosomes. Sex ratios are sometimes environmentally regulated. Protandry, or reversal of the functional sex of an organism, occurs in several phyla.

4.4.2 Comparative Anatomy for Chordates

Chordates are distinguished by a dorsal, hollow nerve cord, gill slits in the throat region, and a notochord. They are classified as vertebral chordates (e.g., tunicates, acorn worms, amphioxus) and vertebrates. Vertebrates have a vertebral column, a closed circulatory system that permits large growth, a better developed nervous system, and improved sensory apparatus. Fish include the classes Agnatha (jawless species), Chondrichthyes (species with all cartilage, except the inner ears), and Osteichthyes (bony species). The pectoral fins, pelvic fins, and lateral line system are important for balance.

Lobe-fin fish, or crossopterygians (e.g., latimeria), invaded land, had lungs, and had stubby fins. The evolution of bones into fins was a crucial step for land invasion. These fish gave rise to amphibians. Amphibians (e.g., frogs, toads, salamanders) are still linked to water because their eggs are easily desiccated. Reptiles (e.g., snakes, turtles, crocodiles) arose from amphibians. Land life was possible because of the amniotic egg, which did not desiccate and which had a sufficient food supply. Reptiles are also advanced beyond amphibians because of their internal fertilization by copulation and the small cerebral hemispheres in their brains.

Pterosaurs, which are now extinct, gave rise to birds. Aves (i.e.,birds) can fly because they have special feathers (e.g., large quills for the flying surface, fan-like tail feathers for stabilization, contour and down feathers for insulation), a light skeleton, and a breast bone that is adapted for flight muscles. In addition, these warm-blooded animals have efficient respiration, a four-chambered heart, and advanced sight and muscular coordination.

Mammals arose from a different type of reptile. Key distinguishing features of mammals are the internal development of the young and nutrition by mammary glands; a strong jaw and differentiated teeth; a diaphragm that separates the thorax and abdomen and is used in breathing; legs that are swung underneath the body; and a large brain.

4.4.3 Vertebrate Chordates

Vertebrates are multicellular animals that are derived from embryos. They have three tissue, or germ, layers, the ectoderm, mesoderm, and endoderm. The body has bilateral symmetry; a body cavity, or coelom, lined by mesoderm; and a complete gut (i.e., separate openings for mouth and anus). The anus is derived from an opening in the surface of the early embryo (i.e., the blastopore), or a point near the blastopore. The internal skeleton is derived from the mesoderm, and the mesoderm is formed, at least in part, by tissue derived from the embryonic gut.

4.4.4 Integuments

Vertebrate skin consists of a stratified, nonvascular epidermis and a vascular dermis. The epidermis of fish and aquatic amphibians is covered with a thin basic coat of mucus. In fish, this coat is produced by otherwise undifferentiated cells at the surface of the epidermis. Stratum corneum results from keratinization of the epidermal cells as they approach the surface. In fish, the epidermis has many mucous glands, many unicellular glands, and no stratum corneum. Semiterrestrial amphibians have few mucous glands, fewer unicellular glands, and a thin covering of cornified cells. Terrestrial vertebrates have few mucous glands, no unicellular glands, and a well-defined stratum corneum. The surface of terrestrial vertebrates is covered with a stratum corneum that inhibits dehydration. The stratum corneum of amniotes forms epidermal scales, scutes, crests, claws, nails, hooves, horns, baleen, rattles, horny teeth, beak coverings, feathers, hair, and other structures.

Feathers consist of a shaft and vanes and are elevated by smooth arrector muscles. There are contour and down feathers as well as filoplumes. Modifications of hair include spines, quills, bristles, vibrissae, scales of anteaters, and perhaps rhinoceros horns. Hairs are elevated by smooth arrector muscles. The principal components of dermis are collagen and fibrin. The dermis supports blood vessels, lymphatics, chromatophores, the bases of multicellular epidermal glands, hair and feather follicles, and muscles. It also contains other connective tissues, including bony plates and scales. Epidermal structures that invade the dermis receive nutrition from the surrounding capillaries.

Bone in the dermis is a primitive and generalized condition; its absence is a specialization. Bone was the chief component of the dermis of the earliest fish and tetrapods; it is still present in nearly all fish and some toads. Most reptiles as well as armadillos, which are mammals, form broad plates, smaller bony scales, flexible modern fish scales, osteoderms, and shells. Bony scales and plates are ganoid (e.g., holosteans), placoid (e.g., elasmobranchs), or centoid and cycloid (e.g., teleosts).

Chromatophores are pigment-containing cells that originate from the neural crest and have branching extensions of the cell body. Physiologic color changes are rapid and result from the movement of pigment granules into or out of the processes. Morphologic color changes are slow, depend on melanin synthesis, and are often modified by molting, shedding, or aging.

4.4.5 Skeletal System

The skeleton protects the viscera, stores minerals, contributes rigidity to an otherwise soft body, and provides the series of firm, hinged segments that are essential, in conjunction with the muscles, for locomotion. In amniotes, the skeleton aids in ventilation of the lungs. An external skeleton (e.g., insect, crab) also aids in locomotion. An internal skeleton also permits the reception of external stimuli, thermoregulation by homeotherms, and integumentary respiration by certain aquatic forms. For large animals, particularly terrestrial animals, an external skeleton would be prohibitively heavy.

4.4.6 Muscular System

The muscular system is important in the analysis of locomotor mechanisms and the establishment of phylogenetic relations. Homologies are usually evident among the muscles of related orders and lower taxa. Homologies often can be established among related classes. Nearly all functions of the body are in part muscular. Without muscles, vertebrates could not move, their tissues soon would be starved or poisoned, and the products of their glands could not be distributed. Humans could not read, speak, or write. Muscles accomplish these tasks by creating tension along the axis of their fibers, which tends to shorten their substance. Active muscles usually shorten, moving a bone or constricting a space. They may also prevent motion by opposing gravity, or the pull of other muscles. With little or no motion, a part of the body may become rigid. Further, muscles offer controlled resistance to extrinsic forces that tend to stretch them.

The muscular system also helps to maintain the body temperature of homeotherms and, because of its bulk, distributes the weight of the body, affects the contours of the body, and protects the viscera.

Study nervous control of muscles. Compare and contrast the characteristics of motor and sensory control. Distinguish between the control mechanisms for voluntary and involuntary muscles. Understand the sliding filament theory and the mechanisms of muscular contraction, with an emphasis on the myosin-binding mechanism in the contractile process. Review the differences between isotonic and isometric contractions. Understand that there are 700 skeletal muscles, but do not memorize them. Focus on their location, shape, and size.

4.4.7 Circulatory System

Unless their size and structure place all of their cells in close proximity to an aqueous environment, animals must have a system of internal transport. Vertebrates, which are large and solid, have the most highly evolved circulatory system in the animal kingdom. This system transports respiratory gases, nutrients, metabolic wastes, hormones, and antibodies and also maintains the internal environment. It removes toxic and pathogenic materials from the body and helps to regulate temperature. Further, the circulatory system repairs leaks, compensates for damage, and responds to the varying requirements of the body.

The vertebrate circulatory system consists of the heart, blood vessels, and blood. Arteries distribute blood from the heart to tissues, and veins return blood from the tissues to the heart. Physiologic exchange between blood and tissues occurs through the thin walls of capillaries. At several locations in the body, blood that has passed a capillary bed enters a second capillary bed before reaching the heart. The veins between two capillary networks form a portal system. The circulatory system of vertebrates is a continuum of vessels and is considered closed.

Identify the complex structures and functions of contractile cells and tissues, with emphasis on the cardiac muscle. Identify the thermoregulatory function of the cardiovascular system and its components: heart, blood, arteries, veins, and capillaries. Visit a hospital or clinic to learn about heart transplants, artificial heart machines, and blood bank operations.

Learn the following laws, their limitations, and the stated and unstated assumptions behind them as applied to the circulatory system:

1. Marey's law: If blood pressure decreases, the heart beats faster (an inversely proportional relation).
2. Starling's law: The length of stretched cardiac muscle fibers is related to their strength of contraction (a directly proportional relation).
3. Frank-Starling law: The heart automatically adjusts its pumping capability according to the blood volume to be pumped (a directly proportional relation).

Understand these laws and under what conditions they are valid. Remember that cardiac muscle is not plastic, but that the tone of the heart makes it contract continuously. Also review animal circulatory systems.

4.4.8 Respiratory System

All vertebrate cells use oxygen and release carbon dioxide. These gases are moved into and out of tissues by diffusion. Because all vertebrates are too large for each cell to interact directly with the environment, certain organs, known as the respiratory system, are specialized to accomplish the essential gaseous exchange with the environment. This exchange, known as external respiration, occurs in certain fetal membranes, at the surface of the skin, in gills, in lungs, or elsewhere. Ozygen and carbon dioxide are transported between respiratory organs and other tissues by the circulatory system. These gases are then exchanged with the tissues in the respective capillary beds, a process known as internal respiration.

Diffusion of gases in the respiratory system is increased by (1) providing a large surface of contact between the environmental medium and the blood; (2) reducing the thickness of the barrier between the medium and blood; (3) maintaining the contact of each blood cell with the medium for an adequate time; and (4) for each gas, establishing a large diffusion gradient between the medium and blood. The respiratory organ provides the first three requirements. The fourth requirement is met by behavioral and structural adaptations for moving both medium and blood to, from, and within the respiratory system.

4.4.9 Digestive System

The digestive system receives ingested food, stores it temporarily, reduces it physically, further reduces it chemically, absorbs the products of digestion, holds them temporarily, and eliminates wastes. The structure of the gut relates to its function and to the contours of the body, especially in fish. Food is taken into the mouth with aid of the teeth and jaws; the tongue in some agnaths and tetrapods; the forefeet in some mammals; the lips in some mammals; the beak in birds; or pharyngeal suction in many fish, amphibians, and turtles.

Most vertebrates are intermittent feeders; when food is available, it must be taken into the body faster than it can be digested. If the food is bulky, or if feeding and drinking are infrequent and rapid, food and water must be stored temporarily. The principal storage organ is the stomach. Some birds have a storage sac near the esophagus. Many rodents and some other mammals have internal or external cheek pouches that open, respectively, inside or outside the lips. If digestion is slow (e.g., for diets of coarse vegetation), much digesting food must be retained, and the storage capacity of the digestive tract is greatly increased.

Physical reduction of food, especially roughage, is necessary to release nutrients from indigestible components and to increase the surface contact between food and digestive juices. Physical reduction of food is accomplished in several ways. Food is chewed, rasped, or ground by the oral teeth, the pharyngeal teeth in some fish, the stomach or, in many birds, the gizzard. The food is moistened, softened, and dissolved by fluids of the mouth, stomach, and intestines. In the stomach and small intestine, food is also churned and mixed by anterior to posterior waves of contraction, or peristalsis; reverse peristalsis; and dividing motions, or segmentation. Liver secretions emulsify fats.

Chemical reduction of food occurs principally in the stomach and small intestine by enzymes produced in those organs or in the pancreas. Because most animals eat foods of similar chemical composition, the enzymes and the glands that secrete them are similar. Animals that digest food through bacterial fermentation (e.g., ungulates, some marsupials) store food in the stomach or cecum for long periods. Absorption of the end products of digestion requires significant surface contact between the digested food and the intestinal epithelium. This contact is achieved by a long intestine, folds or pleats in the lining of the gut, microscopic villi on the lining of the digestive tract, and smaller microvilli, visible electron microscopically, in portions of the tract.

Understand the histologic features and mechanisms associated with the digestive system. For example, the gastrointestinal tract has the peritoneum and other muscular control layers, such as the tunica serosa, tunica muscularis, tunica submucosa, and tunica mucosa. Review the microscopic structure of the muscularis mucosa, lamina propria, and circular and longitudinal muscles to understand the role and mechanisms of digestion. Integrate the histologic features of the digestive system with the biochemical and muscular actions performed within the system.

4.4.10 Excretory System

Kidneys are the primary excretory organs of vertebrates. Other organs that aid in the elimination of wastes are gills, lungs, skin, parts of the digestive system, and salt glands. Together, these organs perform two essential functions: they remove the nitrogenous waste products of protein metabolism and other harmful substances, and they eliminate controlled amounts of water and salts to maintain the internal environment within narrow limits.

The functional unit of a kidney is a nephron. Each kidney contains 1 million nephrons, and each nephron is composed of a glomerulus and a tubule. The tubule is composed of renal corpuscles, podocytes, and distal and proximal tubules.

Understand the histologic features of podocytes, and examine sample electron micrographs. Identify various types of nephrons (e.g., juxtamedullary, cortical) and their functions. Review tubular reabsorption, both active and passive, the definition and use of the milliosmole as a unit of concentration, and the hydrostatic forces involved in effective filtration. Use numerical problems to apply various concepts to experimental data on kidneys and filtration rates.

4.4.11 Nervous System

Nerve cells conduct stimuli from one place to another. They are activated by sensory cells or other nerve cells. A stimulus is usually carried to many other nerve cells before it reaches the muscle or gland that responds. Messages are diminished, reinforced, selected, stored, blocked, or integrated within the nervous system. The nervous system determines the response of the body to changes in the internal and external environments. It is the messenger and coordination system of the body.

The four major components of the nervous system are the central nervous system; the peripheral nervous system; the autonomic nervous system, including the sympathetic and parasympathetic systems; and the sense organs (i.e., eyes, nose, ears). The central nervous system is the command center. Messages or impulse arrive there and are sent to the glands, organs, and muscles.

The motor system is also known as the efferent system, and the sensory system is also known as the afferent system. The efferent system is divided into the autonomic and somatic nervous systems.

The most efficient way to review the nervous system is to understand the function and physiologic role of each component. An important principle is that each type of sensory nerve fiber transmits only one modality of sensation.

4.4.12 Endocrine System

The endocrine glands are ductless and secrete hormones that are discharged into the circulatory system for distribution. Specific tissues of the body respond to each hormone. The response may be morphologic (e.g., sex hormones that affect the development of secondary sexual characteristics) or physiologic (e.g., an adrenal hormone that affects kidney function). Many hormones act directly on tissues that are receptive to their messages. However, the action is usually indirect. For example, when a hormone secreted by the hypothalamus is released by the hypophysis, the ovary secretes a hormone that affects the lining of the uterus.

The function of the endocrine glands is similar to that of the nervous system in several respects. Each system controls and integrates bodily functions, each mediates control through the release of chemicals, and each interacts within its own system to coordinate its activities. Endocrine control is slower and more sustained than nervous control. The functions of the two systems often merge.

Endocrine glands are small and highly vascular. They are often diffuse in lower vertebrates, but tend to be discrete in tetrapods. Most are constructed of cords of cuboidal cells that are arranged among sinusoids and supported by a matrix of connective tissue. Several endocrine glands are constructed of thin, attenuated cells, although the thyroid gland is composed of follicles. The hormones of glands of mesodermal origin (e.g., gonads, adrenal cortex, placenta) are steroids; the hormones of glands of ectodermal or endodermal origin are proteins, peptides, or other derivatives of amino acids. Because endocrine glands transmit signals through the circulatory system, their shape is of little importance, and a gland may be single, multiple, or diffuse without relation to its function. Only the aggregate volume of cells is critical. Even the secretions have been remarkably constant over the ages, with some exceptions. Responses to the secretions are varied. Endocrine glands have diverse developmental origins, are usually unrelated in space, and are incompletely related in function. These glands do not form an organ system in the usual sense. Endocrine function in most lower vertebrates is inadequately known.

Knowing the cellular mechanisms of hormone action aids in understanding the specificity and target tissues of each hormone. Review and memorize the organic structure and physical and chemical properties (e.g., molecular weight, density, melting or boiling point) of the major hormones.

4.4.13 Lymphatic and Immune Systems

Without drainage by the lymph system, fluids would accumulate in the tissues and cause swelling. Tissue fluids enter netlike or blindly ending lymphatic capillaries, where they form lymph. Lymph passes slowly into larger and larger lymphatic vessels, until it is discharged into the venous system at several points. Lymphatic capillaries in the gut are known as lacteals.

Although some classifications of immunity are complex and confusing, the simple classification of innate and acquired immunity is useful. Innate immunity is nonspecific and common to a species or race. Because of innate immunity, humans do not have blackleg of cattle, and cattle do not have typhoid fever. All members of a species or race are innately susceptible or innately immune to a given disease, but occasionally, immune individuals are found in a susceptible species.

Acquired immunity is specific and develops during the lifetime of a person or an animal. For example, a person may have been susceptible to smallpox at birth, but an acquired immunity developed because the person had the disease or was vaccinated. Immunity may be acquired in two ways:

1. In active immunity, the body develops immunizing antibodies as a result of a stimulus received from the entrance of a foreign substance known as an antigen (e.g., pathogenic bacteria). Through metabolism, the living cells of the body produce one or more chemicals that injure the pathogens or neutralize their products. Because the body produces these antibodies through its own activity, this type of acquired immunity is known as active.
2. In passive immunity, the body that is immunized plays no active part. It receives an injection of antibody or another protective substance that was previously formed by an animal with active immunity. Some of the antibodies of the immune animal are deposited in the serum of the blood. If injected into a susceptible person or animal, the serum confers passive immunity.

The ways in which the body protects itself from disease when pathogens are introduced and the way in which it recovers and rids itself of pathogens have been the subject of much study.

More than one mechanism operates in immunity. In some diseases, at least two actions must be taken to protect the body: (1) The toxins that have been released in the body must be neutralized, or they will do harm independently of the organisms that produced them. (2) The organisms must be destroyed or eliminated. These activities require different agents, although they are all considered antibodies. Antibacterial agents do not destroy toxins, and antitoxins do not destroy bacteria and complement fragments.

The presence of antibodies in the blood permits phagocytes to engulf bacteria more rapidly. These antibodies are known as opsonins. They are specific, which means that the opsonin of one disease has no effect on the bacteria of another disease. If serum containing opsonin is added to a bacterial culture, the organisms are not killed or injured. However, the organisms are affected so that if leukocytes are added, the bacteria are attracted to them and are more easily ingested. The opsonins also may cause other changes in the bacterial cells. In some diseases, the amount of opsonin, or the opsonic index, is increased as immunity develops and the patient recovers.

The blood and other body fluids of healthy animals can dissolve bacteria. This process is known as bacteriolysis, and it is one example of the more general phenomenon of cytolysis, or dissolution of foreign cells, such as red and white blood corpsucles from other animals. In certain diseases, bacteriolysins that destroy the causative bacteria are found in the bloodstream of immune individuals.

This phenomenon has been the subject of extensive research that shows that two substances in the blood act jointly to destroy bacterial cells. One substance, known as complement, is a regular constituent of the normal blood of vertebrates. Complement is nonspecific, with one type aiding in the destruction of all types of bacteria, and thermolabile, destroyed by heating at 56° C for 30 minutes. The level of complement in the blood does not increase as the body becomes immune to disease. The other immunizing substance that participates in bacteriolysis is amboceptor, or sensitizer. It is specific: a particular amboceptor is produced by the body in response to a particular type of bacteria and reacts only with that type of bacteria. The amboceptors are thermostable at 56° C for 30 minutes. The normal body has little amboceptor, but produces it as immunity develops during the course of a disease or after successful vaccination.

If the blood or serum of an animal containing an antibody is mixed in the presence of an electrolyte, such as sodium chloride, with a laboratory culture of the type of organism that stimulated its formation, the combination causes the cells to clump, or agglutinate, although they do not die. This agglutination reaction is used to diagnose typhoid fever, brucellosis in cattle and humans, and several other diseases. For example, in Widal's serum test for typhoid fever, if the blood serum of a patient causes agglutination of a laboratory culture of *Salmonella typhi* under proper conditions, the patient has formed typhoid agglutinin. In the presence of suggestive symptoms, the disease is diagnosed as typhoid fever. Because the cells of a killed culture clump as readily as those of a living culture, the agglutination is not caused by locomotion, but by the effect of the antibody on the cell surface. The principles of this reaction were used to determine the potency of influenza virus vaccine and the amount of antibody in the serum of a previously inoculated animal.

Precipitins are closely related to agglutinins. Precipitins cause molecules of protein or other substances to form a fine precipitate. In the precipitin reaction, bacteria clump. The precipitin reaction is helpful in the serologic identification of soluble proteins in medicine, industry, and chemistry.

Early studies showed that some types of bacteria, notably *Corynebacterium diphtheriae* and *Clostridium tetani,* produce deadly toxins. The blood serum of people who have recovered from the diseases produced by these organisms contains a specific antibody, antitoxin, that neutralizes the toxin. The effect of the antitoxin on the toxin is not known, but their union is physical rather than chemical. The toxin is not irretrievably destroyed; to some extent, it can be separated from a mixture of toxin and antitoxin. Antitoxins are specific for their respective exotoxins.

A common misconception about immunity is that good general health protects against disease, whereas poor health increases susceptibility. In reality, good health does not protect people from most infectious diseases. Healthy people readily contract smallpox, measles, or typhoid fever if they are properly exposed. People in poor physical condition do not contract these diseases if they have active immunity against them. However, a person who is in poor physical condition is less likely than a healthier person to recover from prolonged, severe illness.

Two infectious diseases, pneumonia and tuberculosis, support the popular idea that illness is more likely to occur in people who are in good health than in those who are undernourished or otherwise weakened (e.g., by previous disease). Many noninfectious diseases, such as rickets and scurvy, are the direct result of malnutrition and other debilitating conditions.

4.4.14 Methods of Conferring Immunity

Immunity is conferred in several ways. Invasion of living, fully virulent organisms produces the typical pattern of infection, illness, and recovery. Introduction of living, attenuated organisms causes a mild form of disease and confers immunity. Organisms may be attenuated by heat, with chemicals, or by passage through the body of an animal. Active immunization against smallpox is accomplished by this method.

Injection of the dead bodies of some pathogenic organisms into a susceptible host stimulates the host to produce active immunity. Because the organisms cannot multiply, this method is safe. It is used to protect people against several diseases, including typhoid fever, whooping cough, and Rocky Mountain spotted fever.

Bacterial toxins are poisonous substances, but they can be used in two ways to confer active immunity. One method is to inject a small dose into the host, with increasing doses used for subsequent injections. The other method is to treat the toxin first with a chemical that weakens it. The product is known as a toxoid. The toxin of scarlet fever and the toxoid of diphtheria are examples.

Passive immunity is acquired in only one way. Antibodies or other protective substances that have been formed by another person or animal and deposited in its blood serum are injected into the host. Passive immunity is successfully conferred in few diseases; they include diphtheria, tetanus, some types of pneumonia, meningitis, and gas gangrene.

Confusion surrounds the role of vaccines and that of serums as agents for conferring immunity. Both agents are injected hypodermically with a small syringe, and the patient normally does not know what substance is injected.

Like many terms, "vaccine" has both a broad and a restricted meaning. In its broad use, a vaccine is any biologic material injected into the body to stimulate active immunity (e.g., living or dead microorganisms, toxin). In its more restricted sense, a vaccine is material containing living attenuated organisms (e.g., virus). Smallpox vaccine is a common example. Those who use the term in its restricted sense usually refer to dead bacteria used for the same purpose as "bacterins."

Immunizing the body by vaccination is usually performed for prevention rather than cure. The vaccine is administered before exposure occurs to allow the body to establish active immunity before invasion by the organisms occurs. An exception is the use of autogenous vaccines. These vaccines are prepared by culturing the organisms from the lesions of the patient, killing them, and injecting them into the same patient. This method is used for such localized conditions as boils, in which the bacteria are so located that they do not stimulate active immunity. Such immunity occurs when large numbers of bacteria are injected under the skin.

An immunizing serum is the blood serum of a person or animal. It contains an immunizing material, or antibody. In many cases, the specific antibody is antitoxin. The antibody may be obtained by withdrawing blood from a person who is recovering from a disease, such as measles, or by injecting the toxin into an animal, usually a horse. After active immunity is established, some blood is withdrawn from the animal. The blood corpuscles are removed from the serum, and the serum is standardized as to the strength of the antitoxin. The serum is stored in sterile tubes or bottles. It is not practicable, on a commercial scale, to obtain chemically pure antitoxin free from serum, although the usual practice is to concentrate it by removing inert materials.

Antitoxin serums are used for cure rather than prevention. They may be given for prevention after exposure occurs, but their immunizing effects are the same as those of the disease. In active immunity, the antitoxin or other immunizing material is diminished or eliminated slowly and is constantly renewed. In passive immunity, renewal does not occur, and the host soon becomes susceptible again. As a curative agent, the action of the antitoxins is rapid unless the damage has already occurred (e.g., the toxin has reached the nervous system).

Review the structures and functions of the lymphatic and immune systems. Understand the mechanisms that these systems use to regulate various processes in the human body. Study the composition of blood on both a physical and a chemical basis as well as the mechanisms that control the flow of lymph at various lymph nodes.

Review the physical structure, physical properties, chemical properties, and stereochemistry of helper T-cells, killer T-cells, suppressor T-cells, and T-cell receptors. Review autoimmunity, active immunity, and passive immunity. Read current research reports on bone marrow transplants and spleen and thymus surgical procedures. Use your knowledge of microbiology, especially the life history of viruses and bacteria, to understand the response of the immune system.

4.4.15 Allergic Reactions

Humans and other mammals usually tolerate the introduction of many foreign substances, including most proteins. However, sometimes they are sensitive to minute doses taken through the stomach or respiratory tract. Two types of hypersensitivity, anaphylaxis and allergy, are recognized. They are similar, and some authorities consider anaphylaxis a form of allergy.

Anaphylaxis occurs when a normally harmless protein or other substance enters the body. A small dose is sufficient to cause this reaction. No symptoms occur, but in approximately 10 days, the body becomes so sensitive to this protein that another minute dose causes anaphylactic shock. In guinea pigs, which are particularly responsive, anaphylactic shock occurs within a few minutes of the second injection. Anaphylactic shock causes sneezing followed by a spasm in which the animal gasps for breath. The animal usually dies of suffocation in a short time. The symptoms are the same in each animal within a species, regardless of the protein used, but vary in different species. In guinea pigs, the shock is caused by persistent contraction of the involuntary muscles of the bronchioles of the lungs; in rabbits, the right side of the heart dilates. In humans, these disturbances of the involuntary muscles are less pronounced, and usually only a rash occurs.

An important manifestation of hypersensitivity is serum sickness. After an immunizing serum is introduced, the body becomes sensitized to a protein that is part of the serum, but not to the antitoxin. A later injection of serum from the same type of animal (e.g., a horse) causes serum sickness. This illness may occur as anaphylactic shock, but the symptoms are usually different and much milder. After approximately 10 days, the patient experiences an increase in temperature, pain similar to mild arthritis, and an extensive itchy rash. The term "serum sickness" is often restricted to these later manifestations, although similar symptoms may occur after the initial contact with a foreign serum.

The tuberculin test for the presence of tuberculosis is a delayed hypersensitivity reaction. The proteins from *Mycobacterium tuberculosis* are released within the body of the patient and cause sensitization.

All types of hypersensitivity may be considered allergies, but discussion of allergies is often restricted to abnormal sensitivity to natural substances, such as pollen, feathers, hair, dandruff, insect bites, bee stings, and food (e.g., milk, eggs, vegetable proteins). Some confusion exists between ordinary allergy, in which hypersensitivity is caused by the initial dose of a foreign substance, and atopy, in which hypersensitivity is present without the introduction of a foreign substance. Some cases classified as atopy may be caused by unrecognized exposure.

A striking feature of allergies is the range of individual reactions. After exposure to the same substance, some people are atopic, others are sensitized, and still others are immune. Allergy in humans causes hay fever, asthma, and rashes.

4.5 EFFECTS OF DISEASE ON ANIMAL BODY SYSTEMS

Some diseases are more prevalent among younger animals than among older animals. Many viral, bacterial, and parasitic diseases and nutritional deficiencies are more severe in young animals. Young animals require a balanced diet to help them resist disease or parasitic infestation and to meet the demands of growth.

Regardless of the cause of disease and the age, sex, or species of the animal, the severity of a disease is determined by the number of cells affected in a tissue, organ, or organ system; the degree of cell damage; and the importance of the cells.

A disease that affects only one important organ or tissue can cause death. For example, diabetes occurs in dogs, humans, and other animals. In animals with diabetes, the blood sugar level is increased, and sugar cannot be used properly. Diabetes is caused by malfunction of a type of cell in the pancreas. Untreated diabetes can cause death.

Injury to highly specialized cells, such as those of the brain or nervous system, causes more severe damage than injury to less specialized cells. Severe damage of the nerve cells is permanent, although some repair occurs in the peripheral nerves. Examples of poor repair of nervous tissue include paralysis in a human after polio and incoordination or paralysis in a dog after distemper.

Table 4-3 shows diseases that occur in both humans and animals.

4.5.1 Mechanisms of Disease

When infectious agents enter the animal body, they attempt to multiply. The increase in their numbers can cause mechanical injury to the cells and tissue. The effect is cell degeneration and cell death, or necrosis.

Toxins, or harmful by-products, may damage blood vessels, causing hemorrhage; destroy red blood cells, causing anemia; obstruct small blood vessels, cutting off the blood supply to an area of the body; or lead to cell, tissue, organ, or organ system malfunction.

Invasion of the body by disease agents stimulates protective reactions. Increased numbers of white blood cells search for and destroy the invading disease organisms. Protective substances (i.e., antibodies) are produced and cause clumping of the disease agents, allowing the white blood cells to engulf and destroy them. Inflammation is a complex local vascular and cellular response of the body to an irritant. The blood supply to the infected area is increased, and this increased blood supply attempts to dilute, localize, and destroy the invading agents.

In the early days of veterinary medical research, veterinarians were limited to observations of the external appearance and manifestations of disease. For example, the lesions of cowpox and the soft and bent bones of rickets were readily observed. Early veterinarians did not understand the causes of disease, but they observed consistent signs with specific diseases.

When veterinarians began to perform postmortem examinations on animals, they associated internal changes with outward signs of specific diseases. For example, the lesions of tuberculosis were seen in

TABLE 4-3. ***Diseases Common to Animals and Humans***

Bacterial diseases	Viral Diseases
Leptospirosis	B virus
Rat-bite fever	Rabies
Tuberculosis	Cat-scratch fever
Salmonellosis	Newcastle disease
Fungal diseases	Parasitic diseases
Ringworm	Roundworms
Aspergillosis	Ascaridosis
Histoplasmosis	Hookworms
Coccidioides	Strongyloidosis
Cryptococcosis	

the lungs. Examination of animals that died of a chronic respiratory condition showed characteristic lung lesions. The tubercle-like lesions gave tuberculosis its name, but the specific cause of the disease was not known for many years.

Further observation and research were required to associate definite functional and structural changes with symptoms. Through observation, veterinarians attempted to identify the cause and treatment of a variety of diseases. For example, the symptoms of drinking large quantities of water, frequent urination, and sweet-smelling urine were associated with diabetes. These symptoms can be produced experimentally by removing the pancreas.

The following questions are helpful in determining the cause of symptoms: What could be the likely cause of the signs and symptoms? Are they related to a specific body system? Are they likely to be associated with infectious agents, heredity, nutrition, or a combination of factors? Complete laboratory examination and testing may be necessary to identifiy the cause.

Diseases can be classified in many ways. This chapter uses the anatomic method, in which diseases are classified according to the body system that is affected.

4.5.2 Diseases of the Circulatory System

The mammalian circulatory system consists of two separate pumps (i.e., the left and right sides of the heart) and a series of blood vessels. Large, elastic vessels known as arteries carry blood from the left side of the heart. They divide into smaller vessels known as arterioles, which gradually diminish in size to become minute blood vessels, or capillaries, which supply blood to the cells. A second set of blood vessels originate from the capillaries. These vessels are the venules that unite to form larger blood vessels known as veins. Veins carry blood back to the right side of the heart. Blood that contains food and oxygen leaves the left side of the heart through a large artery known as the aorta. The blood is pumped to the capillary beds, which are located in tissues and organs. Blood flows slowly through the capillary bed, from arteries to veins, diffusing the food and oxygen into the surrounding cells. The blood also removes the carbon dioxide and waste materials that are produced by the cells.

Some bacteria damage the inner lining of the blood vessels. The damage may cause debris to accumulate and form a plug. This plug, or clot, may break away from the lining and flow with the blood through the blood vessel. When the clot reaches smaller blood vessels, it may become lodged, obstructing circulation. Cells that receive their blood supply from the affected blood vessel are deprived of nourishment and may die. If these cells are important to a vital organ, such as the heart, brain, or kidney, the animal may die.

The brain is harmed by severe toxic injury to the blood vessels. Damage can be so severe that small blood vessels dissolve, depriving a portion of the brain of blood. Death may also result from internal bleeding or hemorrhaging in the brain or elsewhere.

Injuries and toxic materials also affect the veins. Because these thin-walled vessels are near the skin, they are easily injured. Blood from injured veins escapes into the surrounding tissues. Bruises and blood blisters are common examples of damaged veins. This blood is broken down and reabsorbed, and the waste products are excreted through the kidneys.

The lymph vessels are also connected to the circulatory system. These vessels begin as small capillary-type tubes in the tissues. They join to form larger and larger vessels as they approach the heart. Usually, their course parallels that of the arteries and veins.

The dissolved nutrients in the blood leak through the capillary walls to supply the tissue cells. The lymph system collects the fluid that surrounds the cells and returns it to the circulatory system. The large collecting lymph vessels join a large vein near the heart.

Collections of tissue known as lymph nodes are situated along the lymphatic system. These nodes filter foreign material from the lymph. Organisms and foreign material are phagocytized by the white blood cells. When bacterial organisms overwhelm the protective white blood cells, infection occurs. A common example of infected lymph glands is cervical abscesses, or lump throat, in guinea pigs.

Another problem of the circulatory system is anemia. "Anemia" means "without blood." The quantity or the quality of the blood may be deficient. The animal may have a reduced amount of hemoglobin or a reduced number of red blood cells.

The symptoms of anemia are caused by the destruction of red blood cells. The animal is pale, and mucous membranes (i.e., lining of the mouth, throat, inner surface of the eyelids), which normally appear pink, appear white. Blood cells are found in the urine. The animal huddles, appears cold, is weak, and may have swollen legs.

4.5.3 Diseases of the Digestive System

Digestion is the process by which ingested food is reduced into a form that can be used by the cells. Digestion occurs in a long tube known as the alimentary tract. This name is derived from a Latin word meaning "nourishment," or nutrition. The alimentary tract has two openings to the external environment, the mouth and the anus.

Other than airborne diseases and those transmitted by mosquitoes and blood-sucking insects, most infectious agents are acquired through ingestion. Appropriate sanitation prevents exposure to infectious agents that are present in food and water.

Symptoms of diseases of the digestive tract are visible to careful observers. Lesions of the mouth, such as tumors, sores of the lips or tongue, or increased salivation, are easily detected. Some of these signs suggest a specific disease. For example, in Rhesus monkeys, ulcers of the lip and tongue indicate infection with herpes B virus. Excessive salivation may be a sign of disease or may result from uneven wear of the teeth. A condition in rabbits, known as wet dewlap, is caused by overfeeding or feeding too much green, succulent food. This type of feed is easily fermented and may irritate the stomach and cause increased salivation. The saliva wets heavy folds of hair on the neck, providing a moist, warm site that is ideal for bacterial or fungal infection.

4.5.4 Vomiting

Vomiting is a sign of irritation in the first portion of the alimentary tract, the stomach, or a portion of the small intestine. Liver infection or dysfunction can also cause vomiting. In older dogs and cats, vomiting often results from kidney malfunction. Vomiting may occur when young dogs and cats start to eat solid food. It may result from simply overloading the stomach. Sometimes the esophagus is constricted or contains a large diverticulum, or pouch. These conditions are often congenital and interfere with normal passage of food through the alimentary tract. Vomiting is persistent in animals with this condition. In dogs, foreign objects or masses of roundworms in the stomach or small intestine cause vomiting. The obstruction interferes with the passage of food from the stomach. Because vomiting does not always indicate disease, the clinical history of the animal must be considered during evaluation.

4.5.5 Elimination

The stools are affected by diseases of the digestive system. The color, consistency, odor, and content of the stools often indicate the origin of the problem. For example, in dogs, cats, and monkeys, greasy-appearing gray or white stools indicate improper digestion of fats and possible pancreas disease.

Disease injures the lining of the alimentary tract, removing the natural barrier to microorganisms and allowing them to penetrate the tissues and enter the bloodstream. Irritated tissues produce excessive amounts of mucus. Excessive mucus appears as a glistening jelly-like substance in the stools. In rabbits, mucoid enteritis is characterized by loss of flesh, thirst, abdominal bloating, roughened hair coat, and accumulation of mucus in the posterior gut. This condition usually occurs within the first 6 months of life. Affected animals have either constipation or diarrhea, and the feces contain mucus.

The appearance of mucus in the stools aids in determining which part of the alimentary tract is damaged. Small particles of mucus that are well mixed with feces suggest infection in the small intestine; large pieces of mucus suggest infection in the colon, cecum, or rectum. When severe damage occurs, pieces of the intestinal lining may appear in the stools.

The color of the stools also provides diagnostic information. Severe injury to the digestive system causes hemorrhage. Bright red feces indicate bleeding in the large intestine. Dark tan stools usually indicate bleeding in the stomach or small intestine; the color difference is caused by digestion of the blood.

The consistency of animal stools aids in determining the condition of the digestive system. Diarrhea, or frequent discharge of watery stools, is a common and important symptom that accompanies many infections and noninfectious conditions. Diarrhea is caused by an increased rate of passage, which reduces absorption and increases the passage of fluid with fecal wastes. Diarrhea commonly indicates inflammation of the intestines, or enteritis, and may occur after unusual stress (e.g., shipment of an animal). Diarrhea also may be caused by bacteria, viruses, parasites, or protozoan disease agents that damage the small intestine. In analyzing the cause of enteritis, many factors must be considered, including age of the animal, adequacy of nutrition, species, number of animals infected, appetite, possible stresses, and possible infectious agents. A complete laboratory examination may be necessary to determine the differential diagnosis. Many infectious causes of enteritis are not known.

4.5.6 Diseases of the Respiratory System

The cells, tissues, and organs of the animal body are more dependent on oxygen than on any other substance from the external environment. Animals can survive for weeks without food and for days without water by using stored carbohydrates, proteins, fats, and water. However, animals can survive without oxygen for only a few minutes. If deprived of oxygen for more than 6 minutes, some nerve cells in the brain are severely damaged and cannot be repaired. Because most animals cannot store oxygen, a continual source is necessary.

Some diseases interfere with the delivery of oxygen to animal tissues. Because the respiratory system is responsible for the oxygen supply and the removal of gaseous wastes, diseases that affect this vital system may cause rapid death.

The acquisition of oxygen from the air requires little effort. Unless impairment occurs, breathing is a smooth, rhythmic process that is executed unconsciously. In many animals at rest (e.g., dogs, cats, monkeys), breathing is barely perceptible and usually goes unnoticed.

In animals, elastic lungs are located in a vacuum within a rib cage. The diaphragm is a muscle that separates the chest cavity from the abdominal cavity. The muscles of the rib cage and diaphragm alter the size of the chest cavity. As the size of the cavity changes, air is forced into and out of the lungs. Air is taken into the lungs through the nose, nasal passages, and windpipe. The mouth provides a supplementary intake passage if the quantity taken in through the nose is insufficient. The nose and mouth are equipped with filters, or hairlike cilia, and associated mucous glands. These structures prevent the introduction of foreign particles into the respiratory tract. The mucus traps these particles, and the beating cilia move them outward.

The lungs contain many microscopic air pockets, or alveoli. The exchange between the carbon dioxide carried in by the venous blood and the oxygen in inhaled air occurs in the alveoli. These anatomic features are important because they are related to the signs and symptoms of respiratory diseases.

The primary causes of respiratory disease are viruses, bacteria, fungi, and parasites. These organisms usually enter the nose or mouth along with air. Modifying factors, such as temperature, nutrition, and various stresses, contribute to disease outbreaks and affect the severity of infection. Drafts and sudden changes of temperature predispose animals to pneumonia. Because animals are sensitive to stresses caused by sudden changes in the external environment, conditions must be kept as constant as possible. If conditions fluctuate significantly, respiratory disease can affect the entire herd or colony.

Identification of the causative agent usually requires a complete laboratory examination. Symptoms of respiratory infection include coughing, sneezing, difficult or abdominal breathing, conjunctivitis (i.e., red eyes and lids), and nose and eye discharge.

The suffix -itis denotes inflammation or disease in a specific area of the body. For example, "pneumonic" refers to the lungs. When the lungs are inflamed, veterinarians use the terms "pneumonitis" and "pneumonia."

Respiratory infections affect the lungs and upper respiratory respiratory passages, such as the nose and trachea, or windpipe. In cats, common causes of lung infections are viruses and virus-like agents that cause sneezing, salivation, running nose and eyes, and loss of appetite. Most of these symptoms are caused by irritation of the lining of the lungs and increased production of mucus. The additional mucus and cells are carried from the lungs by the cilia. As the infection progresses, the discharge from the nose and eyes becomes thicker and changes from colorless to yellow-gray. This thick, yellow-gray discharge is known as mucopurulent, or containing mucus and pus.

Cats also have respiratory infections that primarily involve the upper respiratory tract. One cause of these infections is a virus that produces a disease known as feline viral rhinotracheitis. In this disease, the nose and pharynx are coated with cellular debris that causes sneezing and violent coughing. In addition, because the normal air pathway to the lungs is blocked, the cat breathes through the mouth. The amount of debris increases during the course of the infection, and the nares, or openings of the nose, and eyelids close. The veterinarian may relieve the effects of this disease by frequently opening the nares and eyelids and using cotton soaked in warm, mild salt solution to gently remove the caked exudate. Cats with this condition usually refuse to eat; good nutrition may be aided by coaxing the animal to eat with favorite tidbits, such as liver, kidney, or spleen.

Respiratory symptoms are usually the first signs of distemper in dogs. Dogs with distemper usually have a running nose and eyes and frequent sneezing. The watery discharge from the nose and eyes becomes thicker and may block the entrance to the nose and the eyelids. Dogs seldom recover. Vaccines prevent this serious disease.

Snuffles is a common disease of rabbits that is characterized by inflammation of the upper respiratory tract. Affected animals sneeze, cough, and have a profuse nasal discharge. Pneumonia frequently develops. This disease is similar to a cold in humans. A number of organisms cause the disease, either individually or in combination. *Pasteurella multocida* is the organism most often isolated from affected rabbits. In monkeys, respiratory infections are caused by a variety of agents, such as bacteria, viruses, and worms.

In smaller animals, such as rats, mice, and guinea pigs, infections of the respiratory tract are caused by viruses or bacteria. The signs of respiratory infection in these animals are similar to those of cats and dogs: noisy or difficult breathing and nasal exudate. In rats with enzootic murine pneumonitis, a red-tinged discharge accumulates around the nose and eyes. In rat colonies in which this infection is endemic, a high percentage of the rats may be affected without showing any of the typical signs of the disease. When these rats are unduly stressed, either experimentally or environmentally, the disease occurs. On postmortem examination, the lungs appear spotted with solid gray areas, and sometimes a gray coating covers the heart.

4.6 PLANT BIOLOGY

Plants are classified into the kingdoms Protista, Fungi, Plantae, and Monera as follows:

Kingdom Protista
- Phylum Chlorophyta (green algae)
  - Class Chlorophyceae
    - Order Volvocales
    - Order Ulotrichales
    - Order Ulvales
    - Order Oedogoniales
    - Order Conjugales
    - Order Chlorococcales
    - Order Dasycladales
  - Class Charophyceae

- Phylum Euglenophyta (euglenoids)
  - Class Euglenophyceae
- Phylum Pyrrophyta (dinoflagellates)
  - Class Dinophyceae
- Phylum Chrysophyta (yellow-green and golden-brown algae; diatoms)
  - Class Xanthophyceae
  - Class Chrysophyceae
  - Class Bacillariophyceae
- Phylum Phaeophyta (brown algae)
  - Class Phaeophyceae
    - Order Ectocarpales
    - Order Laminariales
    - Order Fucales

Kingdom Fungi

- Phylum Schizomycophyta
  - Class Schizomycetae
  - Class Actinomycetae
- Phylum Myxomycophyta
  - Class Myxomycetae
  - Class Acrasieae
  - Class Plasmodiophoreae
- Phylum Eumycophyta
  - Class Phycomycetae
  - Class Ascomycetae
  - Class Basidiomycetae
  - Class Deutoeromycetae
  - Class Chytridiomycetae
  - Class Oomycetae
  - Class Zygomycetae

Kingdom Plantae

- Subkingdom Bryophyta (nonvascular plants)
- Phylum Bryophyta (bryophytes)
  - Class Hepaticae (liverworts)
    - Order Marchantiales
    - Order Jungermanniales
  - Class Anthocerotae (hornworts)
  - Class Musci (mosses)
    - Order Sphagnales
    - Order Bryales
- Phylum Tracheophyta (vascular plants)
- Phylum Psilophyta (whisk ferns)
  - Class Psilopsidae
    - Order Psilotales
    - Order Psilophytales
- Subphylum Lycopododiophyta (club mosses)
  - Class Lycopodineae
    - Order Lycopodiales
    - Order Selaginellales
    - Order Lepidodendrales
    - Order Isoetales
    - Order Pleuromeiales
- Subphylum Rhyniopsida
- Subphylum Zosterophyllopsida
- Subphylum Trimerophytopsida

Subphylum Progymnospermopsida
Subphylum Filicopsida
Subphylum Sphenopsida
Class Equisetineae
Order Hyeniales
Order Sphenophyllales
Order Calamitales
Order Equisetales
Subphylum Peteropsida
Class Filicineae
Order Coenopteridales
Order Ophioglossales
Order Marattiales
Order Filicales
Class Gymnopsermae
Subclass Cycadopsidae (cycads)
Subclass Coniferopsida (conifers)
Subclass Gnetopsida (gnetophytes)
Class Angiosperm
Subclass Dicotyledonae
Subclass Monocotyledonae
Order Anthocerotales

Kingdom Monera
Phylum Scizonta or Schizophyta (bacteria)
Class Archaebacteria
Class Eubacteria
Class Actinobacteria
Phylum Cyanonta or Cyanophyta (blue-green algae)
Phylum Prochloronta or Prochlorophyta

4.6.1 Plant Tissues and Growth

Most of the thousands of plant species are flowering plants. Despite their diversity, flowering plants are composed of only three types of tissue: dermal, ground, and vascular. Dermal tissues form a protective cover at the surface of the plant. Ground tissues account for most of the plant body. Vascular tissues are similar to pipelines that run through the ground tissues. They distribute water, dissolved minerals, and the products of photosynthesis through the roots, stems, and leaves of the plant.

Plants grow at the tips of their roots and shoots. Each tip has a region of undifferentiated cells. These cells divide repeatedly, elongate, and develop into the specialized types of cells that form the dermal, ground, and vascular tissues. The growth that originates at the root and shoot tips produces the primary tissues of the plant body. Many plants also show secondary growth that increases the diameter of the roots and stems. The regions that are responsible for secondary growth are not found at the tips of the roots and shoots. A fully developed lateral meristem is a long, thin cylinder that produces new cells along the length of an older root or stem. Extensive secondary growth produces wood.

4.6.2 Reproduction and Development

For flowering plants, sexual reproduction requires the production of spores as well as gametes. The spores form in specialized reproductive structures known as flowers. In many species, the flowers coevolved with insects, birds, and other animals that assist in pollination and seed dispersal. Male floral structures produce haploid microspores that develop into immature male gametophytes. Sperm form inside pollen grains. Female floral structures produce haploid megaspores that develop into female gametophytes. Eggs form inside the female gametophytes. Pollen grains are released from the parent plant and are adapted for traveling to the eggs. Female gametophytes remain attached to the parent plant and are nourished by it. After fertilization occurs, seeds develop. Each seed contains an embryo saprophyte and tissues that aid in nutrition, protection, and dispersal.

Many plants also reproduce asexually. Sexual reproduction requires the formation of gametes, followed by fertilization. Two sets of genetic instructions, from two gametes, are present in fertilized eggs. Asexual reproduction occurs through mitosis, and individuals of the new generation are clones (i.e., genetically identical to the parent plant).

4.7 EVOLUTION AND GENETICS

Molecular genetics, mutations, and comparative chordate anatomy are elements of the evolutionary process. The history and mechanisms that control evolution for various organisms can be directly applied to solving problems in the areas of gene flow, genetic drift, and genetic, or chromosomal, mapping.

Genetic variation among individuals occurs as a result of five types of events: (1) gene mutation; (2) abnormal changes in chromosome structure or number; (3) crossing over and genetic recombination during meiosis; (4) independent assortment of chromosomes during meiosis; and (5) fertilization between different gametes. Only mutation creates new molecular forms of a gene. The other types of events simply shuffle existing genes into new combinations. Chapter 5 discusses problem solving and probability mathematics.

4.7.1 The Mechanisms of Evolution

Evolution is the study of the changes that occur in organisms. Minor changes lead to better adaptation to an environment, whereas major changes lead to the formation of a new species. Changes occur when organisms survive because of phenotypic differences. These phenotypic differences are based on underlying genetic differences, as found in the germ cells. The survival of selected organisms causes alterations in the gene frequencies and combinations in the population. These changes lead to alterations in phenotypic characteristics and, hence, evolution.

4.7.2 Evolution of Species

The effects of evolution are seen in the changes that occur in a given species. Minor changes, or clines, are gradual variations that are caused by geographic, or environmental, variations, such as altitude or latitude. Subspecies, or races, are formed when an abrupt environmental change is associated with an abrupt change in characteristics. Finally, some evolutionary changes are so great that they result in a new species. This process is known as speciation.

A species is a set of genetically distinct organisms that share a gene pool (i.e., gene flow is possible between them) and are reproductively isolated from all other groups. The first step in speciation is usually geographic isolation of two populations of the same species. A barrier (e.g., river, canyon, mountain) prevents the populations from coming together to mate. The separate populations differ for several reasons: (1) the gene frequencies usually differ; (2) each population experiences different mutations; (3) the different environments exert different selection pressures; and (4) if small, genetic drift can cause changes. The second step in speciation is reproductive isolation. The populations differ so that gene flow between them is no longer possible, even if they are brought together. This change occurs through intrinsic reproductive isolating mechanisms that act at all of the steps of reproduction These mechanisms are: (1) ecogeographic isolation (i.e., the organisms can no longer survive in each other's environment); (2) habitat isolation (i.e., the organisms occupy different habitats within the same range); (3) seasonal isolation (i.e., the breeding periods occur at different times); (4) behavioral isolation (i.e., mating rituals differ); (5) mechanical isolation (i.e., nonfitting of genitals); (6) gametic isolation (i.e., fertilization cannot occur); (7) hybrid inviability (i.e., the offspring cannot reproduce); and (8) developmental isolation (i.e., fertilization occurs, but the embryo dies). By geographic isolation followed by reproductive isolation, the mechanisms of evolution lead to the creation of new species.

General patterns of evolution are divergent (i.e., moving from one species to a different species, the typical pattern), convergent (i.e., moving from separate to common species), or parallel (i.e., two species

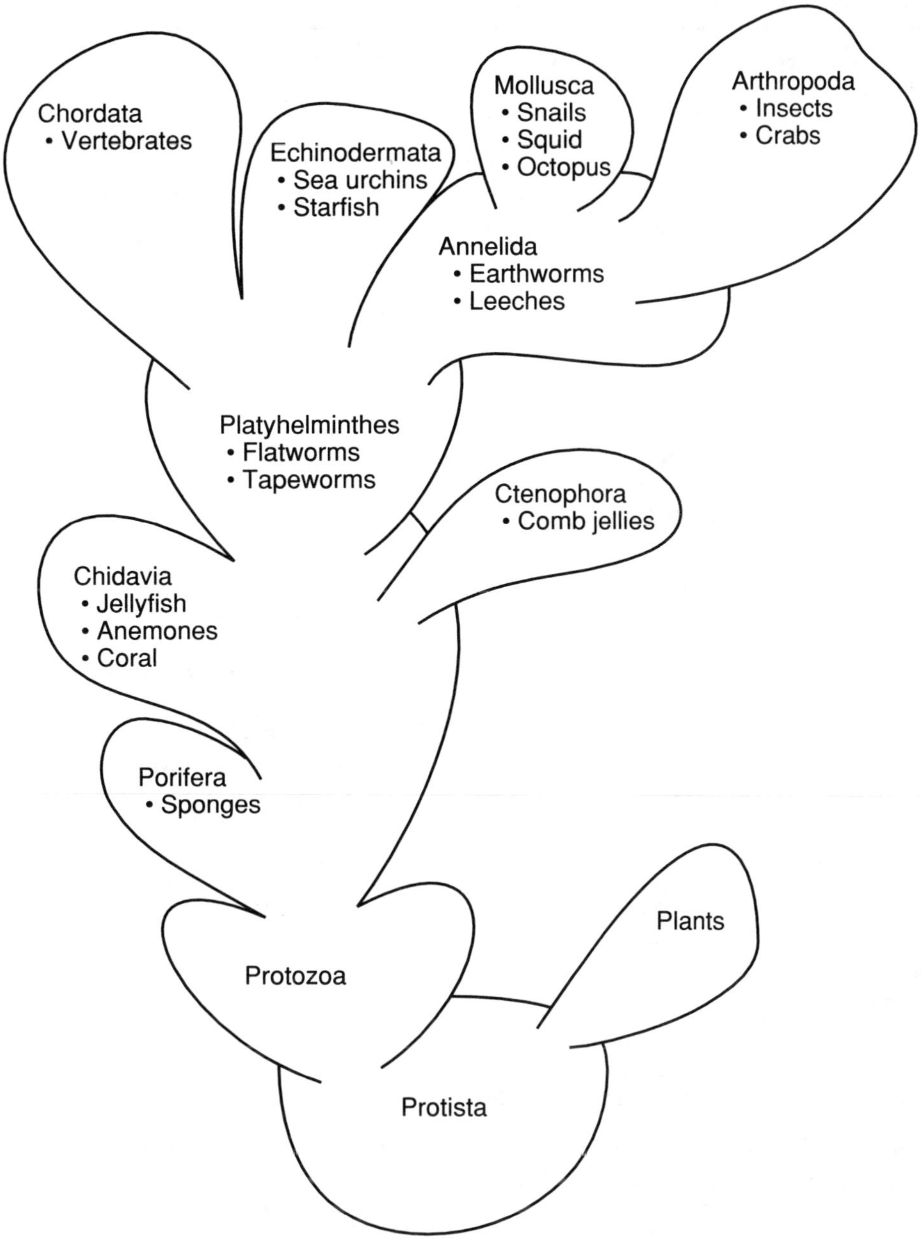

Figure 4.3. The phylogenetic tree.

resulting from one species, but evolving in parallel). Adaptive radiation is the gradual divergent differentiation of a species, usually in response to environmental variations. Homologous structures arise from a common structure, even though their functions may differ. Analogous structures have common functions, but arise from different structures. Table 4-4 shows the evolutionary timetable.

4.8 TAXONOMY

The hierarchical classification of organisms is primarily the result of work by Linnaeus. At each level, organisms are grouped on the basis of their similarities. At higher levels, the characteristics are more general. A well-known mnemonic is often used.

Kings	Kingdom
Play	Phylum

TABLE 4-4. ***Evolutionary Timetable***

Geologic Era	Period	Time (millions of years ago)	Features
Precambrian	. . .	2700	Origin of nonshelled invertebrates and eukaryotic cells
Paleozoic	Cambrian	600	Trilobites; brachipods
	Ordovician	500	First fish (jawless); age of invertebrates
	Silurian	430	First air-breathing animals; first insects; age of fish
	Devonian	410	First amphibians; sharks; sea lilies
	Carboniferous	350	First reptiles appear; age of amphibians
	Permian	275	Expansion of reptiles; decline of amphibians
Mesozoic	Triassic	225	First dinosaurs
	Jurassic	175	Age of dinosaurs; first birds
	Cretaceous	130	Primitive mammals; first modern birds; dinosaurs become extinct
Cenozoic	Tertiary	60	Rapid development of higher mammals and birds
	Quaternary	2	Age of human civilization; extinction of giant mammals

Chess	Class
On	Order
Fine	Family
Grain	Genus
Sand	Species

All organisms have a two-component Latin name. The first is the genus name, which is capitalized, and the second is the species name, which is not capitalized. The names of the genus and species are italicized.

For example:

Yucca is commonly called soaptree, palmilla, and Spanish bayonet. In scientific terminology, it belongs to each of the following categories:

Subkingdom	Embryophyta
Phylum	Tracheophyta
Subphylum	Pteropsida
Class	Angiospermae
Subclass	Monocotyledonae
Order	Liliales
Family	Liliaceae
Genus	*Yucca*
Species	*elata*

For a long time, all organisms were classified as either animals or plants. However, to classify certain microorganisms, biologists now use the following five-kingdom system:

Kingdom Protista
Organisms are algae or protozoa. Protozoa are classified into four phyla based on their method of movement: Paramecium, Flagellate, Amoeba, and Malaria Plasmodium. Algae are classified into eight phyla.

Kingdom Fungi
Fungi do not contain chlorophyll. Common examples are molds, mildews, yeasts, and mushrooms. They are subclassified as threadlike fungi, sac fungi, club fungi, and imperfect fungi.

Kingdom Monera
Organisms include bacteria and blue-green bacteria. The classification is based on the shape, type of nutrition, oxygen requirements, and other characteristics of these organisms.

Kingdom Plantae
The two major phyla in the plant kingdom are nonvascular and vascular plants. Nonvascular plants belong to the phylum Bryophyta and include mosses and liverworts. Vascular plants belong to the phylum Tracheophyta and include ferns and seed plants. Seed plants are grouped as angiosperms and gymnosperms. Angiosperms produce fruit to cover their seeds. Gymnosperms have uncovered seeds (e.g., pines, spruces, cedars).

Kingdom Animalia

Invertebrates include eight phyla: Platyhelminthes (e.g., blood flukes, tapeworms), Porifera (e.g., sponges), Coelenterata (e.g., jellyfish, anemones, corals), Nematoda (e.g., roundworms, *Trichinella*), Annelida (e.g., earthworms, leeches), Mollusca (e.g., clams, octopuses, squids), Echinodermata (e.g., sand dollars, sea urchins), and Arthropoda (e.g., crabs, spiders, insects).

Vertebrates include eight classes: Agnatha (i.e., jawless fish), Placodermi (i.e., placoderms), Chondrichthyes (i.e., cartilaginous fish), Acanthodii (i.e., acanthodians), Amphibia (i.e., amphibians), Reptilia (i.e., reptiles), Aves (i.e., birds), and Mammalia (i.e., mammals).

The class Agnatha contains subclasses Ostracodermi (i.e., ostracoderms) and Cyclostomata (e.g., lampreys, hagfish). The class Chondrichthyes includes subclasses Elasmobranchii (e.g., sharks, rays) and Holocephali (e.g., chimeras, ratfish). The class Amphibia contains subclasses Labyrinthodontia (i.e., extinct hard-skinned amphibians) and Lissamphibia (e.g., salamanders, frogs). The class Reptilia includes subclasses Anapsida (e.g., turtles, stem reptiles), Euryapsida (e.g., ichthyosaurs), Synapsida (i.e., mammal-like reptiles), Lepidosauria (e.g., tautaras, lizards, snakes), and Archosauria (e.g., alligators, crocodiles).

The class Aves includes subclasses Archaeornithes (i.e., ancestral birds) and Neornithes (i.e., modern birds). The class Mammalia contains subclasses Prototheria (e.g., platypuses) and Theria (i.e., live-bearing mammals).

4.9 SAMPLE TEST

Select the one best answer for each question.

1. Autotrophic organisms:
- **A.** must obtain all organic molecules from their environment.
- **B.** are capable of nitrogen fixation.
- **C.** belong to the kingdom Plantae.
- **D.** can synthesize organic molecules from inorganic raw materials.

2. Which substance is NOT an electron carrier in cellular energy production?
- **A.** Adenosine triphosphate
- **B.** NAD^+
- **C.** FAD
- **D.** Ubiquinone

3. The conversion of the code sequence in DNA to a code sequence in mRNA is:
- **A.** secretion.
- **B.** transcription.
- **C.** translation.
- **D.** condensation.

4. Which substance is NOT ordinarily found in cell membranes?
- **A.** Globular proteins
- **B.** Phospholipids
- **C.** DNA
- **D.** All of the above

5. The main difference in the outcome of mitosis versus meiosis is:
   A. meiosis produces identical daughter cells, and mitosis produces different daughter cells.
   B. mitosis occurs only in vertebrates.
   C. meiosis produces somatic cells.
   D. meiosis results in haploid cells, and mitosis results in diploid cells when the parents are diploid.

6. Which substance probably would NOT cross a membrane by simple diffusion?
   A. Ethanol
   B. Chloride ion
   C. Glucose
   D. Water

7. The function of molecular oxygen in cellular respiration is to:
   A. oxidize the fuel molecule.
   B. combine with carbon to form carbon dioxide.
   C. generate adenosine triphosphate.
   D. serve as a final hydrogen acceptor.

8. All of the following hormones are secreted by the anterior pituitary gland EXCEPT:
   A. oxytocin.
   B. prolactin.
   C. luteinizing hormone.
   D. thyroid-stimulating hormone.

9. Factors important in the differentiation of cells include:
   A. cytoplasmic composition and distribution of constituents.
   B. characteristics of neighboring cells.
   C. physical environmental agents.
   D. all of the above.

10. The control center of respiration is in the:
    A. cerebrum.
    B. cerebellum.
    C. diaphragm.
    D. medulla.

11. The secretion of pepsinogen is stimulated by:
    A. enterogastrone.
    B. secretin.
    C. gastrin.
    D. enterokinase.

12. The doctrine that living things arise from other living things is:
    A. biogenesis.
    B. cellularity.
    C. development.
    D. heredity.

13. The tropic level with the largest biomass in a natural ecosystem is formed by:
    A. decomposers.
    B. primary consumers.
    C. producers.
    D. secondary consumers.

14. Below are the structures of a typical fatty acid and a hexose.

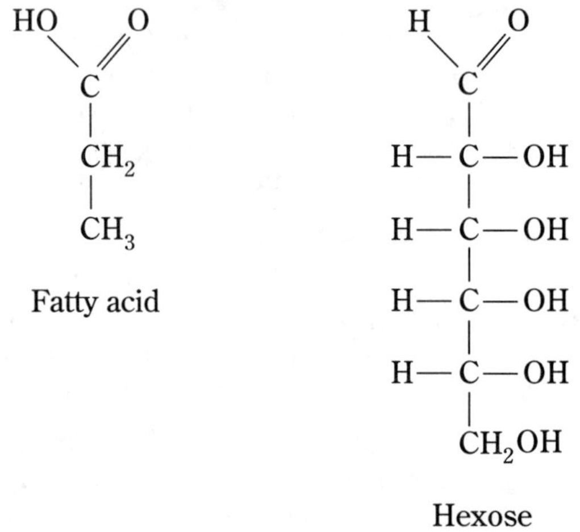

If both were degraded bioenergetically to CO_2 and H_2O, equal weights of fatty acid would yield:
    A. more energy because it is more reduced than hexose.
    B. less energy because it is more reduced than hexose.
    C. less energy because it is more oxidized than hexose.
    D. more energy because it is more oxidized than hexose.

15. Sex-linked traits:
    A. are found more in females than in males.
    B. are found on the X and Y chromosomes.
    C. allow recessive alleles to be expressed when one such allele is present in the male.
    D. occur in males who have a 50% chance of receiving sex-linked alleles from the father.

16. Because enzymes are proteins, they are affected by the same factors that affect proteins. An enzyme functions under a

certain set of conditions. Which of the following conditions would be most conducive to the normal function of a human cellular enzyme?
A. Temperature of 25°C
B. Temperature of 37°C
C. pH of 1.0
D. pH of 7.0

17. Fungi:
A. are prokaryotes.
B. may be unicellular.
C. contain chlorophyll.
D. are not saprophytic.

18. What probably limits the size a cell may attain?
A. Surface area
B. Cell volume
C. Balance of surface area and volume
D. Osmotic pressure

19. Which type of muscle is a syncytium?
A. Skeletal
B. Cardiac
C. Smooth
D. All of the above

20. Lymph nodes:
A. are found in veins.
B. contain lymphocytes only.
C. may contain lymphocytes and macrophages.
D. are not directly important in protecting the body against disease.

21. Which statement concerning bile salts is INCORRECT?
A. They break down, or digest, lipids.
B. They emulsify and solubilize lipids.
C. They are synthesized in the liver.
D. They are stored in the gallbladder.

22. During inspiration of air into the lungs:
A. the chest cavity has a positive pressure.
B. the diaphragm moves upward.
C. the diaphragm contracts.
D. all of the above.

23. All of the following are part of the human kidney EXCEPT the:
A. glomerulus.
B. loop of Henle.
C. malpighian tubules.
D. collecting ducts.

24. All of the following are specifically associated with a neuron EXCEPT:
A. lack of a nucleus.
B. Nissl bodies.
C. dendrite.
D. axon.

25. Which of the following pairs is NOT a hormone and related disease or abnormal process?
A. growth hormone: acromegaly
B. insulin: diabetes mellitus
C. cortisol: abnormal calcium/phosphate metabolism
D. thyroxin: altered metabolic rate

26. One of the scientists who helped to disprove spontaneous generation was:
A. Leeuwenhock.
B. Redi.
C. Einstein.
D. Miller.

27. According to Linnaeus, the five major categories to which most living things belong are the Animalia, Plantae, Protista, Fungi, and Monera:
A. kingdoms.
B. species.
C. classes.
D. grouped phyla.

28. Diseases such as blights, wilts, and galls are caused by:
A. fungi.
B. viroids.
C. bacteria.
D. virions.

29. NAD^+ is a noncovalently bound coenzyme for the enzyme α-glycerol-phosphate dehydrogenase. NAD^+ picks up an H^{-1} (hydride) and becomes NADH; the enzyme is not affected by the reaction. The activation energy is decreased by the system.
A. This process is not true catalysis because the NAD^+ is changed in the reaction.
B. This process is true catalysis because the NAD^+ is not covalently bound to the enzyme.
C. This process is true catalysis because the activation energy of the reaction is decreased by the enzyme, which is unchanged in the reaction.
D. This process is true catalysis because the activation energy of the reaction is increased by the enzyme, which is unchanged in the reaction.

30. What type of neuron allows for one-way conduction of impulses in the nervous system?
- **A.** Axons
- **B.** Dendrites
- **C.** Synapses
- **D.** Somas

31. Melatonin is produced by the:
- **A.** pineal gland.
- **B.** skin.
- **C.** liver.
- **D.** pituitary gland.

32. Lymph moves toward the veins as a result of:
- **A.** tissue pressure.
- **B.** muscle action.
- **C.** pumping action of the heart.
- **D.** gravity.

33. Iron is absorbed in the:
- **A.** stomach.
- **B.** jejunum.
- **C.** ileum.
- **D.** duodenum.

34. The autonomic nervous system includes:
- **A.** the sympathetic system.
- **B.** the parasympathetic system.
- **C.** the somatic nervous system.
- **D.** both A and B.

35. Which type of tissue secretes hormones?
- **A.** Pancreas
- **B.** Ovaries
- **C.** Gastrointestinal tract
- **D.** All of the above

36. Filtration of blood occurs in which structure in the kidney?
- **A.** Loop of Henle
- **B.** Collecting ducts
- **C.** Tubules
- **D.** Glomerulus

37. Heterotrophs are organisms that:
- **A.** feed on inorganic compounds.
- **B.** feed on organic molecules.
- **C.** use anaerobic fermentation of nitric acid.
- **D.** use aerobic fermentation of nitric acid.

38. Mollusks are most closely related to:
- **A.** roundworms.
- **B.** coelenterates.
- **C.** annelids.
- **D.** flatworms.

39. Which of the following is a viral disease?
- **A.** Anthrax
- **B.** Syphilis
- **C.** Polio
- **D.** Tuberculosis

40. All of the following are associated with reproductive functions in fungi EXCEPT:
- **A.** conidia.
- **B.** sporangium.
- **C.** basidium.
- **D.** mesenchymal.

41. The A-band of striated muscle represents:
- **A.** myosin only.
- **B.** actin only.
- **C.** both A and B.
- **D.** calcium channels.

42. An enlarged lymph node may mean:
- **A.** infection.
- **B.** inflammation.
- **C.** metastasis.
- **D.** all of the above.

43. The enzyme responsible for the activation of trypsinogen in the intestine is:
- **A.** pepsin.
- **B.** enterokinase.
- **C.** chymotrypsin.
- **D.** carboxypeptidase.

44. What structures are used to prevent the bronchi from collapsing?
- **A.** Cartilage rings
- **B.** Bony rings
- **C.** Fibrous tissue
- **D.** All of the above

45. Which statement about the antidiuretic hormone is correct?
- **A.** It is synthesized in the posterior pituitary gland.
- **B.** It acts on the collecting duct of the kidney.
- **C.** It is also known as aldosterone.
- **D.** All of the above.

46. Reabsorption of most of the water, glucose, amino acids, sodium, and other nutrients occurs at the:
- **A.** loop of Henle.
- **B.** collecting duct.
- **C.** proximal convoluted tubule.
- **D.** distal convoluted tubule.

47. Myelin sheaths are found:
   A. surrounding tendons.
   B. covering the brain.
   C. covering muscles.
   D. around axons of neurons.

48. All of the following hormones are correctly paired with one of their major functions EXCEPT:
   A. thyroxin: increases metabolic rate.
   B. glucocorticoids: increase blood sugar levels.
   C. aldosterone: role in the fight or flight sympathetic response.
   D. parathyroid hormone: regulates calcium/phosphorous metabolism.

49. Ethyl alcohol is converted into lactic acid during the process of:
   A. aerobic respiration.
   B. excretion.
   C. coenzyme production.
   D. anaerobic respiration.

50. All of the following are vertebrates EXCEPT the:
   A. sponge.
   B. cow.
   C. shark.
   D. eagle.

51. Which of the following is a fungal disease?
   A. Influenza
   B. Pneumonia
   C. Both A and B
   D. Ringworm

52. What is the correct sequence of filtered blood through the kidney?
   A. Bowman's capsule, glomerulus, tubules, collecting ducts
   B. Glomerulus, Bowman's capsule, collecting ducts, tubules
   C. Bowman's capsule, collecting ducts, glomerulus, tubules
   D. Glomerulus, Bowman's capsule, tubules, collecting ducts

53. In the fungus:
   A. the haploid phase tends to dominate.
   B. the diploid phase tends to dominate.
   C. only asexual reproduction occurs.
   D. spores are sexual structures only.

54. Which structure does NOT play a part in the motion of cells?
   A. Microvilli
   B. Cilia
   C. Flagella
   D. Pseudopods

55. The products of triglyceride hydrolysis by lipases in the intestine may include:
   A. fatty acids.
   B. monoglycerides.
   C. diglycerides.
   D. all of the above.

56. All of the following may cause an increase in respiratory rate EXCEPT:
   A. increased hydrogen ion concentration.
   B. increased carbon dioxide tension.
   C. increased oxygen tension.
   D. decreased oxygen tension.

57. The acidity of plasma is caused by:
   A. oxidation of glucose and fat.
   B. metabolism of sulfur-containing amino acids.
   C. production of CO_2 by the tissues.
   D. all of the above.

58. Which ion determines the resting potential of a nerve cell?
   A. Sodium
   B. Potassium
   C. Calcium
   D. Both A and B

59. All of the following are arthropods EXCEPT:
   A. jumping spiders.
   B. dragonflies.
   C. snails.
   D. soft-shell crabs.

60. Infectious diseases:
   A. are inherited.
   B. are caused by pathogens.
   C. are caused by rickettsiae.
   D. are never easy to cure.

61. All of the following substances are filtered at the glomerulus EXCEPT:
   A. platelets.
   B. proteins.
   C. glucose.
   D. sodium.

62. Secretion of bicarbonate and fluid from the pancreas is stimulated by:
   A. secretin.
   B. cholecystokinin.
   C. enterokinase.
   D. gastrin.

63. All of the following are functions of the medulla EXCEPT:
   A. voluntary movements.
   B. respiratory regulation.
   C. circulatory regulation.
   D. the cough reflex.

64. In the hypothalamic-pituitary-adrenal axis, if the long feedback loop holds:
   A. corticotropin inhibits the production of corticotropin-releasing factor by the hypothalamus.
   B. cortisol inhibits the production of corticotropin by the pituitary.
   C. cortisol inhibits the corticotropin-releasing factor produced by the hypothalamus.
   D. all of the above.

65. Urea:
   A. is a product of protein metabolism.
   B. contains only carbon, hydrogen, and oxygen.
   C. is excreted by the lungs.
   D. all of the above.

66. During the early phase of the action potential:
   A. only Na^+ moves.
   B. only K^+ moves.
   C. only Ca^{++} moves.
   D. Na^+ moves into the cell, and K^+ moves out.

67. All of the following are types of bacteria EXCEPT:
   A. metatrophic.
   B. parasitic.
   C. autotrophic.
   D. tsutsugamushi.

68. Which of the following is the correct sequence of the meninges from outside inward?
   A. Arachnoid, dural, pial
   B. Dural, pial, arachnoid
   C. Pial, arachnoid, dural
   D. Dural, arachnoid, pial

69. A vaccine primarily results in:
   A. passive immunity.
   B. active immunity.
   C. production of antibodies.
   D. both B and C.

70. An organism makes and gives off useful chemical compounds. It is carrying on the life process of:
   A. secretion.
   B. photosynthesis.
   C. catalysis.
   D. cellular respiration.

71. Calcitonin:
   A. decreases the serum calcium level.
   B. has no effect on the serum calcium level.
   C. is produced in the parathyroid gland.
   D. is a steroid.

72. All of the following are families in the suborder Eubacteriineae EXCEPT:
   A. Rhizobiaceae.
   B. Chlamydobacteriales.
   C. Achromobacteriaceae.
   D. Parvobacteriaceae.

73. Which statement about the parasympathetic system is INCORRECT?
   A. Ganglia are located near the end organ.
   B. The parasympathetic system increases the heart rate.
   C. The parasympathetic system maintains homeostasis.
   D. The parasympathetic system increases digestive action.

74. All of the following are infections EXCEPT:
   A. typhoid.
   B. botulism.
   C. common flu.
   D. strep throat.

75. Which statement about gene mapping is correct?
   A. Only three-factor crosses may be used to sequence gene loci.
   B. The recombination frequencies are always representative of the recombination rates of the gene loci.
   C. The recombination frequency is equal to the map units.
   D. Viral DNA is used for gene mapping.

76. Which statement about cytoplasmic inheritance is correct?
   A. Cytoplasmic interitance does not follow mendelian laws.
   B. The maternal cytoplasm plays the dominant role.
   C. Replication of mitochondria is an example.
   D. All of the above.

77. Homozygous refers to:
A. similar types of chromosomes.
B. having similar functions on an evolutionary basis.
C. particles in a solution that are not separable microscopically.
D. identical alleles for a given trait.

78. Which statement about X and Y chromosomes is INCORRECT?
A. X is larger than Y.
B. They are not homologous.
C. XY is a genotypic male.
D. Traits that appear on X, but not on Y, are called sex-linked traits.

79. Which statement is INCORRECT?
A. Genotype is the set of alleles for a given trait in an individual.
B. Phenotype is the expression of the genotype.
C. A given genotype gives rise to different phenotypes.
D. Different genotypes may give rise to the same phenotype.

80. Which animal is NOT affected by cold temperatures and other seasonal changes?
A. Rabbit
B. Robin
C. Weasel
D. Groundhog

81. Which animal has the longest average life span?
A. Hippopotamus
B. Giraffe
C. Human
D. Parrot

82. Which animal can live underwater without going to the surface?
A. Penguin
B. Dolphin
C. Shark
D. Sperm whale

83. Fungi and plants are classified into separate kingdoms based on the presence or absence of chloroplasts, mode of nutrition, and:
A. presence or absence of chloroplasts.
B. motility (9+2 cilia).
C. material in the cell wall.
D. presence of nuclear membrane.

84. If one species freely exchanged genes, or interbred, with another, then each species would:
A. lose its unique characteristics.
B. produce more adaptive offspring.
C. ultimately become extinct.
D. none of the above.

85. Which is a correct descending order (largest to smallest group) of taxa?
A. Division, phylum, order, family
B. Class, family, order, genus
C. Family, order, genus, species
D. Division, order, family, genus

86. Organisms that show many homologous structures:
A. are unrelated.
B. have different phylogenetic histories.
C. have a common evolutionary origin.
D. have adapted to the same conditions.

87. The evolutionary history of a group or species is known as:
A. homology.
B. otogeny.
C. taxonomy.
D. phylogeny.

88. Enzymes, or proteins that regulate chemical reactions in living systems, are always:
A. fibrous proteins.
B. complex carbohydrates.
C. globular proteins.
D. necessary.

89. Proteins whose secondary structure consists largely of a helical or pleated-sheet form are known as:
A. fibrous proteins.
B. globular proteins.
C. enzymes.
D. polypeptides.

90. The fats, or lipids, that are most important for structural purposes are:
A. nonpolar.
B. mostly steroids.
C. neutral fats.
D. phospholipids.

91. When phospholipids associate with water, the hydrophobic ____________ protrudes away from the water.
A. phosphate
B. fatty acid

C. nitrogenous base
D. glycerol

92. If a 2.5-g hummingbird stores 2.0 g fat, it has enough energy to fly from Florida to Yucatan. How much glycogen would it need to store to make the same flight?
A. 5 g
B. 4 g
C. 3 g
D. 2 g

93. Cellulose, the most common organic molecule in the biosphere, makes up __________% of young cell walls.
A. 27
B. 40
C. 48
D. 32

94. Metabolically active cells are small because they:
A. require less surface area in relation to their volume.
B. must be specialized for many different functions.
C. require large surface areas for efficient membrane exchange.
D. must withstand the force of gravity.

95. Smooth endoplasmic reticulum:
A. produces cytoplasmic proteins.
B. produces lipids, such as steroids.
C. detoxifies drugs, such as phenobarbital.
D. provides a molecular passage to the Golgi bodies.

96. The pectins and other polysaccharides that cement adjacent plant cells together are known as:
A. cell walls.
B. cell membranes.
C. middle lamellae.
D. cellulose.

97. Integral membrane proteins are primarily concerned with:
A. catalyzing metabolic reactions.
B. intercellular recognition.
C. transporting polar molecules.
D. reducing membrane permeability.

98. If water and blood flowed in the same direction through the gills of a fish, the:
A. countercurrent effect would be improved.
B. efficiency of oxygen uptake would decrease.
C. efficiency of oxygen uptake would increase.
D. fish could pump less water over its gills without decreasing the amount of oxygen taken in.

99. The total of chemical reactions involved in molecular synthesis is known as:
A. metabolism.
B. anabolism.
C. catabolism.
D. metabolic pathways.

100. The plant pigment directly involved in transforming light energy to chemical energy is:
A. beta carotene.
B. chlorophyll a.
C. chlorophyll b.
D. xanthophyll.

101. In the dark reactions of photosynthesis:
A. light energy is used to form adenosine triphosphate from adenosine diphosphate.
B. electron carrier molecules are reduced.
C. CO_2 is reduced to form a simple sugar.
D. a simple sugar is oxidized to form CO_2.

102. To produce a six-carbon sugar such as glucose, how many revolutions of the Calvin cycle are required?
A. 1
B. 3
C. 6
D. 9

103. Which of the following can operate independently?
A. Photosystem I
B. Photosystem II
C. Both
D. Neither

104. What drives the diffusion of CO_2 in leaves?
A. Water evaporation
B. The chemiosmotic gradient
C. A concentration gradient of CO_2
D. Ambient air flow

4.10 ANSWER KEY

1. **D.** [Topic: diversity of life]
2. **A.** [Topic: cell and molecular biology]
3. **B.** [Topic: cell and molecular biology]
4. **C.** [Topic: cell and molecular biology]
5. **D.** [Topic: cell and molecular biology]
6. **C.** [Topic: cell and molecular biology]
7. **D.** [Topic: cell and molecular biology]
8. **A.** [Topic: vertebrate anatomy and physiology]
9. **D.** [Topic: developmental biology]
10. **D.** [Topic: vertebrate anatomy and physiology]
11. **C.** [Topic: vertebrate anatomy and physiology]
12. **A.** [Topic: cellular and molecular biology and origin of life]
13. **C.** [Topic: evolution, ecology, and behavior]
14. **A.** [Topic: cellular and molecular biology]
15. **C.** [Topic: genetics]
16. **B.** [Topic: enzymology]
17. **B.** [Topic: organelle structure and function]
18. **C.** [Topic: organelle structure and function]
19. **D.** [Topic: structure and function of the muscular system]
20. **C.** [Topic: structure and function of the immunologic system]
21. **A.** [Topic: structure and function of the digestive system]
22. **C.** [Topic: structure and function of the respiratory system]
23. **C.** [Topic: structure and function of the urinary system]
24. **A.** [Topic: structure and function of the nervous system]
25. **C.** [Topic: structure and function of the endocrine system]
26. **B.** [Topic: origin of life]
27. **A.** [Topic: biologic organization and relation of major taxa]
28. **C.** [Topic: structure and function of the immunologic system]
29. **C.** [Topic: cell metabolism]
30. **C.** [Topic: structure and function of the nervous system]
31. **A.** [Topic: structure and function of the endocrine system]
32. **B.** [Topic: structure and function of the immunologic system]
33. **D.** [Topic: structure and function of the digestive system]
34. **D.** [Topic: structure and function of the nervous system]
35. **D.** [Topic: structure and function of the endocrine system]
36. **D.** [Topic: structure and function of the urinary system]
37. **B.** [Topic: structure and function of the immunologic system]
38. **C.** [Topic: relation of the major taxonomic groups]
39. **C.** [Topic: structure and function of the immunologic system]
40. **D.** [Topic: major differences between eukaryotic and prokaryotic cells]
41. **C.** [Topic: structure and function of the muscular system]
42. **D.** [Topic: structure and function of the immunologic system]
43. **B.** [Topic: structure and function of the digestive system]
44. **A.** [Topic: structure and function of the respiratory system]
45. **B.** [Topic: structure and function of the endocrine system]
46. **C.** [Topic: structure and function of the urinary system]
47. **D.** [Topic: structure and function of the nervous system]
48. **C.** [Topic: structure and function of the endocrine system]
49. **D.** [Topic: cell metabolism, photosynthesis]
50. **A.** [Topic: biologic organization of chordates]
51. **D.** [Topic: immunology, basic pathology]
52. **D.** [Topic: structure and function of the renal system]
53. **A.** [Topic: reproduction in eukaryotic cells]
54. **A.** [Topic: characteristics of prokaryotic and eukaryotic cells]
55. **D.** [Topic: structure and function of the digestive system]
56. **C.** [Topic: structure and function of the respiratory system]
57. **D.** [Topic: structure and function of the circulatory system]
58. **D.** [Topic: structure and function of the nervous system]
59. **C.** [Topic: biologic classification]
60. **B.** [Topic: infectious diseases]
61. **A.** [Topic: structure and function of the renal system]

62. **A.** [Topic: structure and function of endocrine glands]
63. **A.** [Topic: structure and function of the nervous system]
64. **C.** [Topic: structure and function of the nervous and endocrine system]
65. **A.** [Topic: structure and function of the urinary system]
66. **A.** [Topic: modes of cellular transport]
67. **D.** [Topic: bacteria types and origins]
68. **D.** [Topic: structure and function of the nervous system]
69. **D.** [Topic: structure and function of the immune system]
70. **A.** [Topic: cellular metabolism]
71. **A.** [Topic: structure and function of the endocrine system]
72. **B.** [Topic: bacterial classification]
73. **B.** [Topic: structure and function of the parasympathetic system]
74. **B.** [Topic: infectious diseases]
75. **D.** [Topic: genetics]
76. **D.** [Topic: eukaryotic cells]
77. **D.** [Topic: genetics]
78. **B.** [Topic: genetics]
79. **C.** [Topic: genetics]
80. **A.** [Topic: animal biology, skin systems]
81. **C.** [Topic: animal biology]
82. **C.** [Topic: animal biology]
83. **C.** [Topic: plant biology]
84. **A.** [Topic: genetics and speciation]
85. **D.** [Topic: taxonomy]
86. **C.** [Topic: homology]
87. **D.** [Topic: taxonomy]
88. **C.** [Topic: enzymes, proteins]
89. **A.** [Topic: protein structure]
90. **D.** [Topic: fats, or lipids]
91. **B.** [Topic: fatty acids]
92. **A.** [Topic: glycolysis]
93. **B.** [Topic: cellulose, plant cell structure]
94. **C.** [Topic: cell characteristics]
95. **D.** [Topic: cell structure and function]
96. **C.** [Topic: plant cells]
97. **B.** [Topic: cell membrane]
98. **B.** [Topic: transport in fish gills]
99. **B.** [Topic: cellular metabolism]
100. **B.** [Topic: photosynthesis]
101. **C.** [Topic: photosynthesis]
102. **C.** [Topic: glucose, Calvin cycle]
103. **A.** [Topic: photosystems]
104. **C.** [Topic: photosynthesis, diffusion in plants]

4.11 REFERENCES

Hoar WS: *General and Comparative Physiology*, 3rd ed. Englewood Cliffs, NJ, Prentice-Hall, 1983.

Jackson JD, Taylor JB: *Study Guide for Starr's Biology Concepts and Applications*. Belmont, CA, Wadsworth, 1991.

Kaufman B, et al. *Practical Botany*. Reston, VA, Reston, 1983.

Kaufman PB, et al. *Plants: Their Biology and Importance*. New York: Harper & Row, 1989.

Noggle GR, Fritz GJ: *Introductory Plant Physiology*, 2nd ed. Englewood Cliffs, NJ, Prentice-Hall,1983.

Rayle DL,Wedberg HL: *Botany: A Human Concern*, 2nd ed. Philadelphia,WB Saunders, 1980.

Schmidt-Nielsen K: *Animal Physiology*, 3rd ed. Engelwood Cliffs, NJ, Prentice-Hall, 1970.

Schmidt-Nielsen K: *Animal Physiology: Adaptations and Environment*, 4th ed., New York, Cambridge University Press, 1990.

Starr C: *Biology: Concepts and Applications*. Belmont, CA, Wadsworth, 1991.

Ville CA, Solomon EP, Davis WP: *Biology*, 2nd ed. Philadelphia, WB Saunders, 1985.

Wilkins M: *Plantwatching: How Plants Remember, Tell Time, Form Partnerships & More*. New York, Facts on File, 1988.

5

CHAPTER

Developing Quantitative Reasoning Skills for the VETs

5.0 QUANTITATIVE REASONING AND THE VETs

The quantitative ability section of the VETs includes arithmetic, algebra, geometry, trigonometry, and basic statistics. This section tests the ability to reason with numbers, manipulate numerical relations, and apply information in situations involving numbers. Speed and accuracy are necessary for proficiency on this section of the VETs. Because no aids (e.g., mathematical tables, rulers, calculators) are allowed inside the testing center, you should prepare for the VETs without them.

The quantitative ability sections of the Veterinary College Admission Test (VCAT) and Graduate Record Examination (GRE) General Test have two types of questions: mathematical operations and applied mathematics problems. Mathematical operations questions test knowledge of arithmetic, algebra, geometry, and trigonometry. Applied mathematics problems are practical word problems. The Physical and Biological Sciences Subtests of the Medical College Admission Test (MCAT) evaluate knowledge of mathematical concepts. Table 5-1 compares the quantitative ability sections of the VCAT, GRE, and MCAT. These tests do not require knowledge of differential or integral calculus.

5.1 QUANTITATIVE APPROXIMATION

The ability to approximate, estimate, and round off numbers in mathematical calculations is useful for the VETs. However, these skills must be used carefully because estimating may not provide enough information to allow differentiation between similar answer choices. While preparing for the VETs, compare your estimated answers with actual answers. Experience and practice will improve your performance.

Rounding is expressing a number in fewer digits. Rounding allows rapid mental calcuation of a problem. Numbers may be rounded down, rounded up, or rounded to the nearest specified unit (e.g., hundred).

When a number is rounded down, if the first digit to be dropped is less than 5, the last retained digit is unchanged (e.g., 3.1416 rounded to two decimal places is 3.14). When a number is rounded up, if

TABLE 5-1. ***Comparison of the VCAT, GRE, and MCAT Quantitative Ability Sections***

VCAT	GRE	MCAT
Arithmetic concepts Discrete mathematics Ratio, proportion, percentage, rate Powers and logarithms Algebra and analytic geometry Euclidean geometry and trigonometry	Arithmetic Mathematical operations, percentages, averages, factors, counting probability Algebra Equations, factors, word problems Geometry Parallel lines, circles, inscribed and central angles, triangles, rectangles, polygons, special triangles Quantitative comparison problems Data interpretation problems	Arithmetic calculations Ratio, proportion, percentages, square roots Algebra Exponentials, logarithms, quadratic and simultaneous equations, data, functions Basic trigonometric and inverse trigonometric functions Conversion factors between British and metric units Algebra of physical units Experimental error effect of propagation of error, estimations Mathematical probability calculations for an event Arithmetic mean, range, statistical association, correlation Vector algebra

the first digit to be dropped is 5 or greater, then the last retained digit is increased by 1 (e.g., 0.4536 rounded to three decimal places is 0.454).

Numbers may be rounded to the nearest ten, hundred, thousand, and so on (e.g., 246 rounded to the nearest ten is 250; 246 rounded to the nearest hundred is 200). Sums are estimated by rounding to the nearest convenient unit.

For example:
$789 + 42 = 831$
$790 + 40 = 830$

or

$428 + 583 = 1011$
$400 + 600 = 1000$

Numbers can be added or multiplied by simplifying them, or rewriting each number as a sum or difference of equivalent numbers (e.g., $58 = 50 + 8$ and $66 = 60 + 6$).

For example:

$$\begin{aligned} 789 + 42 &= (700 + 89) + (40 + 2) \\ &= (700 + 40) + (89 + 2) \\ &= (740 + 80) + 9 + 2 \\ &= 820 + 11 = 831 \end{aligned}$$

or

$$\frac{89}{58} \approx \frac{90}{60} \approx 1.50$$

$$\frac{89}{58} = 1.53$$

Example: Using the form:

$$(a + b)(a + b) = a^2 + 2ab + b^2$$

$$\begin{aligned} 58 \times 66 &= (50 + 8)(60 + 6) \\ &= 3000 + 300 + 480 + 48 \\ &= 3000 + 300 + 400 + 80 + 40 + 8 \\ &= 3700 + 128 \\ &= 3828 \end{aligned}$$

$$\begin{aligned} 58 \times 66 &\approx 60 \times 65 \\ &\approx 3900 \end{aligned}$$

5.2 FRACTIONS AND FACTORS

A fraction is a ratio of two numbers expressed as a/b, where a is any positive or negative number and b is any positive or negative number except 0. A fraction has two parts, the numerator and the denominator. For example, in 3/7, the numerator is 3, which indicates how many of the 7 equal parts are considered. In 5/6, 6 is the denominator, which indicates the number of equal parts. Factors are associated with fractional operations and interpretations.

5.2.1 Interpreting Fractions

In a proper fraction, the numerator is less than the denominator (e.g.,1/2, 7/9, 11/13). A fraction whose numerator is greater than or equal to the denominator is known as an improper fraction (e.g., 6/6, 8/5, 10/5). A mixed number contains a whole number and a fraction (e.g., 3-1/4). Equivalent fractions have the same value, but different numerators and denominators (e.g., 2/6 and 1/3). Multiplying a numerator and denominator by the same whole number produces equal fractions (e.g., 1/2 = 3/6 because 3/3 × 1/2 = 3/6). Reciprocal fractions are two fractions whose numerators and denominators are reversed. Their product is always 1 (e.g., 3/4 and 4/3 are reciprocals because 3/4 × 4/3 = 1).

5.2.2 Determining Factors

The factors of a whole number are whole numbers that divide evenly into it. A whole number is even if it can be divided evenly by 2.

For example:
Write all of the factors of 8.
8: 1, 2, 4, 8

Two is a factor of a number if the last digit in the number is even. Three is a factor of a number if the sum of the digits is divisible by 3. Four is a factor of a number if the sum of the last two digits is divisible by 4. Five is a factor of a number if the last digit in the number is 0 or 5. Six is a factor of a number if the last digit is even and the sum of the digits is divisible by 3.

Common factors are identical factors that occur in two or more numbers.

For example:
Write all of the factors of 8 and 28.
8: 1, 2, 4, 8
28: 1, 2, 4, 7, 14, 28
The common factors are 1, 2, and 4.

The greatest common factor is the greatest of the common factors found in two or more numbers.

For example:
Write the greatest common factor of 24 and 32.
24: 1, 2, 3, 4, 6, 8, 12, 24

32: 1, 2, 4, 8, 16, 32
The common factors are 1, 2, 4, and 8.
The greatest common factor is 8.

A fraction is expressed in its simplest form when the greatest common factor of the numerator and denominator is 1. Dividing the numerator and denominator by the greatest common factor does not change the value of a fraction.

For example:
$\frac{6}{8} = \frac{6}{8} \div \frac{2}{2} = \frac{3}{4}$

6: 1, 2, 3, 6
8: 1, 2, 4, 8
The greatest common factor is 2.

Example: Reduce $6\frac{8}{12}$ to its simplest terms.

Solution: $6 + \frac{8}{12} \div \frac{4}{4} = 6 + \frac{2}{3} = 6\frac{2}{3}$

A multiple is the product of a number and a whole number. To find the multiples of a number, multiply it by each integer (e.g., 1, 2, 3).

For example:
The multiples of 3 are 3, 6, 9, 12, 15, . . .
The multiples of 4 are 4, 8, 12, 16, 20, . . .

If one number is divisible by another, it is a multiple of that number. When the multiples of two or more numbers have a value in common, this value is known as a common multiple.

For example:
Find a common multiple of 3 and 5.
3: 6, 9, 12, 15
5: 10, 15
A common multiple is 15.

The smallest common multiple of two or more numbers is known as the least common multiple.

For example:
Find the least common multiple of 2, 3, and 4.
2: 2, 4, 6, 8, 10, 12
3: 3, 6, 9, 12
4: 4, 8, 12
The least common multiple is 12.

The least common denominator of two or more fractions is the least common multiple of the denominators.

For example:
Find the least common denominator of $\frac{1}{4}$ and $\frac{1}{5}$.
4: 4, 8, 12, 16, 20, 24
5: 5, 10, 15, 20, 25
The least common denominator is 20.

5.3 MATHEMATICAL OPERATIONS WITH FRACTIONS

Mathematical operations include addition, subtraction, multiplication, and division. Special rules apply to these operations when they involve fractions.

5.3.1 Adding Fractions

To add fractions that have common denominators, add their numerators. The denominator does not change.

For example:

Add $\frac{1}{4} + \frac{5}{4} + \frac{3}{4}$

Add the numerators $1 + 5 + 3 = 9$

Retain the common denominator 4:

$\frac{1}{4} + \frac{5}{4} + \frac{3}{4} = \frac{9}{4} = 2\frac{1}{4}$

To add fractions with unlike denominators, determine the least common denominator. Express each fraction in equivalent form with the least common denominator. Then perform the addition.

For example:

Add $\frac{1}{2} + \frac{3}{4} + \frac{2}{8}$

The least common denominator is 8:

$\frac{4}{8} + \frac{6}{8} + \frac{2}{8} = \frac{12}{8} = \frac{3}{2} = 1\frac{1}{2}$

To add mixed numbers, calculate the sum of the integers separately from the sum of the fractions. Then add the sums.

For example:

Add $7\frac{1}{6}$ and $2\frac{3}{4}$

First, add the integers:

$7 + 2 = 9$

Then add the fractions:

$\frac{1}{6} + \frac{3}{4} = \frac{2}{12} + \frac{9}{12} = \frac{11}{12}$

Add the sum of the integers to the sum of the fractions:

$7\frac{1}{6} + 2\frac{3}{4} = 9\frac{2 + 9}{12} = 9\frac{11}{12}$

5.3.2 Subtracting Fractions

Before two fractions can be subtracted, they must have a common denominator.

For example:

Subtract $\frac{3}{4} - \frac{2}{3}$

The least common denominator is 12.

Subtract with the fraction in equivalent form:

$\frac{3}{4} \times \frac{3}{3} - \frac{2}{3} \times \frac{4}{4} = \frac{9}{12} - \frac{8}{12} = \frac{1}{12}$

5.3.3 Multiplying Fractions

To multiply fractions, multiply the numerators to obtain the numerator of the product. Multiply the denominators to obtain the denominator of the product.

For example:

Multiply $\frac{3}{7} \times \frac{2}{5}$

$\frac{3 \times 2}{7 \times 5} = \frac{6}{35}$

Express all of the numerators and denominators in factored form, cancel the common factors, and multiply the remaining factors. Cancellation decreases the chance of error because it permits the simplest forms of the fractions to be used.

For example:

Multiply $\frac{2}{5} \times \frac{10}{3} \times \frac{6}{7}$

$$\frac{2}{5} \times \frac{2 \times 5}{3} \times \frac{2 \times 3}{7} = \frac{8}{7} = 1\frac{1}{7}$$

Every integer a/b where $b \neq 0$, can be written as a fraction. An integer divided by 1 is equal to the integer.

For example:

Multiply $\frac{3}{5} \times 6$

$$\frac{3}{5} \times 6 = \frac{3}{5} \times \frac{6}{1} = \frac{3 \times 6}{5} = \frac{18}{5} = 3\frac{3}{5}$$

To multiply mixed numbers, convert them into improper fractions and multiply the fractions.

For example:

Multiply $1\frac{3}{4} \times 3\frac{1}{7}$

Convert $1\frac{3}{4}$ and $3\frac{1}{7}$ into improper fractions and multiply them:

$$1\frac{3}{4} = \frac{4}{4} + \frac{3}{4} = \frac{7}{4}$$

$$3\frac{1}{7} = \frac{21}{7} + \frac{1}{7} = \frac{22}{7}$$

$$\frac{7}{4} \times \frac{22}{7} = \frac{7}{2 \times 2} \times \frac{2 \times 11}{7} = \frac{11}{2} = 5\frac{1}{2}$$

5.3.4 Dividing Fractions

Division by zero is impossible, and a fraction cannot have zero as a denominator. To divide one fraction by another, invert the second fraction to produce its reciprocal, and multiply the fractions. The reciprocal of a/b is b/a, where $a \neq 0$ and $b \neq 0$ (e.g., the reciprocal of 3/2 is 2/3). To find the reciprocal of a whole number, convert the whole number to a fraction with a denominator of 1, and find the reciprocal of that fraction (e.g., the reciprocal of 5 is 1/5 because 5 = 5/1). The reciprocal of a number is 1 divided by the number. The product of a number and its reciprocal is 1.

For example:

The reciprocal of $\frac{a}{b}$ is $\frac{b}{a}$

Therefore $\frac{a}{b} \times \frac{b}{a} = \frac{ab}{ab} = 1$

Example:

Divide $\frac{3}{5} \div 7$

Solution: Rewrite 7 as $\frac{7}{1}$

Divide $\frac{3}{5} \div \frac{7}{1}$

Apply the rule for dividing fractions:

$$\frac{3}{5} \div \frac{7}{1} = \frac{3}{5} \times \frac{1}{7} = \frac{3}{35}$$

To divide mixed numbers, convert them to fractions, and apply the rule for division.

Example:

What is the value of $\frac{1}{6} - \frac{3}{8} - \frac{2}{3} + \frac{3}{4}$

A. $\frac{1}{24}$

B. $\frac{3}{24}$

C. $\frac{21}{24}$

D. $\frac{1}{24}$

The answer is **B**.

Solution: To identify the least common denominator, find the least common multiple of 6, 8, 3, and 4.

6: 6, 12, 18, 24

8: 8, 16, 24

3: 3, 6, 9, 12, 15, 18, 21, 24

4: 4, 8, 12, 16, 20, 24

The least common denominator is 24.

$$\begin{aligned}\frac{1}{6} - \frac{3}{8} - \frac{2}{3} + \frac{3}{4} &= \frac{4(1) - 3(3) - 8(2) + 6(3)}{24}\\ &= \frac{4 - 9 - 16 + 18}{24}\\ &= \frac{-5 - 16 + 18}{24}\\ &= \frac{-21 + 18}{24}\\ &= -\frac{3}{24}\end{aligned}$$

5.4 PERCENTS, DECIMALS, AND FRACTIONS

Figure 5-1 shows a conversion model for percents, decimals, and fractions.

Percent means "part of 100," or 1/100. A quantity is a certain number of 100 equal parts. The word "rate" is sometimes used to express this concept. Thus, a percent is a fraction: 25% is 25 parts of 100, or 25/100, or 1/4.

Percentage is a specified percent of a quantity. The use of percent in calculations is known as percentage operations. "Base" is the number of which a percent is calculated.

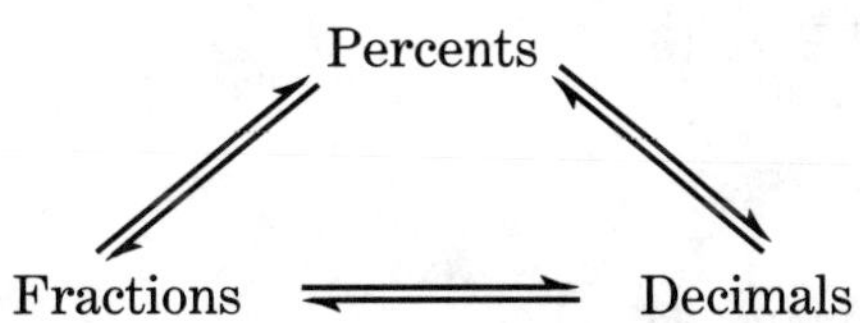

Figure 5-1 Conversion Model for Percents, Decimals, and Fractions

5.4.1 Converting Percents, Decimals, and Fractions

Percent can be expressed as a fraction with 100 as a denominator. The symbol for percent is %. Thus, 20% means 20/100, and 60% means 60/100. A percent may be reduced to a fraction, and a fraction may be expressed in decimal form. Thus, 25% is the same fractional measure as 25/100, or 1/4, or the same decimal measure as 0.25. A fractional measure is expressed as a percent by writing an equivalent fraction with 100 as its denominator. Thus, 0.24 = 24/100 = 24%, and 1.15 = 115/100 = 115%.

To convert a decimal fraction to the equivalent percent, multiply the decimal fraction by 100. The decimal point moves two places to the right. For example, to express 2.15 as a percent, multiply it by 100, or move the decimal point two places to the right (i.e., 2.15 × 100 = 215%).

To convert a fraction to a decimal, divide the numerator by the denominator. For example, express 1/4 as a decimal by dividing 4 into 1. Because 4 does not divide into 1, add a 0 and add a decimal point to the quotient to obtain 1.0/4 ≈ 0.2. Add another 0 to obtain 1.00/4 = 0.25. Memorize a few common conversions for standarized tests: 1/4 = 0.25; 1/2 = 0.50; 3/4 = 0.75; 1/8 = 0.125; 3/16 = 0.1875; 3/8 = 0.375.

To convert a fraction to a percentage, convert the fraction so that its denominator is 100. The numerator of the new fraction is the percentage.

For example:
Express $\frac{6}{25}$ as a percentage by multiplying the fraction by $\frac{4}{4}$.

$$\frac{6}{25} \times \frac{4}{4} = \frac{24}{100}$$

The answer is 24%.

A fraction also may be converted into its decimal equivalent with long division.

For example:
Express $\frac{3}{7}$ as a percentage by converting $\frac{3}{7}$ to its decimal equivalent,

$$\frac{3}{7} = 3 \div 7 = 0.42857\ldots \approx 42.86\%.$$

5.4.2 Percentage Problems

Percentage problems are of three types: (1) calculating the percent of a given quantity, or percentage; (2) determining the rate, or percent rate; and (3) calculating the base, or quantity. Most percentage problems involve three quantities: the rate R, which is followed by a percent (%) sign; the base B, which usually follows the word "of" or a preposition; and the percentage P, which usually follows the word "is" or a verb. A basic equation, or formula, can be used to solve most percentage problems:

$$\frac{R}{100} = \frac{P}{B}$$

For example:
What is 5.7% of 160?

Solution: Using the formula $\frac{R}{100} = \frac{P}{B}$

$R = 5.7\%$, $P =$ unknown, and $B = 160$

$$\frac{5.7}{100} = \frac{P}{160}$$

$$100P = 160\,(5.7)$$

$$P = \frac{10 \times 16\,(5.7)}{10 \times 10} = \frac{91.2(10)}{10 \times 10} = 9.12$$

The answer is 9.12.

Example: 72 is what percentage of 120?

Solution: Using the formula $\frac{R}{100} = \frac{P}{B}$

R = unknown, P = 72, and B = 120

$$\frac{R}{100} = \frac{72}{120}$$

$$120R = 72\ (100)$$

$$R = \frac{72\ (10)\ (10)}{12\ (10)} = \frac{720}{12} = 60$$

The answer is 60%.

Example: A compound contains 80% copper by weight. How much copper is contained in a 1.95-g sample?

A. 15.60
B. 156
C. 1.56
D. 15.0

The answer is **C.**

Solution: Using the formula $\frac{R}{100} = \frac{P}{B}$

R = 80%, P = unknown, and B = 195

$$\frac{80}{100} = \frac{P}{1.95}$$

$$100P = 80\ (1.95)$$

$$P = \frac{(10)\ (8)\ (1.95)}{(10)}\ (10)$$

$$P = \frac{15.60}{10} = 1.56$$

The sample contains 1.56 g copper.

5.4.3 Special Percentage Problems

Percent change, percent increase, and percent decrease are special types of percentage problems. The difficulty involves using the correct numbers to calculate the percent. The formula is:

$$\frac{(\text{New amount}) - (\text{Original amount})}{\text{Original amount}} \times 100 = \text{Percent change}$$

When the new amount is less than the original amount, the numerator is a negative number, and the result is a percent decrease. When a decrease is needed, the negative sign is omitted. When the new amount is greater than the original amount, the percent change is positive and is known as a percent increase. The percent increase or decrease is found by creating a fraction with the amount of increase or decrease as the numerator and the original amount as the denominator and multiplying this fraction by 100.

For example:
Joe received a salary increase from \$25,000 to \$27,000. Find the percent increase.
Using the formula:

$$\frac{(\text{New amount}) - (\text{Original amount})}{\text{Original amount}} \times 100$$

$$\frac{27000 - 25000}{25000} \times 100 = \frac{2000}{25000} \times 100$$
$$= \frac{20}{250} \times 100$$
$$= \frac{200}{25} = 8$$

The percent increase is 8%.

A percentage is an alternative way to represent a fraction or ratio. The statement "x is $P\%$ of y" means that:

$$x = \frac{P}{100} \times y$$

or

$$P = \frac{x}{y} \times 100$$

A percentage is a fraction with a denominator of 100 (e.g., a nickel is 5% of a dollar). Percentages are used to express the relation of a part to a whole; for example, if there are 16 women in a class of 25 students, then $P = (16/25)(100)$; in other words, 64% of the students in the class are women. Percentages are also used to express an increase or decrease in quantity. If x_2 is the result when x_1 is increased by $P\%$, then:

$$x_2 = x_1 + \frac{P}{100} \times x_1 = x_1\left(1 + \frac{P}{100}\right)$$

If x_2 is the result when x_1 is decreased by $P\%$, then:

$$x_2 = x_1 - \frac{P}{100} \times x_1 = x_1\left(1 - \frac{P}{100}\right)$$

In both of these definitions, the change in the variable is expressed as a percentage of its original value (x_1), not its final value (x_2).

For example:

What is the percent increase or decrease in a quantity x when its value is: (1) doubled, (2) halved, (3) reduced by a third, (4) reduced to a third of its original value, and (5) reduced to a fifth of its original value?

1. $x_2 = 2x_1$

$$2x_1 = x_1\left(1 + \frac{P}{100}\right)$$

$P = 100\%$increase

2. $x_2 = \frac{1}{2}x_1$

$$\frac{1}{2}x_1 = x_1\left(1 - \frac{P}{100}\right)$$

$P = 50\%$ decrease

3. $x_2 = \frac{2}{3}x_1$

$$\frac{2}{3}x_1 = x_1\left(1 - \frac{P}{100}\right)$$

$P = 33\frac{1}{3}\%$ decrease

4. $x_2 = \frac{1}{3}x_1$

$$\frac{1}{3}x_1 = x_1\left(1 - \frac{P}{100}\right)$$

$$P = 66\frac{2}{3}\% \text{ decrease}$$

5. $x_2 = \frac{1}{5}x_1$

$$\frac{1}{5}x_1 = x_1\left(1 - \frac{P}{100}\right)$$

$$P = 80\% \text{ decrease}$$

5.5 SCIENTIFIC OPERATIONS

Scientific notation is expression of a number as the product of a number between 1 and 10 and some integral power of 10. For example, 1000 is written in scientific notation as 1×10^3 or, more simply, 10^3; 0.0001 is written as 10^{-4}; and 1247 is written as 1.247×10^3.

5.5.1 Converting Numbers to Scientific Notation

Because the decimal point of any number can be shifted to the left or right by multiplying the number by a power of 10, any number n can be written in scientific notation as $n = a \times 10^z$, where a is a number between 1 and 10 and z is a positive or negative integer.

For example:
Write 10,000,000 in scientific notation. The decimal point in 10,000,000 occurs after the last 0. The first significant digit is 1. Move the decimal point to the left seven places (1.0000000). Multiplying the number by 10^7 converts the number to scientific notation: $10{,}000{,}000 = 1 \times 10^7$, usually written as $10^{7.}$

Example: To write 0.005329 in scientific notation, the decimal point is moved to the right three places. The resulting number is 5.329×10^{-3}.

5.5.2 Ten Rules for Exponential Algebra

The three basic rules for mathematical operations with exponentials are:

1. $x^m \times x^n = x^{m+n}$ where m and n are positive integers and $x \neq 0$ — $3^2 \times 3^3 = 3^{2+3} = 243$
2. $\frac{x^m}{x^n} = x^{m-n}$ where m and n are positive integers and $x \neq 0$ — $\frac{3^2}{3^3} = 3^{2-3} = 3^{-1} = \frac{1}{3}$
3. $(x^m)^n = x^{mn}$ where m and n are positive integers and $x \neq 0$ — $(3^2)^3 = 3^6 = 729$

Manipulating these rules shows:

4. $x^0 = 1$; $x^0 = x^{n-n} = \frac{x^n}{x^n} = 1$ where x is any positive real number — $3^0 = 1$
5. $x^{-m} = \frac{1}{x^m}$; $x^{-m} = x^{0-m} = \frac{x^0}{x^m} = \frac{1}{x^m}$ — $3^{-2} = \frac{1}{3^2} = \frac{1}{9}$

This discussion of exponentials can be extended to include nonintegral (i.e., any real number) exponents. A radical is a fractional exponent. It is customary to ignore the 2 in $^2\sqrt{3}$; therefore, $\sqrt{3}$ is the square root of 3.

6. $x^{1/n} = {}^n\sqrt{x}$; $({}^n\sqrt{x})^n = x$ (by definition) $3^{1/2} = \sqrt[2]{3} = \sqrt{3}$
$(x^m)^n = x$ (by letting $x^m = {}^n\sqrt{x}$)
$x^{mn} = x^1$

Thus $mn = 1$; $m = \dfrac{1}{n}$

Therefore:

7. $x^{m/n} = ({}^n\sqrt{x})^m = {}^n\sqrt{x^m}$ $3^{2/3} = (\sqrt[3]{3^2}) = \sqrt[3]{9}$
($\sqrt[3]{9}$ is the cube root of 9)

8. $x^{-m/n} = \dfrac{1}{x^{m/n}} = \dfrac{1}{{}^n\sqrt{x^m}} = \dfrac{1}{(n\sqrt{x})^m}$ $3^{-2/3} = ({}^3\sqrt{3})^{-2} = {}^3\sqrt{\dfrac{1}{3^2}} = {}^3\sqrt{\dfrac{1}{9}}$

At this point, m and n are still positive integers.

The last two exponent rules have an exponent m/n that can be any rational number. Any rational number can be written as a fraction of two integers. Because any irrational number can be approximated by a rational number $y = x^p$, where the base x is any number except 0 and the exponent p is any real number. If p is not an integer, it represents the combined operations of an integral exponent m and an nth root on the number x, where p equals exactly, or approximately, if it is irrational, m/n. The three basic exponent rules apply for m and n, when m and n are real numbers, not just positive integers. Finally:

9. $(x \times y)^n = x^n \times y^n$ $(3 \times 4)^3 = 3^3 \times 4^3 = 27 \times 64 = 1728$

10. $\left(\dfrac{x}{y}\right) n = \dfrac{x^n}{y^n}$ $\left(\dfrac{3}{4}\right)^3 = \dfrac{3^3}{4^3} = \dfrac{27}{64}$

For example:
Evaluate each expression.

(A) $\dfrac{10^2 \times 10^3}{10^{15}} = 10^{2+3-15} = 10^{-10}$

(B) $\left(\dfrac{3^6 \times 3^3 \times 9}{3^0 \times 3^4}\right)^2 = (3^{6+3+2-0-4})^2$
$= (3^7)^2 = 3^{7\times 2} = 3^{14}$

(C) $\left(\dfrac{1}{4}\right)^{-2} = \left(\dfrac{1}{\frac{1}{4}}\right)^2 = \dfrac{1}{\frac{1}{16}} = 16$

Exercise 1. Evaluate each expression.

(A) $\dfrac{4^4 \times 4^8}{4^5}$

(B) $\left(\dfrac{6^4}{6^2}\right)^3 \times 6^{-5}$

(C) $(7^4)^0$

Example: Find the value of each expression.

(A) $8^{4/3} = {}^3\sqrt{8^4} = (4096)^{1/3} = 16$
$= \left({}^3\sqrt{8}\right)^4 = 2^4 = 16$

(B) $(289x)^{3/2} = (289^3)^{1/2}x^{3/2}$
$= (289^{1/2})^3x^{3/2} = 17^3 \times x^{3/2} = 4913x^{3/2}$

(C) $\dfrac{8^6 \times 8^3 \times {}^3\sqrt{8}}{8^{5/3} \times 8^7} = 8^{6+3+1/3-5/3-7}$

$= 8^{2/3} = (8^{1/3})^2 = 2^2 = 4$

Exercise 2. Find the value of each expression.

(A) $216^{4/3}$
(B) $256^{3/4}$
(C) $\dfrac{\sqrt{ab}\times\sqrt[4]{a^3\times b^3}}{\sqrt[3]{a^2\times b^2}}$
(D) $\left(\dfrac{3}{5}\right)^{-8}\left(\dfrac{9}{25}\right)^{3}$

5.5.3 Logarithms

The discussion of exponentials shows that:

$$x^m \times x^n = x^{m+n}$$
$$\frac{x^m}{x^n} = x^{m-n}$$
$$(x^m)^n = x^{mn}$$
$$x^0 = 1$$
$$x^{-m} = \frac{1}{x^m}$$

where x is any number except 0 and m and n are any real numbers. By assuming a specific base x, these exponent rules can be rewritten in terms of the exponents only. The logarithm of a number M is defined as the power (i.e., exponent) m to which a base x must be raised to produce the number M:

If $M = x^m$, then m = logarithm of M with respect to the base x and is usually written as: $m = \log_x M$. If $N = x^n$, then $n = \log_x N$.

Logarithms are simply exponents:

$x^{\log_x M} = M$

For example:

Write each expression in its equivalent logarithmic form.

(A) If $8^3 = 512$, then $\log_8 512 = 3$
(B) If $10^{4.6990} = 50{,}000$, then $\log_{10} 50{,}000 = 4.6990$
(C) If $2^{-2} = \frac{1}{4}$, then $\log_2 \left(\frac{1}{4}\right) = -2$

Example: Find x.

(A) $\log_2 32 = x$	$2^x = 32;\quad x - 5$
(B) $\log_5 1 = x$	$5^x = 1;\quad x = 0$
(C) $\log_m (m^{10}) = x$	$m^x = m^{10};\quad x = 10$
(D) $2\log_2{}^3 = x$	$\log_2 3 = \log_2 x;\quad x = 3$
(E) $4\log_4{}^{16} = x$	$\log_4 16 = \log_4 x\ ;\quad x = 16$

Exercise 3. Find x.

(A) $\log_4 \left(\frac{1}{16}\right) = x$
(B) $\log_z{}^2 (Z^b) = x$
(C) $\log_x 1 = 0$
(D) $5 \log_5{}^{625} = x$
(E) $4 \log_2{}^{16} = x$

5.5.4 Rules of Logarithms

With logarithms, the first five rules for exponentials can be rewritten as:

1. $\log_x M + \log_x N = \log_x (MN)$
2. $\log_x M - \log_x N = \log_x (M/N)$

3. $\log_x (M^n) = n(\log_x M)$
4. $\log_x 1 = 0$
5. $\log_x (1/M) = \log_x (M^{-1}) = -\log_x M$

The expression $\log_{10} M$ is usually written as $\log M$.

For example:

If $\log_2 = 0.3010$ and $\log_3 = 0.4774$, then:

(A) $\log_6 = \log_{(2\times3)} = \log_2 + \log_3 = 0.3010 + 0.4774 = 0.7784$

(B) $\log_5 = \log\left(\frac{10}{2}\right) = \log_{10} - \log_2 = 1 - 0.3010 = 0.6990$

(C) $\log_8 = \log(2^3) = 3(\log_2) = 3(0.3010) = 0.9030$

(D) $\log_{60} = \log(2 \times 3 \times 10) = \log_2 + \log_3 + \log_{10} = 0.3010 + 0.4774 + 1 = 1.7784$

Example: Solve for x.

$$2\log_x = \log_a + \log_b - \log_c$$
$$\log x^2 = \log\left(\frac{ab}{c}\right)$$
$$x^2 = \frac{ab}{c}$$
$$x = \sqrt{\frac{ab}{c}}$$

Exercise 4. Express as a single logarithm.

(A) $\log_M{}^2 + 7\log_N - \frac{1}{3}\log_P$

(B) $\log\sqrt{x^5} - 3\log\sqrt[4]{x} + \log_x{}^3$

Exercise 5. Solve for x.

(A) $\log_9 (x + 1) = \frac{1}{2}$

(B) $3\log_x = 2\log_a + 3\log_b + 4\log_c - 5\log_d$

The two most common bases used for logarithms are 10 (i.e., common logarithms) and e (i.e., natural logarithms). Common logarithms are an extension of scientific notation: the coefficient of the power of 10, which is between 1 and 10, is also written as a power of 10. Thus, the number is written completely as an exponential with the base 10:

$$y = a \times 10^b$$
$$= 10^c \times 10^b = 10^{c+b}$$
$$\log_y = c + b$$

where $a = 10^c$, c is the mantissa, and b is the characteristic

Before the use of calculators, common logarithms were an important tool for solving problems; however, calculators have largely replaced their use. Calculators are not permitted during the VETs; consequently, learning common logarithms is essential for solving science problems. Conceptually, logarithms are important for topics such as pH, sound intensity, and exponential decay and growth. The base of natural logarithms e is an irrational number that is approximately equal to 2.71828. Natural logarithms and the base e play an important part in many scientific problems. Only a basic understanding of logarithms is needed for the VETs.

5.6 CONVERTING UNITS OF MEASURE

A measurement includes a quantity and a unit (i.e., 3 feet, 7 miles, 12 yards). One unit of measure can be converted to another if they both measure the same quality (i.e., length). Equivalence between units is used to convert one unit of measure to another (e.g., 12 inches = 1 foot; 36 inches = 1 yard; 5280 feet = 1 mile).

For example:
Thirty-two bricks, each 8 inches long, are laid end to end to form the base of a wall. Find the length of the wall in feet.

Solution: Convert 8 inches to feet.
12 inches = 1 foot

$$8 \text{ inches} = \frac{8}{12} = \frac{2}{3} \text{ feet}$$

$$\text{Multiply } \frac{2}{3} \text{ feet} \times 32 = \frac{2}{3} \times \frac{32}{1} = \frac{64}{3}$$

$$= 21 \text{ feet, } 4 \text{ inches}$$

The wall is 21 feet, 4 inches long.

5.7 PROBABILITY AND STATISTICS

Probability values range from 1 to 0. A value of 1 represents absolute certainty; 0 indicates that there is no chance that the event will occur. Few events in life are certain, and most events have probability values between 1 and 0.

For example:
If Molly tosses a new coin, the probability of obtaining a head is one of two. This probability can be expressed as $P = 1/2$, or 0.5. The probability of obtaining a tail is also 1/2, or 0.5. In this situation, only one outcome can occur. The sum of the two probabilities is 1. The probability of an event occurring is represented by p, and the probability of it not occurring is represented by q. The sum of $p + q$ is always 1.

Example: Peter tosses a six-sided die into the air. What is the probability of any single side landing face-up? The probability of any single outcome is 1/6, or 0.167. In other words, when Peter tosses the die, the chance of throwing a six is one in six, or there are five chances in six that some other number will appear on the upturned face. In this case, $p = 1/6$ and $q = 5/6$; therefore, $p + q = 1/6 + 5/6 = 6/6 = 1$.

Example: Sara has a bag with 6 yellow marbles and 2 blue marbles. If she draws a marble out of the bag without looking, what are the chances that it will be blue?

A. $\frac{2}{8}$

B. $\frac{6}{8}$

C. $\frac{2}{6}$

D. $\frac{6}{2}$

The answer is **A**.

Solution:
Let p = number of favorable outcomes, which is 2
q = number of unfavorable outcomes, which is 6
$p + q$ = total outcomes

$$\frac{p}{p + q} = \frac{2}{8}$$

5.7.1 Statistical Data Analysis

In elementary statistical analysis, data from two experiments are presented and analyzed.

For example:
Experiments A and B are peformed at a university research center.

Experiment A: To test the difficulty of a maze, 10 rats run the maze. Their solution times to the nearest 0.1 second are:
8.3, 7.1, 8.8, 11.1, 7.0, 13.7, 9.5, 10.3, 10.8, 9.9

Experiment B: Two groups of 35-year-old subjects, one group of men and one group of women, have their blood cholesterol levels measured. The data obtained, rounded to the nearest 1 mg/100 ml, are:
Group I (men): 195, 198, 199, 196, 195, 196, 191, 194, 195, 196
Group II (women): 196, 193, 194, 201, 202, 205, 204, 202, 199, 204

The next step is to organize and analyze the information so that it can be interpreted meaningfully. This example shows two types of raw data (i.e., obtained during an experiment and not manipulated into graphs, means, or ranges). In Experiment A, the data are continuous because all decimal values of time are possible (e.g., 8.003, 9.1083), even though all values are not recorded. Count data are integer values (e.g., age, number of animals in an experimental group, number of times the teeth are brushed each day). In Experiment B, cholesterol level is a continuous variable, but it is rounded to permit comparison between subjects.

When presented with a set of data, simple observations are helpful. One approach is to list the data in ascending or descending order. In ascending order, the data from Experiment A are:

7.0, 7.1, 8.3, 8.8, 9.5, 9.9, 10.3, 10.8, 11.1, 13.7

The data in Experiment A can be analyzed as follows:

Experiment A:
Lowest value: 7.0
Highest value: 13.7
Range: 7.0 − 13.7 (13.7 − 7.0 = 6.7)
Average value: $\approx 10 \left(\frac{13.7 + 7.0}{2}\right) = 10.35$

These observations suggest the limits of the data, the average value of the data, the variability of the data, and the distribution of the data over its possible values.

Exercise 6. Perform this analysis on the data for Experiment B.

5.7.2 Structuring Data

The next step in data analysis is to construct graphs or tables to show general trends as well as more specific findings. Another way to structure a set of data is to determine what percentages, or proportions, meet specific criteria.

For example:
In Experiment A,what percentage of rats have maze times of less than 9.0 seconds?

Solution: Four of the ten rats had times of less than 9.0 seconds. Therefore:
$\frac{4}{10} \times 100 = 40\%$

The answer is 40%.

In Experiment A, 40% of the rats ran the maze in more than 10.0 seconds. What number of rats T ran the maze in more than than 10.0 seconds?

Solution: $T = \frac{40}{100} \times 10 = 4$
The answer is four rats.

Exercise 7. In Experiment B, what respective percentages of subjects in Groups I and II had blood cholesterol levels of 196 or lower?

5.7.3 Statistical Analysis

After a set of data is structured and preliminary analysis is performed, more formal statistical calculations can be performed. Statistically, the two key features of a set of data are its central tendency and its variation.

5.7.4 Central Tendency

The central tendency, or expected value, of a set of data is the value that the data seem to approach. This value represents the entire set of data. The common measures of central tendency are the mode, median, and average, or mean. Only the computation of averages is required for the VETs. Although computing the mode and median is not required, you should be familiar with these concepts.

The average considers the value of each data point It is calculated by adding each data point and dividing the sum by the total number of data points.

$$\text{Average} = x = \frac{x_1 + x_2 + \ldots + x_n}{n}$$

where $x_1, x_2, \ldots\ x_n$ are the individual data points and n is the total number of data points.

For example:
In Experiment A, the average =

$$\frac{7.0 + 7.1 + 8.3 + 8.8 + 9.5 + 9.9 + 10.3 + 10.8 + 11.1 + 13.7}{10}$$

$= (9.65) \approx 9.7$
The estimated average is 10.

The median is the value in a set of data that is positionally halfway between the lowest and the highest values in the set. The median is determined by listing all of the values in the set of data in ascending order and identifying the value that is positionally in the center. When a set of data contains an even number of values, the median is calculated by averaging the middle two numbers.

For example:
In Experiment A, the values in ascending order are:
7.0, 7.1, 8.3, 8.8, 9.5, 9.9, 10.3, 10.8, 11.1, 13.7.
The number of values is even (10), and the two middle values are 9.5 and 9.9.

$$\text{Median} = \frac{9.5 + 9.9}{2} = 9.7$$

The median value is 9.7.

The mode is the value in a set that appears most frequently. A set of data has a mode only if one value occurs more often than any other. In Experiment A, no mode exists because each value occurs only once.

The question naturally arises as to which measure of central tendency is the best. The answer depends on the distribution of data. Figure 5-2 shows three sets of data, where N = the frequency of a specific value of the variable x.

$$\text{Mean} = 2.9 = \frac{7(2) + 1(4) + 1(5) + 1(6)}{7 + 1 + 1 + 1} \approx 3$$

Median = 2
Mode = 2
Data = 2, 2, 2, 2, 2, 2, 2, 4, 5, 6

Histogram I

$$\text{Mean} = 3 = \frac{2(1) + 2(2) + 2(3) + 2(4) + 2(5)}{2 + 2 + 2 + 2 + 2}$$

Median = 3
One mode does not exist
Data = 1, 1, 2, 2, 3, 3, 4, 4, 5, 5

Histogram II

Mean $= 2.9 = \dfrac{7(2) + 1(4) + 1(5) + 1(6)}{7 + 1 + 1 + 1} \cong 3$
Median $= 2$
Mode $= 2$
Data $= 2, 2, 2, 2, 2, 2, 2, 4, 5, 6$

Mean $= 3 = \dfrac{2(1) + 2(2) + 2(3) + 2(4) + 2(5)}{2 + 2 + 2 + 2 + 2}$
Median $= 3$
One mode does not exist
Data $= 1, 1, 2, 2, 3, 3, 4, 4, 5, 5$

Mean $= 3.3 \approx 3 = \dfrac{2(1) + 2(2) + 3(4) + 3(5)}{2 + 2 + 3 + 3}$
Median $= 4$
Two modes $= 4, 5$ (bimodal)
Data $= 1, 1, 2, 2, 4, 4, 4, 5, 5, 5$

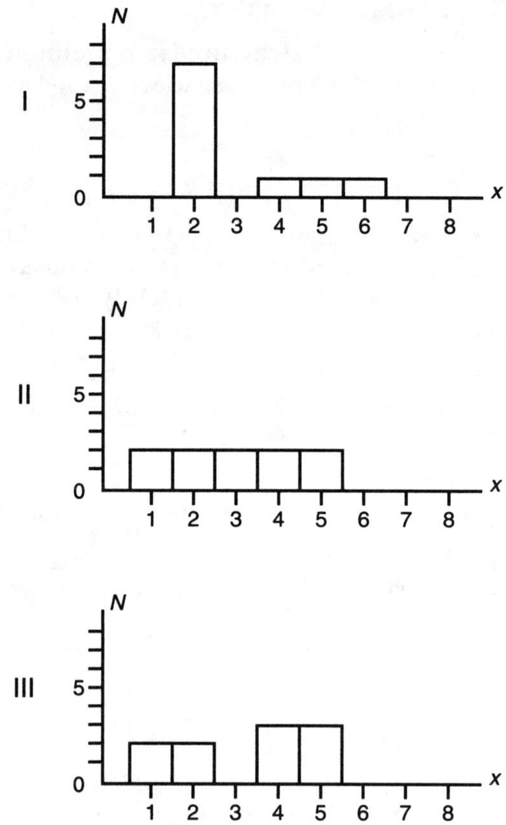

Figure 5-2 Histograms Illustrating Mean, Median, and Mode

$$\text{Mean} = 3.3 \approx 3 = \frac{2(1) + 2(2) + 3(4) + 3(5)}{2 + 2 + 3 + 3}$$

Median $= 4$
Two modes $= 4,5$ (bimodal)
Data $= 1, 1, 2, 2, 4, 4, 4, 5, 5, 5$

Histogram III

For the data in histogram I, both the mode and the median are good measures of central tendency; the average, or mean, probably is not. When the frequency of one value predominates in a set of data, the mode is usually a good measure of central tendency. The data in histograms II and III have no mode. For the data in histogram II, both the average and the median are good measures of central tendency. When the values of a set of data are distributed fairly evenly over the range of the data, as in this case, the average may be a better measure of central tendency because it considers the value of each data point. The median is probably a better measure of central tendency than the average for the data in histogram III. Typically, the median is preferable to the average when the values in a set of data are clustered toward one end of the range, but not when the mode would be a good measure of central tendency, as in histogram I.

Exercise 8. Calculate the mode, median, and average for each group in Experiment B. Identify which measure of central tendency is the best for each group.

5.7.5 Variation From the Average

Each measure of central tendency uses one value to describe a set of data. This one value is inadequate to completely describe the data because it does not consider the variation, or dispersion, of the data around this value. In other words, knowledge of the variation in a set of data is needed to complement knowledge of the central tendency. The common measures of variation are range, variance, and standard deviation. Only the computation of range is required for the VETs. Computing variance and standard deviation is not required; however, you should be familiar with these concepts.

The range is the difference between the highest and lowest values in a set of data. For example, in Experiment A, the range is 13.7 − 7.0 = 6.7. In Experiment B, the range is 90 − 50 = 40. Because the range considers only the highest and lowest values in a set of data, it is a rough measure of variation. When either or both of the extreme values in a set of data are far out of line with the rest of the data, the range is a questionable measure of variation.

In Figure 5-3, N is the frequency of a specific value x. The range of the data in histogram IV shows the variability of the data; the range of data in histogram V does not.

Variance (V) and standard deviation (SD) are intimately related:

$$SD = \sqrt{V}$$

Like mean, variance considers each value in a set of data. It is calculated by determining the average value of the squares of the deviation for each data point from the mean:

$$V = \frac{(x_1 - x)^2 + (x_2 - x)^2 + \ldots + (x_n - x)^2}{n}$$

where $x_1, x_2, \ldots x_n$ are values of individual data points, x is the mean, and n is the total number of data points. The standard deviation is calculated by determining the square root of the variance:

$$SD = \left(\frac{(x_1 - x)^2 + (x_2 - x)^2 + \ldots + (x_n - x)^2}{n}\right)^{1/2}$$

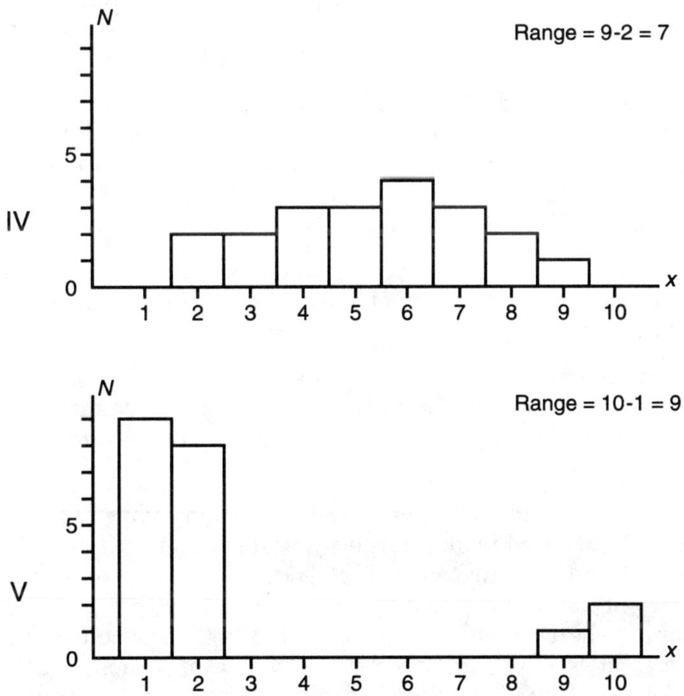

Figure 5-3 Histograms Illustrating Range and Variation in Data

For Experiment A, the standard deviation and variance can be calculated as:

$$V = \frac{(7.0 - 9.7)^2 + (7.1 - 9.7)^2 + \ldots + (11.1 - 9.7)^2 + (13.7 - 9.7)^2}{10}$$

$$= (3.643) \approx 3.6$$

$$SD = \sqrt{V} = \sqrt{3.6} = 1.9$$

The standard deviation of a set of data can be approximated by determining the range and dividing it by 4:

$$SD \approx \frac{\text{Range}}{4}$$

For example:

In Experiment A: $SD \approx \dfrac{13.7 - 7.0}{4} = (1.675) \approx 1.7$

Comparing these estimates of standard deviation with the exact calculations shows that when the range is a good indicator of the variation in a set of data, this approximation of standard deviation is also good.

Some standardized tests require an understanding of these concepts, but complex calculations are not needed. The equations for variance and standard deviation should be reviewed and understood, but not memorized.

Exercise 9. Calculate the range, variance, and standard deviation for each group in Experiment B.

5.7.6 Precision and Accuracy in Measurements

Data analysis involves examining the nature (e.g., limitations) of the measurements. The concept of measurement error stems from the need to know the possible difference between the actual value of a quantity and its measured or calculated value. Section 5.1 describes rounding numbers.

A digit is significant when it has been measured exactly. For example, the number 7.000 has four significant digits because the digits listed after a decimal point are assumed to be accurately measured; the number 7000 has one significant digit because it contains no decimal point; the number 7000. has four significant digits because the decimal point implies that all zeros are accurately measured; and the number 7001 has four significant digits because all zeros between nonzero digits are significant.

When performing an operation (e.g., addition), the result cannot be more precise than the least precise number involved in its calculation. For example, in Experiment A, each data point has two (e.g., 8.3) or three (e.g., 10.3) significant digits. The mean for these data is calculated initially as 9.65 and rounded to 9.7 because some of the numbers used to calculate this mean have only two significant digits. Likewise, the variance is initially calculated as 3.643 and rounded to 3.6, which has two significant digits.

Measurement errors occur because exact numbers cannot be obtained experimentally. In any experiment, the likelihood of obtaining a true value is limited. Several terms are used to describe the error in a measurement or calculation.

The precision, or least count, of a number or an experimental value is the smallest unit of measurement used and is closely related to the number of significant digits in a measured number. For example, in Experiment A, the solution times are recorded to the nearest 0.1 second; therefore, the precision of these measurements is 0.1 second.

The accuracy of a number is how much the measured value may vary from the true value. The true value is normally an average obtained from a large set of data values. For example, in Experiment A, the precision of the watch used to measure each solution time is 0.1 second. If no other sources of error are considered, the accuracy of each time measurement is ± 0.05 second. Specifically, when a measured solution time is 8.8 seconds, the true solution time is 8.8 ± 0.05 seconds. In other words, the true time is between 8.75 and 8.85 seconds. In Experiment B, the precision of the blood cholesterol level measurements is 1 mg/100 ml; therefore, the accuracy of the measurements is ± 0.5 mg/100 ml. A measured value of 196 corresponds to a true value of between 195.5 and 196.5.

When error results from sources other than the limitations of the measuring device, the accuracy and precision are not so simply related. Measurement errors can be classified as mistakes, systematic errors, and random errors. Mistakes are usually nonrepetitive errors that might result from human errors (e.g., misreading an instrument, performing an experimental procedure incorrectly). The error that results from a mistake is largely unpredictable. Unless this error is detected, it may have an unknown effect on the data. A systematic error is a repetitive error caused by human, instrument, or experimental design error. This type of error is repeated in every measurement, usually to the same extent. For this reason, a systematic error that is detected may be corrected to some extent. For example, in an experiment that measures a series of temperatures, if the thermometer is miscalibrated by 2°C, the set of temperature measurements has a systematic error of 2°C.

Investigators always attempt to perform experiments under uniform conditions. Nevertheless, some variability cannot be avoided. Thus, even if all human, instrument, and experimental design errors are corrected, a variability known as random error probably occurs. For example, an experiment is performed to determine the temperature dependence of the solubility of an organic salt in water. The experimental apparatus maintains a constant temperature of ±1°C. The experiment measures the solubility of the salt at 37°C. Although solubility is measured at 37°C each time, the true temperature is actually somewhere between 36°C and 38°C. Because solubility is dependent on the temperature, this variability causes a random error that directly affects the accuracy of the results.

5.8 PLANE GEOMETRY

Geometry deals with the measurement of sides, angles, areas, perimeters, and volumes. It is divided into two branches: plane and solid. Plane and solid geometry are inseparable from two-dimensional and three-dimensional perceptual abilities. Review the principles of plane and solid geometry, and learn the difference between plane angles and dihedral, or solid, angles. Angles in two dimensions (i.e., between two lines or rays) are plane angles. Angles in three dimensions (i.e., between two or three surfaces) are dihedral. For example, in a room, each corner forms dihedral angles. Connect dihedral angles to isometric and perspective views of a solid object, such as the wings of an airplane.

5.8.1 Angles

An angle is formed by two lines that meet at one point. A right angle measures 90°. Complementary angles are two angles, the sum of whose measures is 90°. Supplementary angles are two angles, the sum of whose measures is 180°. An acute angle measures less than 90°. An obtuse angle measures greater than 90°. A straight angle measures 180°. Perimeter is the distance around a plane figure.

5.8.2 Rules and Formulas

1. The sum of the measure of the angles in a triangle is 180°.
2. To find the perimeter p of a figure, add the length of the sides.
   $p = a + b + c$

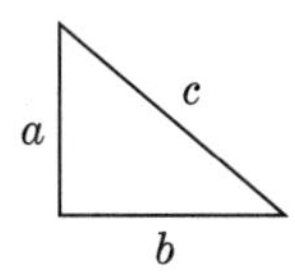

3. Because all sides of a square are of equal length, the perimeter of a square is equal to four times the length of one side s.
   $p = s + s + s + s$
   $p = 4s$

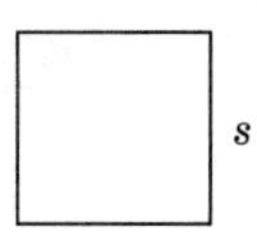

4. A rectangle has two short sides of equal length W and two long sides of equal length L. Therefore, the perimeter is equal to twice the length times twice the width.
$p = 2L + 2W$

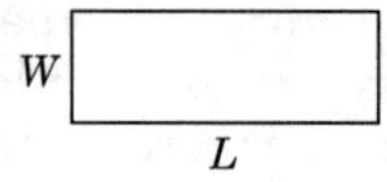

5. The circumference c of a circle is the distance around the circle. The diameter is twice the radius r times π, or π times the diameter d.
$c = 2\ \pi r$
$c = \pi d$
$\pi \approx 3.14 = \frac{22}{7}$

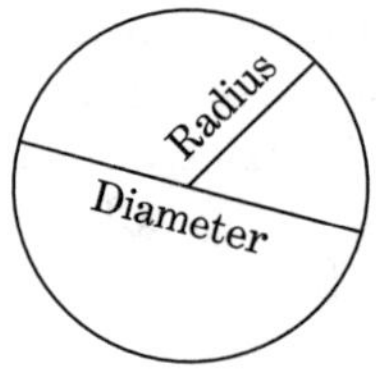

6. Composite geometric figures combine two or more simple geometric figures.

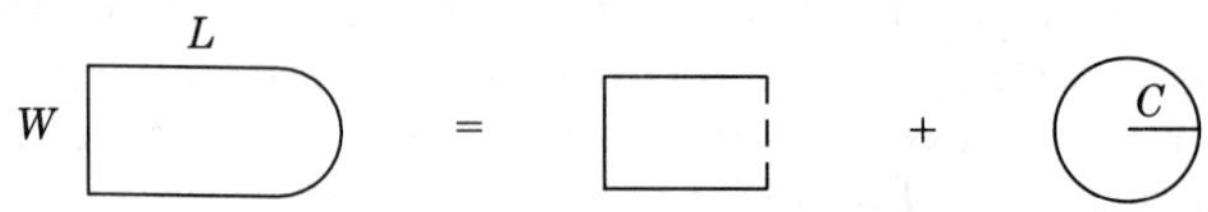

This composite figure is three sides of a rectangle and one-half the circumference of a circle. Its perimeter is twice the length plus the width plus one-half times π times the diameter.
$p = 2L + W + \frac{1}{2} \times \pi \times d$

5.8.3 Triangles

Similar figures have the same shape, but not necessarily the same size. Similar figures have corresponding sides and angles. The relation between the sizes of each of the corresponding sides or angles can be expressed as a ratio, and each ratio is the same.

For example:
Triangles ABC and DEF are similar. The ratios of the corresponding sides are equal.

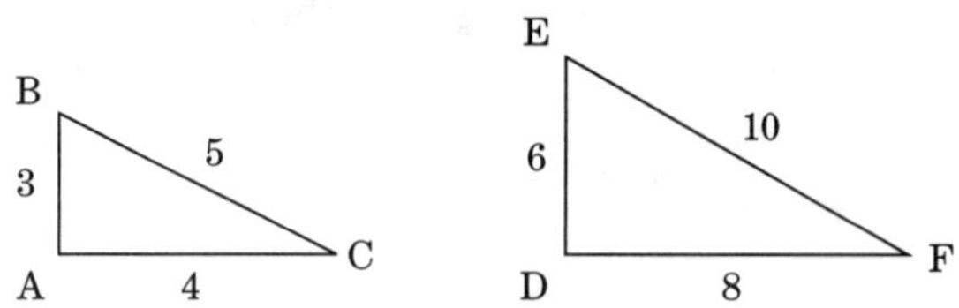

$$\frac{AB}{DE} = \frac{3}{6} = \frac{1}{2}; \quad \frac{BC}{EF} = \frac{5}{10} = \frac{1}{2}; \quad \frac{AC}{DF} = \frac{4}{8} = \frac{1}{2}$$

The ratio of the corresponding sides is 1:2. Because the ratios of the corresponding sides are equal, three proportions can be formed:

$$\frac{AB}{DE} = \frac{BC}{EF}; \quad \frac{AC}{DF} = \frac{BC}{EF}; \quad \frac{AB}{DE} = \frac{AC}{DF}$$

Example: Triangles ABC and DEF are similar. Find the perimeter of triangle ABC.

A. 11
B. 12
C. 14
D. 13

The answer is **B**.

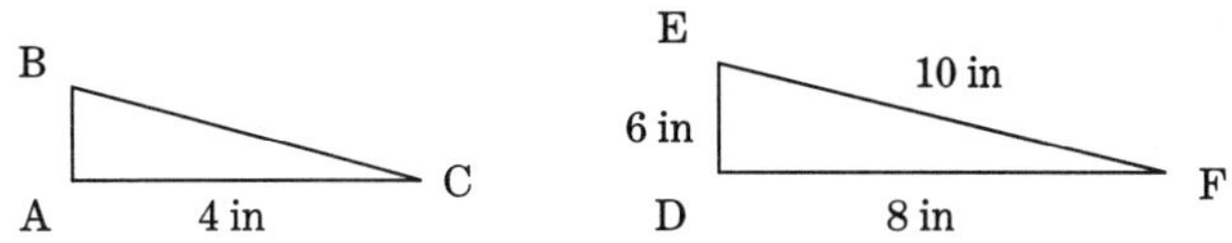

Find the length of BC by using proportion.

$$\frac{AC}{DF} = \frac{BC}{EF}$$
$$\frac{4\text{ in}}{8\text{ in}} = \frac{BC}{EF}$$
$$8\text{ BC} = 40\text{ in}$$
$$BC = 5\text{ in}$$
$$\frac{BC}{EF} = \frac{AB}{DE}$$
$$\frac{5\text{ in}}{10\text{ in}} = \frac{AB}{6\text{ in}}$$
$$10AB = 30\text{ in}$$
$$AB = 3\text{ in}$$
$$\Delta\,ABC = 4 + 3 + 5 = 12$$

The perimeter is 12 inches.

5.8.4 Cartesian Geometry

All graphic representations of data and functions are based on a coordinate system. Even bar graphs, or histograms, and pie graphs have an implicit coordinate system. The most commonly used graphs are based on the rectangular, or Cartesian, coordinate system that consists of two perpendicular axes, each representing a variable (Figure 5-4).

The intersection of the two axes in the Cartesian plane is known as the origin (O). The origin splits each axis into two segments that represent, respectively, positive and negative values of the variable. The ordinate usually represents the dependent variable y, and the abscissa usually represents the independent variable x. The standard positive and negative segments of each axis are labeled in Figure 5-4; the value is also shown by the arrows that indicate the directions of positive change. Each point in the Cartesian plane is represented by a pair of coordinates known as an ordered pair. Each coordinate represents a distance from the origin along one of the axes. In Figure 5-4, $P = (x,y)$; $O = (0,0)$.

5.8.5 Slope

The most important parameter in interpreting the relation between the two variables in a graph is slope. The slope of the line between two points is the ratio of the change in the ordinate to the change in the abscissa.

$$\text{Slope} = \frac{\text{Change in ordinate}}{\text{Change in abscissa}} = \frac{\Delta y}{\Delta x} = \frac{\text{Rise}}{\text{Run}} = \frac{\text{Change in dependent variable}}{\text{Change in independent variable}}$$

As shown in Figure 5-5, slope may be constant (e.g., straight lines, portions of curves that are straight), or it may be constantly changing (e.g., curved lines). Slope is calculated as follows:

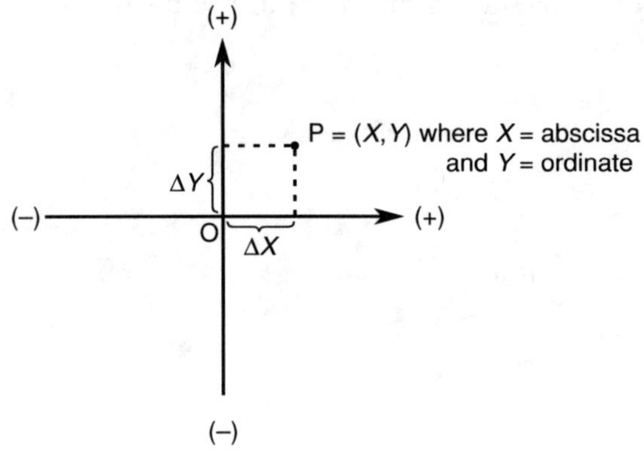

Figure 5-4 Cartesian Coordinate System

For straight lines:

$$\text{Slope} = m = \frac{y_2 - y_1}{x_2 - x_1} = \frac{\Delta y}{\Delta x} = \text{Constant}$$

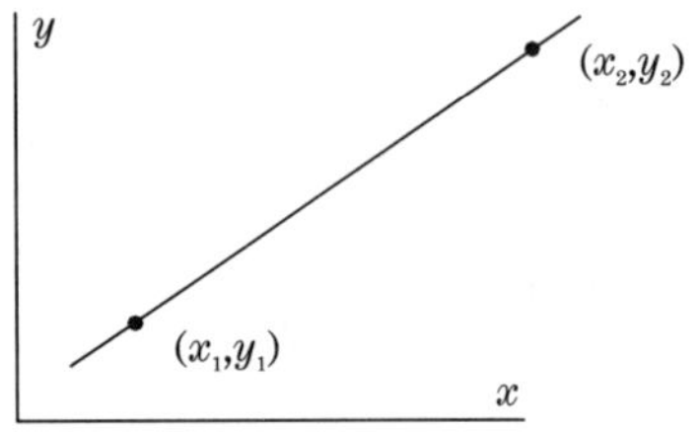

For curved lines:

Measure Δx, Δy for any two points on the tangent.

$$\text{Slope} = m = \frac{\Delta y}{\Delta x} \neq \text{Constant (i.e., changes along the curve)}$$

For example:
Find the slope.

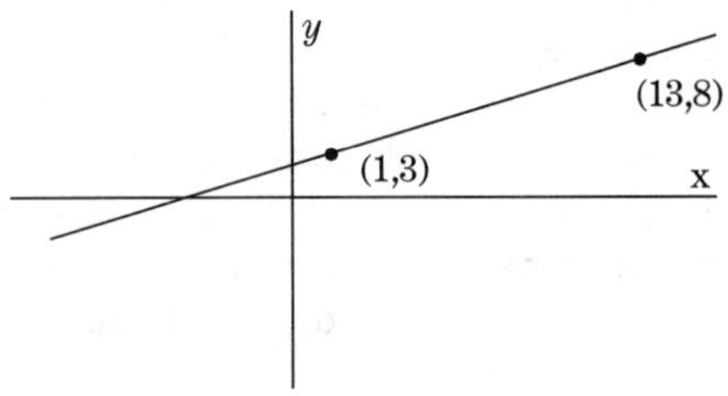

$$m = \frac{y_2 - y_1}{x_2 - x_1} = \frac{8 - 3}{13 - 1} = \frac{5}{12}$$

5.9 ALGEBRAIC EQUATIONS AND PROPORTIONALITY PROBLEMS

Solving a simple equation in one variable usually involves isolating an unknown quantity, or variable, on one side of the equation. Any operation except multiplication or division by zero can be used to isolate the variable as long as it is performed on both sides of the equation. The basic rule for solving equations is that whatever operation is performed on one side must be performed on the other side to maintain the equality of the sides. This concept is similar to a scale with two balanced sides. When an expression is manipulated, regardless of whether it is part of an equation, the order of operations is: (1) parentheses; (2) powers or exponents; (3) multiplication and division, working from the left side of the expression; and (4) addition and subtraction, working from the left side of the expression.

For straight lines: slope $= m = \frac{y_2 - y_1}{x_2 - x_1} = \frac{\Delta y}{\Delta x}$ = constant

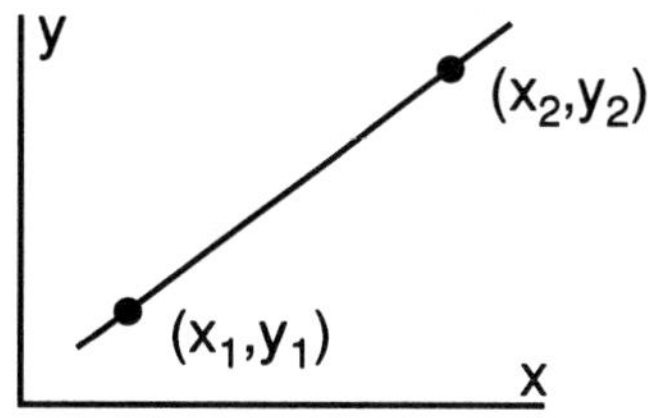

For curved lines: measure $\Delta x, \Delta y$ for any two points on tangent

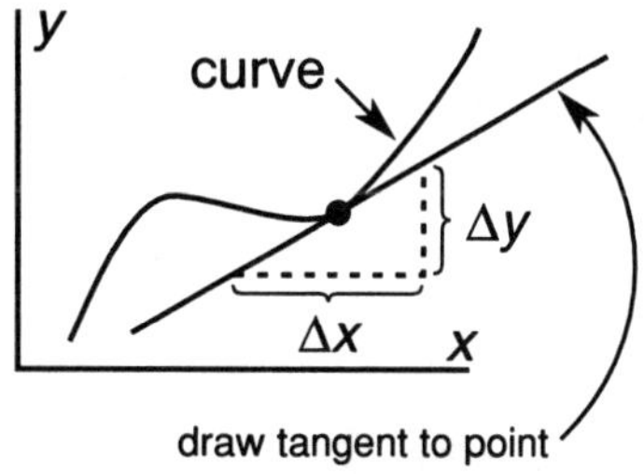

Figure 5-5 Definition Sketch for Slope

For example:

Solve for a.

$$4a + 5 = 13$$
$$4a + 5 - 5 = 13 - 5$$
$$4a = 8$$
$$\frac{4a}{4} = \frac{8}{4}$$
$$a = 2$$

Example: Solve for m.

$$\frac{10}{m} - 8 = \frac{5}{3}$$
$$\frac{10}{m}(3m) - 8(3m) = \frac{5}{3}(3m)$$
$$30 - 24m = 5m$$
$$30 = 29m$$
$$m = \frac{30}{29}$$

Example: Solve for c.

$$3c^2 = 75d^4$$
$$c^2 = 25d^4$$
$$c^2 = \sqrt{25d^4}$$
$$c = \pm 5d^2$$

Example: Solve for q.

$$3[(q + 2)^2 - 4q] = 2q^2 + 13$$
$$3[(q + 2)(q + 2) - 4q] = 2q^2 + 13$$

$$3[q^2 + 4q + 4 - 4q] = 2q^2 + 13$$
$$3q^2 + 12 = 2q^2 + 13$$
$$q^2 = 1$$
$$q = \pm 1$$

Exercise 10. Solve for a.

$$s(a - p) + q = ta + r^2$$

Exercise 11. Solve for d.

$$\frac{1}{d - 2} + \frac{2}{d + 3} = \frac{4}{d - 2}$$

Exercise 12. Solve for x.

$$3\{4x - 2[1 - (x + 5) + 3]\} = 13x + 19$$

Some problems can be solved by recognizing that the quantities are directly or inversely proportional. Two variables, x and y, are directly proportional if their ratio has a constant value a. Figure 5-6 shows proportionality, also known as linear variation.

$$\frac{y}{x} = a$$

or

$$y = ax$$

Consequently, for any distinct values of x, x_1, and x_2, there are corresponding values of y, y_1, and y_2, such that $y_1/x_1 = y_2/x_2$. If three of the terms are known, the fourth term can be determined.

For example:
In a chemical reaction, the quantities of reactants or products are directly proportional. If two moles of compound A react with 5 moles of compound B to form 3 moles of compound C, then how many moles of compound A are required to react completely with 7 moles of compound B?

Let $x_1 = 2$ moles of compound A and $y_1 = 5$ moles of compound B.
Then $x_2 =$ number of moles of compound A and $y_2 = 7$ moles of compound B such that:

$$\frac{5}{2} = \frac{7}{x_2}$$
$$x_2 = 2.8$$

The answer is 2.8 moles.

Exercise 13. In the previous example, how many moles of compound C are formed? Two variables, x and y, are inversely proportional if their product has a constant value b. This variation is nonlinear (Figure 5-7).

$$xy = b$$

or

$$y = \frac{b}{x}$$

Figure 5-6 Linear Variation

$$xy = b \quad \text{or} \quad y = \frac{b}{x}$$

(Nonlinear or hyperbolic variation)

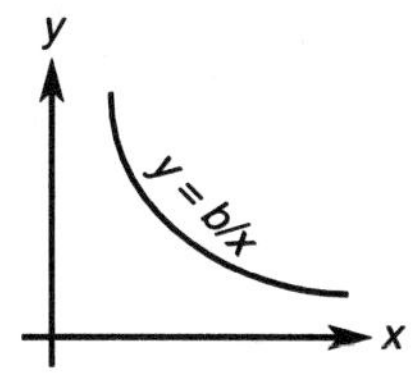

Figure 5-7 Nonlinear Variation

Consequently, for any distinct values of x, x_1, and x_2, there are corresponding values of y, y_1, and y_2, such that:

$$x_1y_1 = x_2y_2$$

or

$$\frac{y_1}{x_2} = \frac{y_2}{x_1}$$

If three of the terms in the equation $x_1y_1 = x_2y_2$ are known, the fourth term can be determined.

For example:
A car traveling at x mph takes 5 hours to go from city A to city B. Traveling at $x - 15$ mph, the car makes the return trip in 6-2/3 hours. What is the speed of the car on the return trip?

Solution: Because distance equals rate times time, $d = rt$, rate and time are inversely proportional for a constant displacement. Let $r_1 = x$ mph and $t_1 = 5$ hours; $r_2 = x - 15$ mph and $t_2 = 6\text{-}2/3$ hours $= 20/3$ hours. Then:

$$5x = (x - 15)\frac{20}{3}$$
$$15x = 20x - 300$$
$$5x = 300$$
$$x = 60$$
$$r_2 = x - 15 = 45$$

The speed is 45 mph.

Exercise 14. Before an engine tune-up, a car with a gas consumption rate of r gallons per mile travels 400 miles on a full tank of gas. After a tune-up, the same car has a gas consumption rate of $r - 0.01$ gallons per mile and travels 500 miles on a full tank of gas. What was the gas consumption rate of the car before the tune-up?

Problem 15. The ideal gas law for 1 mole of any gas is $pV = RT$. Two macroscopic states of 1 mole of a gas are respectively described by:

$$p_1V_1 = RT_1 \quad \text{and} \quad p_2V_2 = RT_2$$

Write an equation that shows the relation between these two states. According to this equation, pressure p is inversely proportional to what quantity?

An important application of proportionality is sensitivity analysis, or the identification of proportional changes in variables that occur when related variables change. This application is an important part of the VETs.

Exercise 16. In 1991, a machine part cost $2500. In 1992, the price increased 20% because materials were scarce. In 1993, the price increased by 10% over the 1992 price. In 1994, an alternate source of materials was found, and the price decreased by 30%. What was the 1994 price?

5.10 TRIGONOMETRY

Trigonometry is concerned with the relations between the angles and sides of triangles. For similar triangles (i.e., triangles that have the same angles, but are not necessarily the same size), the ratios

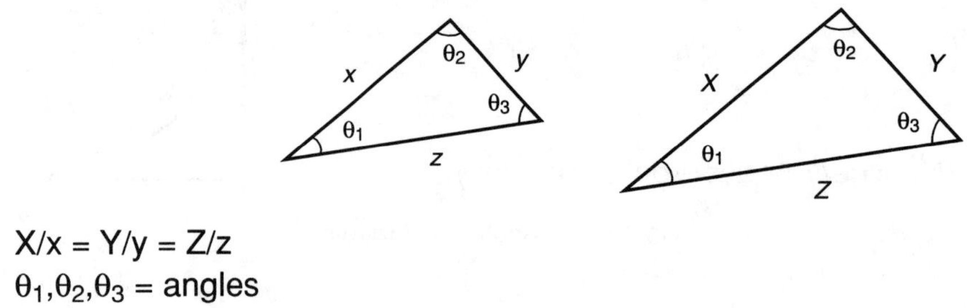

Figure 5-8 Trigonometric Elements of Similar Triangles

of the corresponding sides are equal (Figure 5-8):

$X/x = Y/y = Z/z$
$\theta_1, \theta_2, \theta_3 =$ Angles

The ratio of any two sides of a right triangle is the same for all similar right triangles. In other words, the possible ratios depend only on the angles of the right triangle (Figure 5-9).

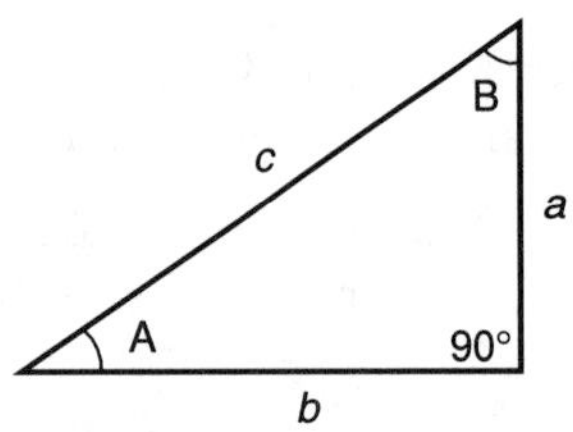

$a, b =$ Legs of the right triangle
$c =$ Hypotenuse of the right triangle
$A, B =$ Angles

Figure 5-9 Definition Sketch Trigonometric Functions

The sine, cosine, and tangent of an angle are defined as:

1. Sine of an angle $= \dfrac{\text{Opposite side}}{\text{Hypotenuse}} \left(\text{i.e., } \sin A = \dfrac{a}{c} \text{ and } \sin B = \dfrac{b}{c}\right)$
2. Cosine of an angle $= \dfrac{\text{Adjacent side}}{\text{Hypotenuse}} \left(\text{i.e., } \cos A = \dfrac{b}{c} \text{ and } \cos B = \dfrac{a}{c}\right)$
3. Tangent of an angle $= \dfrac{\text{Opposite side}}{\text{Adjacent side}} \left(\text{i.e., } \tan A = \dfrac{a}{b} \text{ and } \tan B = \dfrac{b}{a}\right)$

These definitions are interrelated; for example, sin A = cos B, sin B = cos A, and sin A/cos A = tan A. In addition, cot A = 1/tan A; csc A = 1/ sin A, and sec A = 1/cos A.

Exercise 17. Find sin A, cos A, and tan A.

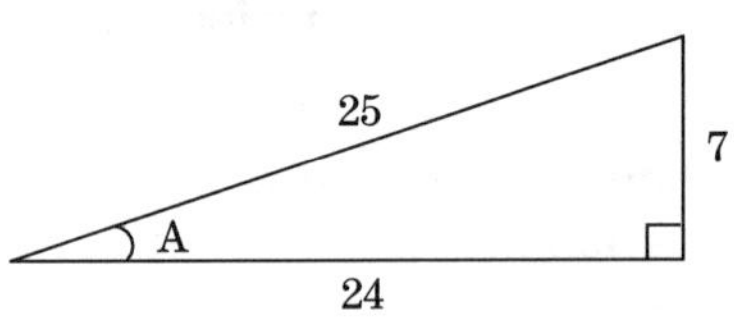

Exercise 18. Find sin B, cos B, and tan B.

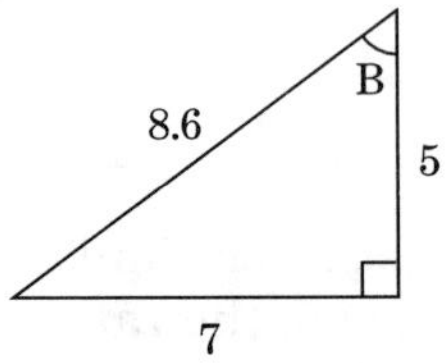

These right triangle definitions of the basic trigonometric functions are restricted to angles between 0° and 90°. However, the definitions of the trigonometric functions can be extended to include all angles. The trigonometric functions for angles between 0° and 360° are shown in Figure 5-10.

Exercise 19. Using the graphs shown in Figure 5-10, find sin θ, cos θ, and tan θ for $\theta = 0°, 90°, 180°$, and 270°.

The trigonometric functions are typically represented graphically for angles between 0° and 360° because they have repeating values (i.e., they are periodic):

$\sin(x + 360°n) = \sin x$
$\cos(x + 360°n) = \cos x$
$\tan(x + 180°n) = \tan x$
where x = angle and n = integer

Trigonometric functions are used to describe quantities that are periodic (e.g., waves). Trigonometry is useful when a quantity is represented as the hypotenuse or a leg of a right triangle. The characteristics of the basic right triangles shown in Figure 5-11, along with the values of the trigonometric functions for their angles, should be memorized for the VETs.

Exercise 20. Using the right triangles in Figure 5-11, find sin θ, cos θ, and tan θ for $\theta = 30°, 45°$, and 60°.

Exercise 21. Find x.

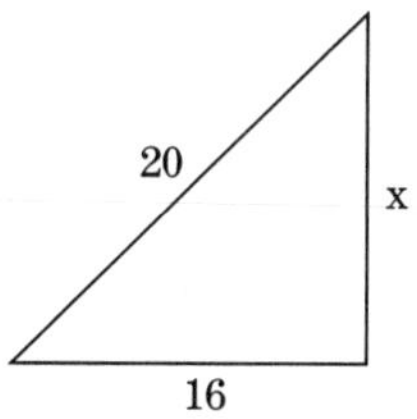

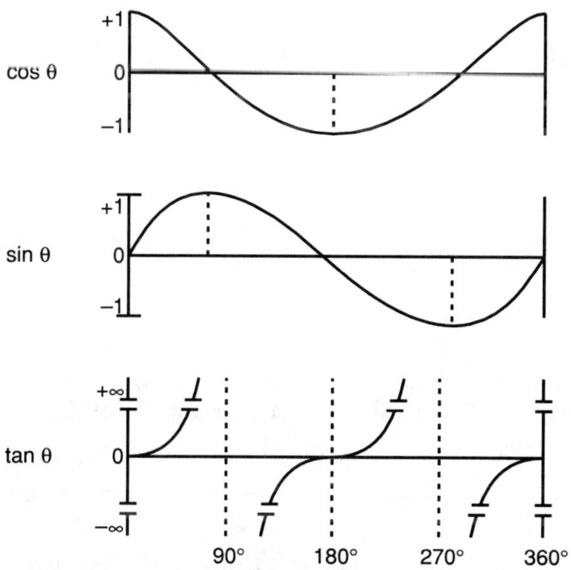

Figure 5-10 Graphical Representation of Trigonometric Functions

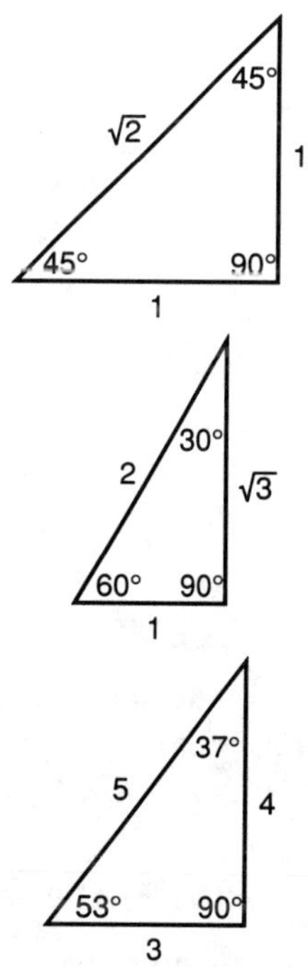

Figure 5-11 Trigonometric Elements for 45° −45° −90°, 30° −60° −90°, and 37° −53° −90° Triangles

Exercise 22. Find x and y.

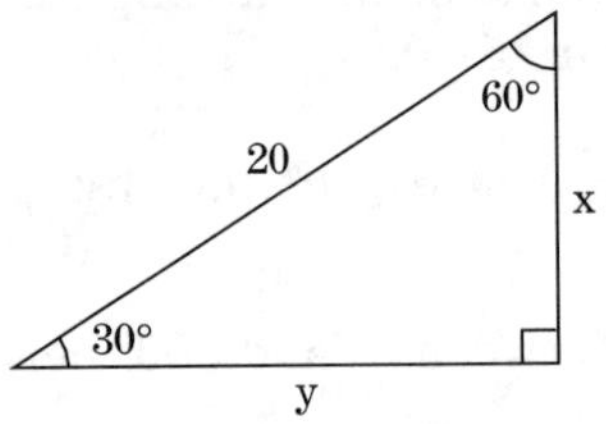

An alternative angular measure is the radian (1 radian = 57.3°). A complete revolution around a point is 360°; the same revolution is represented by 2p radians. Normally, this value is written as 2π; the unit of radians is assumed. The 2π to 360° equivalence determines the proportionality of the two angular measures (e.g., 180° = π, 90° = $\pi/2$, 720° = 4π).

Exercise 23. Express 30°, 45°, and 60° in radian units.

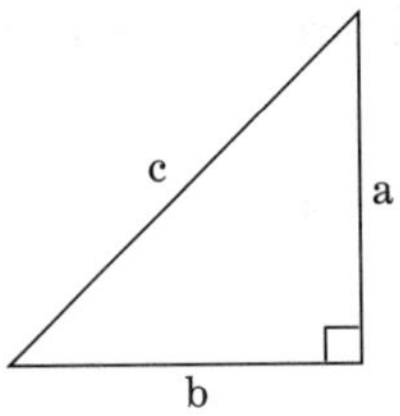

The Pythagorean theorem has many applications in solving problems on the VETs:

$$a^2 + b^2 = c^2$$

Exercise 24. Find b.

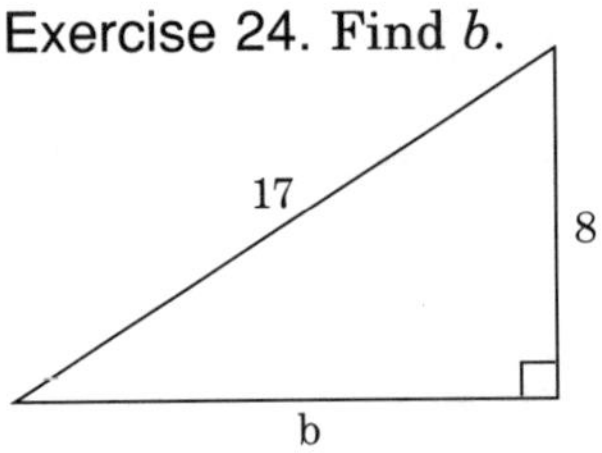

Exercise 25. Evaluate $\sin^2\theta + \cos^2\theta$, and express the answer in simplest form.

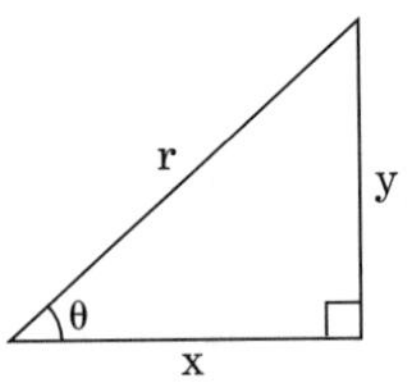

5.11 WORD PROBLEMS

Word problems cause students anxiety because they are often difficult and require multiple steps. In addition to mathematical concepts, word problems require understanding of a specific situation. Science-related problems require basic knowledge of force, weight, or other concepts.

5.11.1 Solving Word Problems

1. Read the problem quickly to familiarize yourself with it. Then read it carefully in detail (i.e., sentence by sentence or phrase by phrase) to identify all of the elements of the problem, their relation, and the information needed to answer the question.

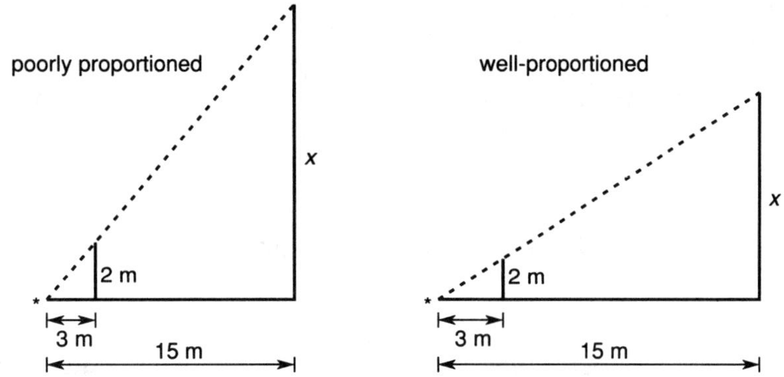

Figure 5-12 Sketching Problem Data

2. Draw a picture to represent the elements of the problem (Figure 5-12).
3. Summarize the problem. It is likely to say that one quantity equals another. Write an equation, using words, not algebraic symbols, to connect or relate the elements of the problem.
4. Use an algebraic symbol (i.e., x, y, or another variable) to represent the unknown element. Clearly state what the symbol represents.
5. Use the unknown variable to construct algebraic statements of the values of other elements of the problem.
6. Write an equation with the algebraic expressions (i.e., variables).
7. Solve the algebraic equation for the numerical value of the variable.
8. Use the value of the variable to answer all of the questions asked in the problem.
9. Check the answers against the statements and data in the original problem.
10. State the required answers in a sentence.

For example:

Use the suggestions for solving word problems to complete the following problem. Write out all of the steps.

A man who is 2 m tall stands 3 m from an intense source of light at the level of his feet. The man's shadow appears on a wall 15 m from the source of light. How tall is the shadow?

A. 6 m
B. 10 m
C. 12.5 m
D. 17.5 m

If you recognize that this problem involves similar triangles, you can create a ratio according to the rule for comparing similar triangles: $3/15 = 2/x$. Because errors are easily made when students work quickly, tests often include an answer choice that reflects a careless error. For example, if your answer was 6, you probably put 12 in place of 15 in the ratio. Solving this problem is simple only if the preliminary steps are completed correctly. This exercise is not difficult in terms of either content or mathematics, but it requires careful thought.

Many students attempt to save time by skipping steps while solving problems; however, skipping steps can lead to errors. Some students draw a diagram accurately and then attempt to solve for the hypotenuse. This complicated and time-consuming task does not yield the correct answer, although a distracter may match this answer.

5.11.2 Percentage Problems

Problems involving percents are described in section 5.4.2.

5.11.3 Ratio and Proportion Problems

A ratio is the comparison by division of two quantities expressed in the same units. For example, if the height of two poles is in the ratio of 3 to 7, one pole may be 3 feet high, and the other may be 7 feet high. A colon (:) is used to indicate ratio. The ratio of the height of the poles is written 3:7 or as the fraction 3/7.

For example:
Ann has $300 saved. Bob has $1200 saved. Compare Ann's savings with Bob's savings.

$$\frac{\text{Ann}}{\text{Bob}} = \frac{3}{12} = \frac{1}{4}$$

A proportion states that two ratios are equal. For example, the ratios 2:3 and 4:6 are equal and form a proportion, which may be written as 2:3 = 4:6, or 2:3::4:6. The proportion 2:3::4:6 is read "2 is to 3 as 4 is to 6." The inside numbers, 3 and 4, are known as the means, and the outside numbers, 2 and 6, are known as the extremes. In any proportion, the product of the means is equal to the product of the extremes. For example, 3:4 = 6:8 is a proportion; the product of the means, 4 and 6, is 24, and the product of the extremes, 3 and 8, is 24.

For example:
Find a if $3:5 = a:15$

$$\frac{3}{5} = \frac{a}{15}$$

$$5a = 3(15)$$

$$a = \frac{45}{5}$$

$$a = 9$$

Example: A blood sample from dog A contains 2850 white blood cells (*WBC*) and 5,000,000 red blood cells (*RBC*). How does this finding compare with a blood sample from dog B that has a 1000:1 ratio of red blood cells to white blood cells?

Solution:

$$\frac{5{,}000{,}000\ RBC}{2850\ WBC} = \frac{\times\ RBC}{1\ WBC}\left[\text{Approximate } \frac{5 \times 10^6}{2850} = \frac{5 \times 10^6}{3000} \approx 1667\right]$$

$$\frac{1754\ RBC}{WBC} = \frac{\times\ RBC}{1\ WBC}$$

The ratio is 1754.

Dog A has a ratio of red blood cells to white blood cells of 1754:1, whereas dog B has a ratio of 1000:1.

5.11.4 Distance, Rate, and Time Problems

Distance problems are solved based on the equation $d = rt$, where d is distance traveled, r is rate of travel, and t is time spent traveling.

For example:
To avoid attack, a gazelle outruns a lion at the rate of 20 mph for 1-1/2 hours. How far does the gazelle travel?

Solution: The distance is the rate traveled multiplied by the time:

$$d = r \times t$$

$$d = \frac{20 \text{ miles}}{\text{hours}} \times 1.5 \text{ hours} = 30 \text{ miles}$$

The answer is 30 miles.

Example: A kangaroo travels 11 miles in 0.5 hours. What is its average speed?

Solution: The rate is the distance divided by the time:
$r = d/t$
$r = 11 \div 0.5$
$r = 22$
The speed is 22 mph.

5.11.5 Motion Problems

Combined quantities involve more than one distance, rate, or time. For example, the rate at which two objects approach each other when traveling toward each other or in directly opposite directions and the rate at which they separate is the sum of their respective rates. The problem may state the total distance traveled by both objects, or it may state that the two objects travel the same distance.

For example:

A car that is traveling at 30 mph leaves Austin, Texas. Two hours later, a second car that is traveling at 50 mph on the same road leaves Austin. In how many hours will the second car pass the first car?

Draw a diagram to illustrate the situation.

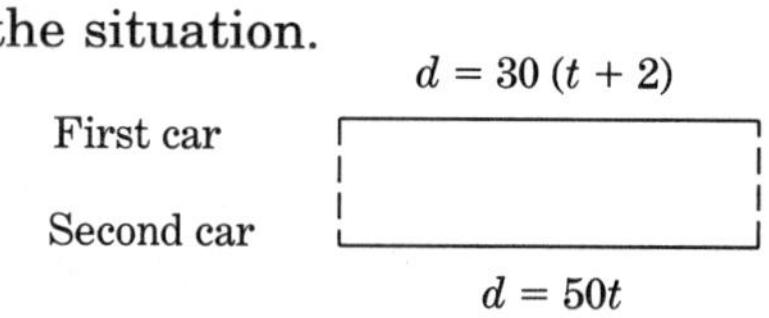

For each object, write a variable expression for the distance, rate, and time. The results can be recorded in a table.

The first car traveled 2 hours longer than the second car.

	Rate	× Time	= Distance
First car	30	$t + 2$	$30\ (t + 2)$
Second car	50	t	$60t$

Determine the relation of the distance traveled by each car.

$30\ (t + 2) = 50t$
$30t + 60 = 50t$
$60 = 50\ t - 30t$
$60 = 20t$
$3 = t$
The second car will pass the first car in 3 hours.

Example: Two runners, Beth and Paul, run the same course. Paul's speed is 2 mph slower than Beth's. Beth finishes the course in 4 hours, and Paul finishes in 6 hours. What is the speed of each runner, and how long is the course?

Solution: Let r = Beth's rate and $r - 2$ = Paul's rate. Since $d = rt$, Beth's distance is $r \times 4$, and Paul's distance is $(r - 2)6$.

	Rate	× Time	= Distance
Beth	r	4	$4r$
Paul	$r - 2$	6	$6(r - 2)$

$4r = 6r - 12$
$12 = 2r$
$6 = r$
Beth's rate is 6 mph, and Paul's rate is 4 mph.

The length of the course can be determined by applying the formula $d = rt$ to either runner's rate.

Using Beth's rate:
$d = rt$
$d = 6 \times 4$
$d = 24$

The course is 24 miles long.

5.11.6 Average Rate Problems

To average two or more rates when the time is the same for both rates, add the rates and divide the sum by the number of rates.

For example:
If Joanne travels at 40 mph for 4 hours, at 50 mph for the next 4 hours, and at 60 mph for the next 4 hours, then her average rate for the 12 hours is $(40 + 50 + 60) \div 3 = 50$ mph.

To average two or more rates when the times are not the same, but the distances are the same, assume the distance to be a convenient length, find the time at each given rate, and find the sum of the distances. Divide the sum by the total time to find the average rate.

For example:
If Steve travels to his brother's house at the rate of 40 mph and returns at the rate of 20 mph, what is the average rate for both trips?

Solution: Assume that the distance is the same for both trips (80 miles).
Time for first trip: $80 \div 40 = 2$ hours
Time for return trip: $80 \div 20 = 4$ hours
Total distance: 160 miles
Total time: 6 hours

Average rate: $160 \div 6 = 26\frac{2}{3}$

Steve's average rate is $26\frac{2}{3}$ mph.

Example: Tom travels 200 miles at 40 mph, 100 miles at 50 mph, and 60 miles at 20 mph. What is the average rate for the three trips?

Solution:
Time for first trip: $200 \div 40 = 5$ hours
Time for second trip: $100 \div 50 = 2$ hours
Time for third trip: $60 \div 20 = 3$ hours
Total distance: $200 + 100 + 60 = 360$ miles
Total time: $5 + 2 + 3 = 10$ hours
Average rate: $360 \div 10 = 36$
The average rate is 36 mph.

Example: If John's car travels 200 miles and uses 8 gallons of gas, what is its gas consumption rate?

Solution: Gas consumption = distance in miles ÷ number of gallons
$200 \div 8 = 25$

The gas consumption rate is 25 miles per gallon.

5.11.7 Work Rate Problems

Work rate problems involve finding the rate at which two or more people working together can complete a task. If the rate at which each person works alone is known, the rate at which they work together can be determined.

To solve work rate problems, find the fraction of the task each person can complete in the time given, multiply each fraction by x, set the sum of the fractions equal to 1, and solve for x. The numerator is the time spent working. The denominator is the total time needed to perform the task if each person works alone.

Example: Working alone, Karen can rake all of the leaves in the front yard in 3 hours. Mark can rake the leaves alone in 2 hours. How long will it take Mark and Karen working together to rake the leaves?

Solution: Express the fraction of the task each can complete in 1 hour. If Karen can complete the entire task in 3 hours, she can complete 1/3 in 1 hour. If Mark can complete the entire task in 1 hour, he can complete 1/2 in 1 hour. Express the fraction of the task each person can complete in x hours, where x = time to complete the task together.

$\frac{1}{3}x$ = fraction of the task Karen can complete in x hours

$\frac{1}{2}x$ = fraction of the job Mark can complete in x hours

Set the sum of the two fractions equal to 1, and solve for x.

$$\frac{1}{2}x + \frac{1}{3}x = 1$$

$$\frac{5}{6}x = 1$$

$$x = \frac{6}{5}$$

Working together, Karen and Mark can rake the leaves in 1.2 hours.

5.11.8 Odd and Even Integer Problems

Integers are real numbers. They consist of negative numbers, zero, and positive numbers. The set of even integers is (. . . −4, −2, 0, 2, 4, . . .). All even integers are divisible by 2. The set of odd integers is (. . . −3, −1, 0, 1, 3, . . .).

Consecutive integers are integers that are listed in consecutive order. If n is even, three consecutive even integers are n, $n + 2$, $n + 4$ (e.g., if $n = 2$, the three consecutive even integers are 2, 4, and 6). If n is an odd integer, three consecutive odd integers are n, $n + 2$, $n + 4$ (e.g., if $n = 1$, then the three consecutive odd integers are 3, 5, and 7).

For example:
Find five consecutive odd integers that have a sum of 45.

Solution:
Let n represent the smallest integer in the series. The other four integers are expressed in terms of n. Consecutive integers differ by 1; therefore, consecutive odd integers differ by 2.

Let n = first odd integer
$n + 2$ = second odd integer
$n + 4$ = third odd integer
$n + 6$ = fourth odd integer
$n + 8$ = fifth odd integer

$$(n) + (n + 2) + (n + 4) + (n + 6) = (n + 8) = 45$$

$$5n + 20 = 45$$

$$5n = 45 - 20$$

$$5n = 25$$

$$n = 5$$

The integers are 5, 7, 9, 11, and 13.

Example: Find three consecutive even integers such that the first equals the sum of the second and third.

A. 0, −2, −4
B. −6, −4, −2
C. 4, 6, 8
D. 8, 10, 12
E. −8, −10, −12

Solution:
Let n = first integer
$n + 2$ = second integer
$n + 4$ = third integer
$n = (n + 2) + (n + 4)$
$n = 2n + 6$
$-6 = n$

The answer is **B**.

5.11.9 Coin or Stamp Problems

To solve coin or stamp problems, convert the value of the coins or stamps to dollars and cents (e.g., multiply the number of nickels by 5 because \$.05 = 1 nickel).

For example: A cash register contains \$30.90 in nickels and quarters. If there are 130 coins in all, how many of each coin are in the cash register?

Solution:
Let x = number of nickels
$130 - x$ = number of quarters
Number of nickels × value of nickels = value in cents
$x \times 5 = 5$
Number of quarters × value of quarters = value in cents
$130 - x \times 25 = 25(130 - x)$
Value of nickels + value of quarters = total value in cents
$5x + 25(130 - x) = 3090$
$5x - 25x + 3250 = 3090$
$-20x = 3090 - 3250$
$20x = 160$
$x = 8$
$130 - x = 130 - 8 = 122$

The answer is 8 nickels and 122 quarters.

Check: $8(0.05) + 122(0.25) = 0.40 + 30.50 = \$30.90$

Example: Michael has 100 stamps with a total value of \$18.00. Some stamps are worth 15¢ each, and the others are worth 30¢ each. How many stamps of each type does he have?

Solution:
Let x = number of 15¢ stamps
$100 - x$ = number of 30¢ stamps
Number of stamps × value of stamps = value in cents
$x \times 15 = 15x$
$100 - x \times 30 = 30\,(100 - x)$

Value of 15¢ stamps + value of 30¢ stamps = total value in cents
$15x + 30(100 - x) = 1800$
$15x + 30\,(100 - x) = 1800$

$$15x + 3000 - 30x = 1800$$
$$15x - 30x = 1800 - 3000$$
$$-15x = -1200$$
$$x = 80$$
$$100x = 100 - 80 = 20$$

Michael has 80 stamps worth 15¢ and 20 stamps worth 30¢.

5.11.10 Age Problems

Age problems compare current, future, and past ages. If current age is represented by x, then future age is found by adding years to x. If current age is represented by x, then past age is found by subtracting years from x.

For example:
Kate is 36 years old when her daughter Laura is born. How old will Laura be when her age is 1/4 of Kate's age? How old will Kate be?

Solution:
Let x = Laura's age
$x + 36$ = Kate's age

$$x = \frac{1}{4}(x + 36)$$
$$x = \frac{x}{4} + 9$$
$$x - \frac{x}{4} = 9$$
$$4x - x = 36$$
$$3x = 36$$
$$x = 12$$
$$x + 36 = 48$$

Laura's age will be 12 years, and Kate's age will be 48 years.

5.12 SOLUTIONS TO EXERCISES

1. (A) $4^7 \ \frac{4^4 \times 4^8}{4^5} = 4^{4+8-5} = 4^7$

(B) $6 \left(\frac{6^4}{6^2}\right) \times 6^{-5} = (6^2)^3 \times 6^{-5} = 6^{6-5} = 6$

(C) $1 \ (7^4)^0 = 1;$ recall $x^0 = 1$

2. (A) $1296 = 216^{4/3} = (\sqrt[3]{216^4}) = 6^4$
$= 216^1 \times (\sqrt[3]{216}) = 216 \times 6$

(B) $64 = 256^{3/4} = (256^{1/4})^3 = 4^3$

(C) $(ab)^{7/12} = \frac{\sqrt{ab} \times \sqrt[4]{a^3b^3}}{\sqrt[3]{a^2b^2}} = \frac{(ab)^{1/2}(ab)^{3/4}}{(ab)^{2/3}}$
$= (ab)^{1/2 + 3/4 - 2/3} = (ab)^{6/12 + 9/12 - 8/12}$

(D) $\frac{25}{9} = \left(\frac{3}{5}\right)^{-8} \left(\frac{9}{25}\right)^3 = \frac{3^{-8}}{5^{-8}} \times \frac{3^6}{5^6} = \frac{3^{-2}}{5^{-2}} = \frac{5^2}{3^2}$

3. (A) $x = -2 = \log_4 \left(\frac{1}{16}\right) = x; \quad 4^x = \frac{1}{16}$

(B) $x = \frac{b}{2} = \log_z{}^2$
$(Z^b) = x; \quad Z^{2x} = Z^b; \quad b = 2x$

(C) x = any real number except zero

$\log_x 1 = 0; \quad x^0 = 1$

(D) $x = 625 = 5^{\log_5 625} = x = \log_5 625 = \log_5 x$

(E) $x = 256 = 4^{\log_2 16}; \quad x = 4^4$

4. (A) $\log\left(\dfrac{M^2N^7}{\sqrt[3]{P}}\right) = \log M^2 + 7\log_N - \dfrac{1}{3}\log_P$

$= \log M^2 + \log_N{}^7 - \log {}_3\sqrt{P}$

(B) $\dfrac{19}{4}\log_x = \log\sqrt{x^5} \quad -3\log\ {}^4\sqrt{x} + \log_x{}^3$

$\log_x{}^{5/2} - \log x^{3/4} + \log_x{}^3$

$= \dfrac{5}{2}\log_x - \dfrac{3}{4}\log_x + 3\log_x$

$= \left(\dfrac{5}{2} - \dfrac{3}{4} + 3\right)\log_x = \dfrac{19}{4}\log_x = \log_x{}^{19/4}$

5. (A) $x = 2 = \log_9(x + 1) = \dfrac{1}{2}; \quad x + 1 = 9^{1/2} = 3$

(B) $x = {}^3\sqrt{\dfrac{a^2b^3c^4}{d^5}} \quad 3\log_x = 2\log_a + 3\log_b + 4\log_c \quad - 5\log_d$

$\log_x = \dfrac{1}{3}(\log_a{}^2 + \log_b{}^3 + \log_c{}^4 - \log_d{}^5)$

$\log_x = \log\left(\dfrac{a^2b^3c^4}{d^5}\right)^{1/3}$

6. For Group I, list the data in ascending order: 191, 194, 195, 195, 195, 196, 196, 198, 199; then determine the smallest value (i.e., 191), largest value (i.e., 199), and range (i.e., 199 − 191 = 8). The data are bimodal (i.e., 195 and 196); therefore, the average is approximately 195 or 196. Few values are found at the extremes of the range (191 and 199), but many are found in the middle (195 and196)

For Group II, list the data in ascending order: 193, 194, 196, 199, 201, 202, 202, 204, 204, 205; then determine the smallest value (i.e., 193), largest value (i.e., 205), and range (i.e., 205 − 193 = 12). The average is approximately (199 + 205)/2 = 199. The values cluster toward the high end of the range.

7. In Group I, the percentage with blood cholesterol levels of 196 or lower = 8/10 × 100 = 80%. In Group II, the percentage with blood cholesterol levels of 196 or lower = 3/10 × 100 = 30%.

8. Group I does not have a unique mode because 195 and 196 both appear three times.

$$\text{Median} = \frac{195 + 196}{2} = 195.5$$

$$\text{Average} = \frac{191 + 194 + 3(195) + 3(196) + 198 + 199}{10} = 195.5$$

Both the average and the median are good measures of the central tendency of the data for Group I.

Group II does not have a unique mode because 202 and 204 both appear twice.

$$\text{Median} = \frac{201 + 202}{2} = 201.5$$

$$\text{Average} = \frac{193 + 194 + 196 + 199 + 201 + 2(202) + 2(204) + 205}{10} = 200$$

Qualitatively, the average reflects the spread of data at the lower end of the range, whereas the median reflects the data at the high end of the range.

9. In Group I, the range $= 199 - 191 = 8$

$$V = \frac{(191 - 196)^2 + (194 - 196)^2 + \ldots + (198 - 196)^2 + (199 - 196)^2}{10}$$

$= 4.5 \approx 5$

$SD = \sqrt{V} = \sqrt{5} = (2.236) \approx 2$

In Group II, the range $= 205 - 193 = 12$

$$V = \frac{(193 - 200)^2 + (194 - 200)^2 + \ldots + 2(204 - 200)^2 + (205 - 200)^2}{10}$$

$= 16.8 \approx 17$

$SD = \sqrt{V} = \sqrt{17} = 4.123 \approx 4$

10. $a = \dfrac{r^2 + sp - q}{s - t}$

$s(a - p) + q = ta + r^2$
$sa - sp + q = ta + r^2$
$a(s - t) = r^2 + sp - q$

11. $d = -13$

$\dfrac{1}{d - 2} + \dfrac{2}{d + 3} = \dfrac{4}{d - 2}$ [Multiply through by $(d - 2)(d + 3)$]

$d + 3 + 2(d - 2) = 4(d + 3)$
$3d - 1 = 4d + 12$

12. $x = \dfrac{13}{5}$

$3(4x - 2[1 - (x + 5) + 3]) = 13x + 19$
$3[4x - 2(4 - x - 5)] = 13x + 19$
$3(4x + 2x + 2) = 13x + 19$
$18x + 6 = 13x + 1$

13. $C = \dfrac{21}{5}$ moles

Let $x_1 = 5$ moles of B and $y_1 = 3$ moles of C
$x_2 = 7$ moles of B and $y_2 =$ number of moles of C
Since B and C are directly proportional:

$\dfrac{y_2}{7} = \dfrac{3}{5}$

$y_2 = \dfrac{21}{5}$

14. $r = 0.05$ gallons/mile
From the problem, $xy = a$, where:
$x =$ gas consumption rate (gallons/mile),
$y =$ number of miles that the car can travel on a full tank of gas
$a =$ number of gallons in a full tank of gas (constant)
Thus, x and y are inversely proportional with $x_1 = r$,
$y_1 = 400$, $x_2 = \mathrm{r} - 0.01$, and $y_2 = 500$
$r(400) = (r - 0.01)500$
$400r = 500r - 5$

15. $\dfrac{p_1V_1}{T_1} = \dfrac{p_2V_2}{T_2}$

$\dfrac{V}{T} p_1V_1 = RT_1$ and $p_2V_2 = RT_2$ can be rewritten as:

$$\frac{p_1V_1}{T_1} = R \quad \text{and} \quad \frac{p_2V_2}{T_2} = R$$

Therefore, the two states are related by:

$$\frac{p_1V_1}{T_1} = \frac{p_2V_2}{T_2}$$

From the definition of inversely proportional variables, if p is one variable, then the other variable is V/T.

16. 1991 cost = $2500

$$\text{1991 cost} = \$2500 + \frac{20}{100} \times \$2500 = \$3000$$

$$\text{1993 cost} = \$3000 + \frac{10}{100} \times \$3000 = \$3300$$

$$\text{1994 cost} = \$3300 - \frac{30}{100} \times \$3300 = \$2310$$

The 1994 price is $2310.

17. Using the right triangle definitions of the trigonometric functions:

$\sin A = \frac{7}{25}$, $\cos A = \frac{24}{25}$, and $\tan A = \frac{7}{24}$

18. Using the right triangle definitions:

$\sin B = \frac{7}{8.6}$, $\cos B = \frac{5}{8.6}$, and $\tan B = \frac{7}{5}$

19. Reading values directly from the graph, the following table can be constructed:

	θ			
Function	**0°**	**90°**	**180°**	**270°**
$\sin\theta$	0	1	0	−1
$\cos\theta$	1	0	−1	0
$\tan\theta$	0	∞	0	∞
	Undefined		Undefined	

20. Using the right triangles shown, the following table can be constructed:

	θ		
Function	**30°**	**45°**	**60°**
$\sin\theta$	$\frac{1}{2}$	$\frac{\sqrt{2}}{2}$	$\frac{\sqrt{3}}{2}$
$\cos\theta$	$\frac{\sqrt{3}}{2}$	$\frac{\sqrt{2}}{2}$	$\frac{1}{2}$
$\tan\theta$	$\frac{1}{\sqrt{3}}$	1	$\sqrt{3}$

21. This triangle is a 3-4-5 right triangle. A 3-4-5 right triangle is recognized by noting a combination of any two sides in the ratio 3:4, 4:5, or 3:5; the third is the missing side. This triangle corresponds to the following known triangle:

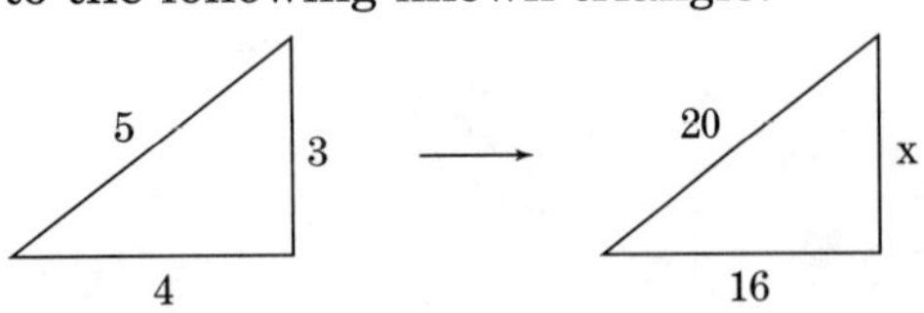

Because these triangles are similar, the corresponding sides are proportional:

$$\frac{x}{3} = \frac{20}{5}$$

or

$$\frac{x}{3} = \frac{16}{4}$$

In either case, $x = 12$.

22. $\sin 30° = \frac{x}{20}$; $x = 20 \sin 30° = 20\left(\frac{1}{2}\right) = 10$

$\cos 30° = \frac{y}{20}$; $y = 20 \cos 30° = 20\left(\frac{\sqrt{3}}{2}\right) = 10\sqrt{3}$

23. Using the proportionality based on the equivalence of 360° and 2π:

$\frac{30°}{360°} = \frac{x}{2\pi} = x = \frac{\pi}{6}$; $30° = \frac{\pi}{6}$

$\frac{45°}{360°} = \frac{x}{2\pi} = x = \frac{\pi}{4}$; $45° = \frac{\pi}{4}$

$\frac{60°}{360°} = \frac{x}{2\pi} = x = \frac{\pi}{3}$; $60° = \frac{\pi}{3}$

24. Using the Pythagorean theorem:

$b^2 + 8^2 = 17^2$

$b^2 + 64 = 289$

$b^2 = 225$

$b = 15$

25. $\sin \theta = \frac{y}{r}$ and $\cos \theta = \frac{x}{r}$

Using the Pythagorean theorem:

$x^2 + y^2 = r^2$

$\sin^2\theta + \cos^2\theta = \frac{y^2}{r^2} + \frac{x^2}{r^2} = \frac{x^2 + y^2}{r^2} = \frac{r^2}{r^2} = 1$

5.13 SAMPLE TEST

1. If $\frac{1}{3}(x - 2) \leq \frac{x + 2}{6}$, then

A. $x \geq 6$
B. $x \leq 6$
C. $x \leq 4$
D. $x \geq 3$

2. Simplify: $\frac{-3}{4} + \frac{1}{6} - \frac{5}{8}$

A. $\frac{5}{4}$
B. $1\frac{5}{4}$
C. $\frac{-5}{4}$
D. $-1\frac{5}{24}$

3. $3\frac{1}{3} \times 2\frac{1}{2} = ?$

A. 6
B. 3
C. $6\frac{1}{6}$
D. $8\frac{1}{3}$

4. Simplify $(a^3b^{-2})^{-2}$ to a form in which the exponents are positive.

A. $\frac{b^4}{a^6}$
B. $\frac{1}{a^2b}$
C. $\frac{a^6}{b^4}$
D. a^2b

5. $\dfrac{\sqrt{12}\,\sqrt{2}}{\sqrt{18}} = ?$

A. $\frac{2}{5}$

B. $\frac{2\sqrt{5}}{5}$

C. $\frac{\sqrt{3}}{6}$

D. $\frac{2\sqrt{3}}{3}$

6. If $\dfrac{x-2}{x+2} = \dfrac{2}{3}$, then $x = ?$

A. 6
B. no value possible
C. 5
D. 10

7. David drives his car until the gas tank is ⅙ full. He fills the tank to capacity by putting in 15 gallons of gas. What is the capacity of the gas tank?

A. 12 gallons
B. 15 gallons
C. 18 gallons
D. 21 gallons

8. Water is 70% of the total body weight of an adult dog. If a dog weighs 60 lb, how much of its weight is water?

A. 36 lb
B. 42 lb
C. 52 lb
D. 58 lb

9. Jeff insures 60% of his property and pays a 2½% premium of $348.00. What is the total value of the property?

A. $19,000
B. $18,000
C. $18,400
D. $23,200

10. If the scale of a blueprint is ⅛ inch = 1 foot, what is the actual length of a wall 8½ inches by scale?

A. 5 ⅔ feet
B. 8.5 feet
C. 102 feet
D. 68 feet

11. A litter of puppies consists of pups with the following weights: 0.2 lb, 0.3 lb, 0.4 lb, 0.5 lb, 0.6 lb, 0.7 lb, 0.7 lb, 0.5.lb, 0.6 lb, 0.6 lb, 0.2 lb. If Matthew chooses a puppy at random, what is the probability that he will choose a 0.6-lb puppy?

A. $\frac{2}{9}$

B. $\frac{3}{11}$

C. $\frac{8}{11}$

D. $\frac{3}{8}$

12. A farmer needs a trough to feed his livestock. Find the perimeter of a trough with the following dimensions (use 3.14 for π).

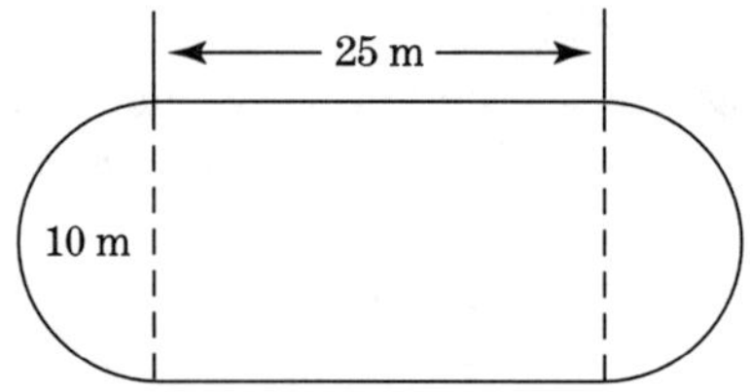

A. 81.4
B. 101.4
C. 112.8
D. 56

13. Find the area of the following figure (use 3.14 for π).

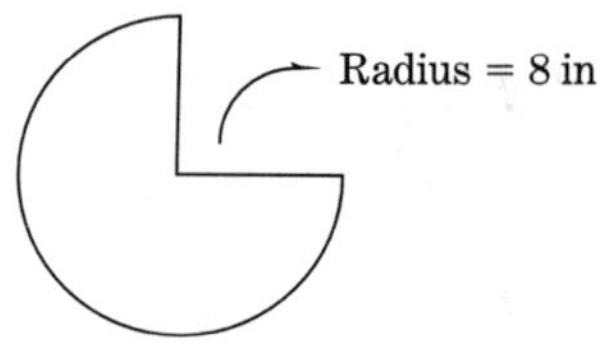

A. 150.72 in^2
B. 200.96 in^2
C. 602.88 in^2
D. 25.12 in^2

14. A 25-foot ladder is placed against a building at a point 20 feet from the ground. Find the distance from the base of the building to the base of the ladder.

A. 25 feet
B. 30 feet
C. 45 feet
D. 15 feet

15. Triangles ABC and DEF are similar. Find the area of triangle DEF.

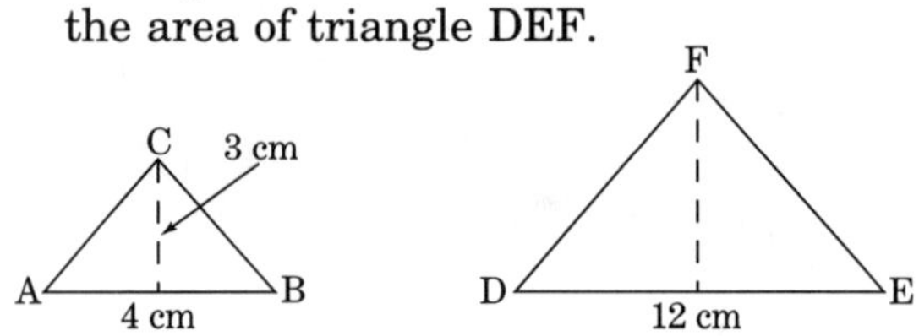

A. 36 cm^2
B. 54 cm^2
C. 48 cm^2
D. 144 cm^2

16. Find the slope of the line whose equation is $y = -\frac{1}{4}x - 1$.
   A. $\frac{1}{4}$
   B. -1
   C. $-\frac{1}{4}$
   D. 1

17. The value of cot q is equal to:
   A. $\sin\theta / \cos\theta$
   B. $\cos q / \sin q$
   C. $1 / \sec\theta$
   D. $1 / \sin q$

18. Determine cos q if P is a point on the terminal side q and the coordinates of P are $P(-3, 4)$.
   A. $\cos q = -\frac{3}{5}$
   B. $\cos q = \frac{3}{5}$
   C. $\cos q = -\frac{4}{3}$
   D. $\cos q = -\frac{5}{3}$

19. If 25% of the dogs in a veterinarian's practice have heartworms, then the ratio of dogs with heartworms to dogs without heartworms is:
   A. 4:1
   B. 10:40
   C. 300:100
   D. 25:1

20. If Chris can finish a job in 3 hours and Kathryn can finish it in 4 hours, how long will it take them if they work together?
   A. $3\frac{1}{2}$ hours
   B. 7 hours
   C. $1\frac{5}{12}$ hours
   D. $1\frac{5}{7}$ hours

5.14 ANSWER KEY

1. B	**6. D**	**11. B**	**16. C**
2. D	**7. C**	**12. A**	**17. C**
3. D	**8. B**	**13. A**	**18. A**
4. A	**9. D**	**14. D**	**19. C**
5. D	**10. D**	**15. B**	**20. D**

5.15 SOLUTIONS TO SAMPLE TEST

1. **[B]** Clear the fraction by multiplying both sides of the inequality by the greatest common denominator, which is 6.

$$6\left[\frac{1}{3}\left(x - 2\right)\right] \leq 6\,\frac{(x + 2)}{6}$$
$$2(x - 2) \leq x + 2$$
$$2x - 4 \leq x + 2$$
$$2x - x \leq 4 + 2$$
$$x \leq 6$$

2. **[D]** Find the least common multiple of 4, 6, and 8.
   4 = 4, 8, 12, 16, 20, 24
   6 = 6, 12, 18, 24
   8 = 8, 16, 24
   Least common multiple: 24

$$\frac{-3}{4} + \frac{1}{6} - \frac{5}{8} = \frac{-18}{24} + \frac{4}{24} - \frac{15}{24}$$
$$= \frac{-18 + 4 - 15}{24}$$
$$= \frac{-29}{24} = -1\frac{5}{24}$$

3. [D] Convert the numbers to improper fractions.

$$3\frac{1}{3} = \frac{9}{3} + \frac{1}{3} = \frac{10}{3}$$

$$2\frac{1}{2} = \frac{4}{2} + \frac{1}{2} = \frac{5}{2}$$

$$\frac{10}{3} \times \frac{5}{2} = \frac{2 \times 5}{3} \times \frac{5}{2} = \frac{25}{3} = 8\frac{1}{3}$$

4. [A] Use the rule for exponential notation and negative exponents.

$$(a^3b^{-2})^{-2} = (a^3)^{-2}(b^{-2})^{-2} = a^{-6}b^4 = \frac{b^4}{a^6}$$

5. [D]

$$\frac{\sqrt{12}\sqrt{2}}{\sqrt{18}} = \frac{\sqrt{2}\sqrt{6}\sqrt{2}}{\sqrt{2}\sqrt{9}}$$

$$= \frac{\sqrt{12}}{3}$$

$$= \frac{\sqrt{3}\sqrt{4}}{3}$$

$$= \frac{2\sqrt{3}}{3}$$

6. [D] $\frac{x - 1}{x + 1} = \frac{2}{3}$

$$2(x + 2) = 3(x - 2)$$
$$2x + 4 = 3x - 6$$
$$2x - 3x = -6 - 4$$
$$-x = -10$$
$$x = 10$$

7. [C] If the gas tank is ⅙ full, then an additional ⅚ capacity is left.

$\frac{5}{6}$ capacity = 15 gallons; therefore

$$15 \div \frac{5}{6} = \frac{15}{1} \times \frac{6}{5}$$

$$= \frac{3 \times 5}{1} \times \frac{2 \times 3}{5} = 18$$

8. [B] 60 lb (0.70) = 42 lb

9. [D] Find the solution in two steps: 2½ % of the insured value = $348.

Find the insured value using the formula $\frac{R}{100} = \frac{P}{B}$

$$R = 2\frac{1}{2}\%$$
$$P = \$348$$

$$\frac{2\frac{1}{2}}{100} = \frac{348}{B}$$

Find B. $2\frac{1}{2}B = 348\ (100)$

$$B = \frac{34800}{5/2}$$

$$B = \frac{34800}{1} \times \frac{2}{5} = 13{,}920$$

The insured value = \$13,920

The insured value (\$13,920) is 60% of the total value. Find the total value:

$R = 60\%$

$\frac{60}{100} = \frac{13920}{B}$

$P = 13{,}920$

Find B.

$60B = 13{,}920 \times 100$

$B = \frac{13920 \times (10)(10)}{(6)(10)}$

$B = \frac{139200}{6} = 23{,}200$

10. **[D]** $\frac{1}{8}$ inch = 1 foot

$8\frac{1}{8}$ inches $\div \frac{1 \text{ inch}}{8 \text{ foot}} = \frac{17}{2}$ inch $\times \frac{8 \text{ foot}}{1 \text{ inch}} = 68$ feet

11. **[B]** Each puppy has an equally likely chance of being chosen. Three puppies weigh 0.6 lb. There are 11 possible outcomes.

Probability of choosing a 0.6-lb puppy $= \frac{\text{Number of 0.6-lb puppies}}{\text{Number of puppies}}$

$P(M) = \frac{3}{11}$

12. **[A]** Perimeter = 2(circumference of semicircle) + (perimeter of rectangle) − 2(width)

$P = 2\frac{(\pi d)}{2} + 2(L + W) - 2W$

$P = 2\frac{[3.14(10)]}{2} + 2(25 + 10) - 2(10)$

$P = 3.14\,(10) + 70 - 20$

$P = 31.4 + 50$

$P = 81.4$ m

13. **[A]** Use the formula: area $= \pi r^2$. The figure is 3/4 of a circle. To find the area of 3/4 of the circle, determine 3/4 of the area. Therefore:

$A = \frac{3}{4}\pi r^2$

$A = \frac{3}{4} \times 3.14(8)^2$

$A = \frac{3}{4} \times 200.96 = \frac{602.88}{4}$

$A = 150.72 \text{ in}^2$

14. **[D]** Draw a figure:

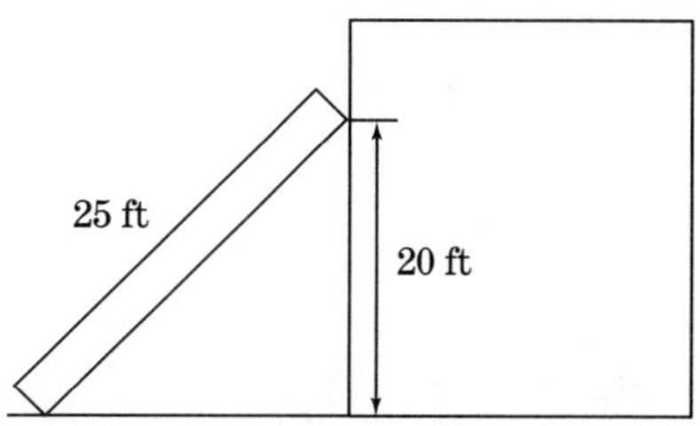

$a^2 + b^2 = c^2$

$(20 \text{ ft})^2 + b^2 = (25 \text{ ft})^2$

$400 \text{ ft}^2 + b^2 = 625 \text{ ft}^2$

$b^2 = 625 \text{ ft}^2 - 400 \text{ ft}^2$

$b^2 = \sqrt{225 \text{ ft}^2}$

$b = 15$

15. **[B]** To find the area of triangle DEF, find the height of triangle DEF, and use the formula: area = 1/2 × base × height.

$$\frac{AB}{DE} = \frac{\text{Height of triangle ABC}}{\text{Height of triangle DEF}}$$

$$\frac{4 \text{ cm}}{12 \text{ cm}} = \frac{3 \text{ cm}}{\text{Height}}$$

$$4 \text{ cm} \times \text{height} = 12 \times 3 \text{ cm}$$

$$4 \text{ cm} \times \text{height} = 36 \text{ cm}^2$$

$$\text{Height} = \frac{36 \text{ cm}^2}{4 \text{ cm}}$$

$$\text{Height} = 9 \text{ cm}$$

$$\text{Area} = \frac{1}{2} \times \text{base} \times \text{height}$$

$$A = \frac{1}{2} BH$$

$$\frac{1}{2} \times 12 \times 9 = 54$$

16. **[C]** Find two ordered pairs that solve the equation:

$$y = -\frac{1}{4}x - 1$$

$$P_1 = (0, -1)$$

$$P_2 = (1, -1\tfrac{1}{4})$$

Using the slope formula:

$$M = \frac{y_2 - y_1}{x_2 - x_1}$$

$$M = \frac{\left(-1\frac{1}{4}\right) - (-1)}{1 - 0} = \frac{-1\frac{1}{4} + 1}{1} = \frac{-1}{4}$$

17. **[C]** $\cot q = \frac{1}{\tan q}$, which is a reciprocal relation.

18. **[A]** $\cos q = \frac{-3}{5}$

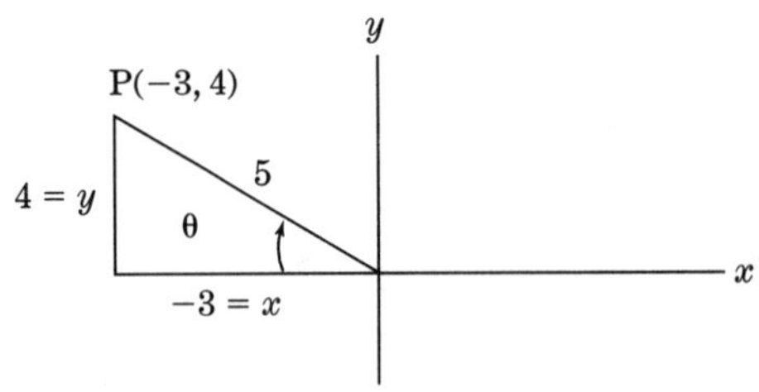

$$r = \sqrt{(-3)^2 + 4^2} = \sqrt{9 + 16} = \sqrt{25} = 5$$

$$\cos q = \frac{\text{Abscissa}}{\text{Distance}} = \frac{x}{r} = \frac{-3}{5}$$

19. **[C]** If 25% of the dogs have heartworms, then 75% are free of heartworms. The ratio of dogs with heartworms to dogs without heartworms is 3:1, or 300:100.

20. **[D]** The correct answer is lower than the shortest time given. No matter how slow a worker is, if he performs part of the task, it will be completed in less time than if he did not perform any of the task.

Let $A = \frac{x}{3}$

Let $B = \frac{x}{4}$

The sum of all individual fractions is 1.
Solve for x.

$$\frac{x}{3} + \frac{x}{4} = 1$$

Find the least common denominator.
Multiply by 12 to eliminate the fraction.

$$4x + 3x = 12$$
$$7x = 12$$
$$x = \frac{12}{7}$$
$$x = 1\frac{5}{7}$$

5.16 REFERENCES

Aufmann RN, Barker VC: *Introductory Algebra: An Applied Approach.* New York, Houghton Mifflin, 1983.

Aufmann RN, Barker VC: *Basic College Mathematics: An Applied Approach, 3rd ed.* New York, Houghton Mifflin, 1986.

Hassan A, Air DH, Bass RG, et al: *A Complete Preparation for the MCAT*, 6th ed. Rockville, MD, Betz, 1995.

Whimbey A, Lochhead J: *Problem Solving & Comprehension,* 5th ed. Hillsdale, NJ, Lawrence Erlbaum Associates, 1991.

Whimbey A, Lochhead J: *Beyond Problem Solving and Comprehension: An Exploration of Quantitative Ability.* Hillsdale, NJ, Lawrence Erlbaum Associates, 1984.

6

CHAPTER

Preparing for the V.E.T.s Chemistry Test

6.0 INTRODUCTION

This chapter describes the topics in general and organic chemistry required for the VETs. The material is divided into content groups, each with a short listing of important topics. The sample test is included to assess understanding of the general and organic chemistry topics required for the VETs and to identify topics that need further review. *A Complete Preparation for the MCAT, Studyware Biology* review software, and the Graduate Record Examination Chemistry Test book are useful resources. Appendixes A through E provide detailed outlines of the material covered in each test. Tables 6-1 and 6-2 compare the chemistry sections of the Veterinary College Admission Test (VCAT), Graduate Record Examination (GRE), and Medical College Admission Test (MCAT).

6.1 GENERAL CHEMISTRY

General chemistry encompasses a wide range of topics.

6.1.1 Basic Concepts and Stoichiometry

Important topics include density, the classification of matter, the law of definite proportions, nomenclature of common polyatomic ions, formula weight of substances, percent composition, moles, empirical formulas, molecular formulas, the law of conservation of mass, balancing chemical equations, the use of balanced chemical equations, and other information needed to calculate the quantities of reactants consumed or products generated in a chemical reaction and to determine a limiting reactant with percent yield.

6.1.2 Gases

Topics to review include Boyle's law, Charles' law, Gay-Lussac's law, Avogadro's law, the ideal gas law, and Dalton's law of partial pressures. Other important topics are gas stoichiometry, standard temperature and pressure, kinetic molecular theory, and diffusion.

TABLE 6-1. ***Inorganic/General Chemistry***

VCAT	GRE	MCAT

Atomic theory
  Structure
  Nuclear Chemistry
  Thermodynamics
  Acids and bases
Bonding theory
  Molecules and compounds
  Chemical reactions
  Oxidation–reduction
  Acids and bases
Physical theory
  Phases
  Solutions
  Kinetics
  Electrochemistry
	Analytical chemistry
	  Classical quantitative analysis
	  Instrumental analysis
	Inorganic chemistry
	  Basic descriptive chemistry of elements
	  Periodic and family trends
	  Electronic and nuclear structure
	  Transition metals/coordination chemistry
	  Special topics
	Physical chemistry
	  General chemistry
	  Classical and status thermodynamics
	  Quantum and structural chemistry
	  Kinetics
		Stoichiometry
		Electronic structure and the periodic table
		Chemical bonding
		Phases and phase equilibria
		Solution chemistry
		Acids and bases
		Thermodynamics and thermochemistry
		Rate processes in chemical reactions: kinetics and equilibrium
		Electrochemistry
		  Electrolytic cell
		  Galvanic cell
		  Concentration cell

TABLE 6-2. ***Topics in Organic Chemistry***

VCAT	GRE	MCAT
Structure and mechanism Simple functional groups Hydrocarbons Oxygen-containing compounds Nitrogen-containing compounds Analysis 50% inorganic chemistry; 50% organic chemistry	Molecular structure Conversion of functional groups Reactive intermediates and reaction mechanisms Special topics Approximately 30% organic chemistry	Molecular structure of organic compounds Biologic molecules Oxygen-containing compounds Amines Hydrocarbons Separations and purifications Use of spectroscopy in structure identification General chemistry is part of the Physical Sciences subtest; organic chemistry is part of the Biological Sciences subtest. MCAT instruments vary from one testing center to another; most items are passage-linked problems.

6.1.3 Liquids and Solids

Important topics include phase changes, intermolecular forces, solutions, colligative properties (e.g., freezing point depression, boiling point elevation, osmotic pressure), hydrogen bonding, and hydrophobic bonding forces.

6.1.4 Solutions

Solution chemistry involves concentration, intermolecular forces, and the properties of solutes and solvents.

6.1.5 Acids and Bases

Important information includes the definition of acids, conjugate acid–base pairs, neutralization reactions, titrations, buffers, and hydrolysis reactions of salts.

6.1.6 Chemical Equilibrium

Important topics include the quantitative treatment of chemical equilibrium and the principles of chemical equilibrium in the gas phase. Other important equilibria are acid–base and solubility.

6.1.7 Thermodynamics

Important topics include spontaneity of a reaction, enthalpy change (ΔH), entropy change (ΔS), and free energy change (ΔG) in terms of the second law of thermodynamics.

6.1.8 Kinetics

To control the rates of reactions, the factors that affect rate must be known. Important factors are the effect of concentration of the reactants, temperature, the presence of a catalyst, and activation energy.

6.1.9 Redox Reactions

Electrical energy produces chemical reactions. Important topics include oxidation numbers, the Nernst equation, and redox chemistry.

6.1.10 Atomic and Molecular Structure

Important topics include electron configuration, Hund's rule, the Pauli exclusion principle, the Aufbau principle, quantum numbers, Lewis dot structures, and the octet rule.

6.1.11 Periodic Properties

Topics to review include named groups (e.g., halogens, alkali metals, noble gases) and periodic trends (e.g., size, ionization potential, electronegativity).

6.1.12 Nuclear Reactions

Topics include balancing nuclear equations, decay processes, and particles.

6.2 ORGANIC CHEMISTRY

Important information includes the International Union of Pure and Applied Chemistry (IUPAC) rules for nomenclature of organic compounds as well as nomenclature, physical properties, preparation, and reactions.

6.2.1 Structure and Stereochemistry

Covalent bonds are formed by two atoms that share a pair of electrons. Covalent bonds usually form between atoms of similar electronegativity. The nearer they are to each other in the periodic table, the farther apart atoms are located; the greater the difference in electronegativity, the greater the likelihood of ionic bonding (e.g., NaCl). The two types of bonds are sigma (i.e., orbital overlap in one area in space) and pi (i.e., orbital overlap in two areas in space). Review the octet rule, resonance structures, dipoles, optical activity, and assignment of configurations.

6.2.2 Alkanes, Alkenes, and Aromatics

For alkanes, the general formula is C_xH_{2x+2}. All names end in -ane, and fragment names end in -yl. The higher the molecular mass, the higher the boiling point. Branched compounds have lower boiling points than related straight-chain compounds. Cyclic compounds have higher boiling points than open-chain compounds. They also have low densities and are nonpolar. The general formula for unsaturated hydrocarbons is C_xH_{2x} for one double bond and C_xH_{2x-2} for one triple bond. Alkenes have the suffix

-ene, and alkynes have the suffix -yne. Geometric isomers are possible for alkenes, cis, and trans, or Z and E. Aromatics are cyclic, planar sp^2, or sp hybrids that obey Hückel's rule. The number of pi electrons = $4n + 2$.

6.2.3 Alcohols, Aldehydes and Ketones, Ethers, and Phenols

Oxygen-containing groups include:

—OH	Alcohols, which have high boiling points, are soluble in water, are polar, and are named for the longest carbon chain plus the suffix -ol.
Ar—OH	Phenols
O ‖ R-C-H	Aldehydes, which are named for the longest carbon chain with the group and the suffix -al. Carbons are numbered beginning at the aldehyde end.
O ‖ R-C-R	Ketones, which are named for the longest chain, numbered to give carbonyl the lowest possible number, and the suffix -one.
R—O—R	Ethers, which are polar and are given two alkyl names plus ether or treated as alkoxy-alkanes.

6.2.4 Carboxylic Acids and Derivatives

Carboxylic acids are named according to the longest carbon chain and the suffix -oic acid. Figure 6-1 shows the amide group.

Anhydrides are formed by the removal of water from two —COOH groups. Anhydrides are more reactive than the corresponding acids. Esters are named by changing the suffix -oic to -ate.

6.2.5 Amines

Amines are weak bases, named either as the organic group amine or using the longest carbon chain numbered to give the amine-N the lowest possible number.

6.2.6 Amino Acids and Proteins

Amino acids can act as zwitterions, ions that have both a cation site and anion site in a single molecule, have a high melting point, and are soluble in water. Proteins are divided into two broad functional classes, fibrous and globular. The structure of proteins is divided into primary, or 1°, secondary, or 2°, tertiary, or 3°, and quaternary, or 4°. The primary structure describes the linkage of the atoms of the protein molecule by covalent bonds. The secondary structure describes the arrangement of the chains in space (e.g., coils, sheets). The tertiary structure describes intramolecular interactions (e.g., hydrogen bonding, van der Waals interactions). The quaternary structure describes intermolecular interactions between protein chains.

6.2.7 Carbohydrates

Carbohydrates are polyhydroxy aldehydes, ketones, or related compounds. Monosaccharides cannot be hydrolyzed to simpler compounds, disaccharides can be hydrolyzed to two, and polysaccharides can

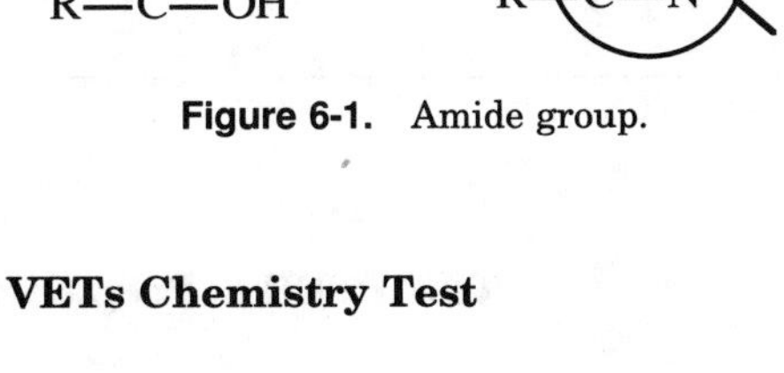

Figure 6-1. Amide group.

be hydrolyzed to many monosaccharides. Aldoses contain an aldehyde group; ketoses contain a ketone group. For example, a five-carbon monosaccharide containing an aldehyde is an aldepentose.

6.2.8 Spectroscopy

Review the identification of organic compounds with infrared (IR) and ^{1}H nuclear magnetic resonance (NMR) data. Important correlations are shown in Tables 6-3 and 6-4.

6.3 Special Topics

This section describes several common topics for the VCAT, GRE, and MCAT: Appendixes A, C, and D describe the tests in greater detail. The major chemistry topics covered on the VETs are outlined as follows:

TABLE 6-3. ***IR NMR***

Functional Group	cm^{-1}	Characteristics
—OH	3640–3610	Usually broad peaks
Amines	3500–3300	1° amines = doublet, 2° amines = singlet
≡C—H	3315–3270	
—C—H	3100–3000	Aromatics
$=CH_2$	3080	
$—CH_3$, $—CH_2—$	2990–2890	Methyl groups have weak intensity; other alkyls are strong
C≡N	2300–2200	
C=O	1750–1740	Ester
	1740–1720	Aldehyde

TABLE 6-4. ***^{1}H NMR***

Group	Chemical Shift (∂ in ppm)	Notes
Methyl	0.9	
Methylene	1.3	
Benzylic	2.3–3	AR—CH
Vinyl	4.5–6.0	C=C—H
Amino	2.0–2.8	RCH_2NH_2
	1–5	RNH_2
Ketone	2.0–2.7	$RCH_2C(=O)R$
Alcohol	3.4–4.0	RCH_2COH
	1–5	RCH_2COH
Ether	3.3–5.0	RCH_2COR
Ester	3.7–4.1	$RC(=O)OCH_2R$
	2.0–2.2	$RCH_2C(=O)OR$
Aromatic	6.0–8.5	Ar—H
Aldehydic	9–10	
Carboxylic acid	10–12	

I. Nuclear chemistry
   A. Types of radiation
   B. Radioisotopes
II. Theories of acids and bases
III. Inorganic polymers
IV. Ionization
   A. Ion separation
   B. Ionic solids
V. Reactive intermediates and reaction mechanisms
   A. Tools of mechanism chemists
   B. Nucleophilic displacement reactions
VI. Structural features of natural products
   A. Special reagents
   B. Synthesis problems

6.3.1 Separations and Purifications

Understand all of the physical and chemical design features of basic instruments and equipment used to separate and purify organic mixtures. Compare laboratory and industrial methods, especially working mechanisms and analytical procedures.

6.3.2 Solvent Extraction

In solvent extraction, a compound is purified by partitioning between two immisicble liquids so that the compound is held strongly in one solvent preferentially over other solutes. Quantitatively, the preference of a solute for solvent A over solvent B is expressed as its partition coefficient:

$$K_{A/B} = [\text{solute}]_A/[\text{solute}]_B = (\text{grams solute/volume A})/(\text{grams solute/volume B})$$

For example, if 1.20 g substance C is partitioned between 50.0 ml CH_2Cl_2 and 50.0 ml H_2O and 0.95 g substance C is found in CH_2Cl_2 and 0.25 g is found in H_2O, the partition is calculated as:

$$K_{CH_2Cl_2}/H_2O = (0.95\text{ g}/50.0\text{ ml})/(0.25\text{ g}/50.0\text{ ml})$$

The greater the partition coefficient, the more soluble the compound is in one solvent versus the other.

It is often useful to separate solutes on the basis of the differences in their acid–base properties. Chemical reactions ionize functional groups in organic molecules and render them soluble in water. Compounds that contain strongly acidic protons (i.e., carboxylic acids) are extracted readily from organic solvents, such as dichloromethane, into aqueous solutions of a weak base, such as $NaHCO_3$. Compounds that contain less acidic protons (i.e., phenols) are extracted from dichloromethane by stronger aqueous bases, such as NaOH. Compounds that are moderately basic (i.e., amines) are extracted from dichloromethane by aqueous hydrochloric acid. Weakly basic compounds (i.e., alcohols, alkenes, carbonyl compounds) are extracted by concentrated H_2SO_4. When the compound of interest is obtained in the aqueous medium to the virtual exclusion of other compounds, the aqueous solution can be brought to neutral pH and back-extracted into an organic solvent. The separation and purification of a mixture of toluene, benzoic acid, phenol, and aniline illustrates this process (Figure 6-2).

6.3.3 Chromatography

Chromatographic separation and purification of compounds is similar to solvent extraction. Chromatographic separations may be viewed as continuous partitions between a mobile phase and a stationary phase. Compounds with different partition coefficients between the mobile and stationary phases are separated because they move at different rates. The more a compound favors the mobile phase, the faster it moves. The greater the difference in partition coefficients between compounds, the greater the difference in their respective velocities and the easier their separation. The generalization "like dissolves like" applies to chromatographic separations.

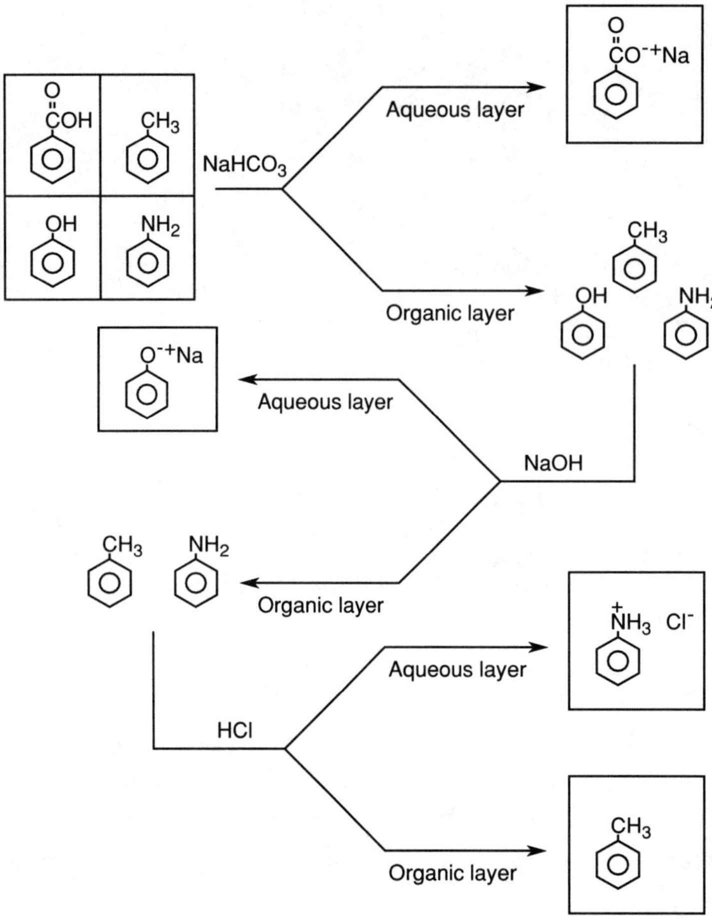

Figure 6-2. Separation of benzoic acid, toluene, phenol, and aniline by solvent extraction.

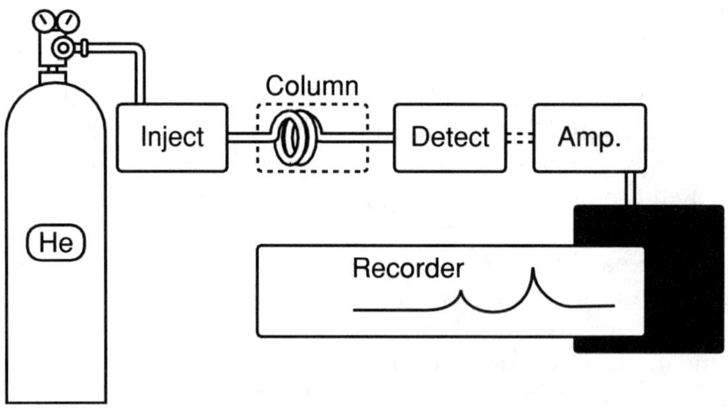

Figure 6-3. Gas chromatography.

Gas–liquid chromatography, or gas chromatography, permits quantitative separation of mixtures of compounds that can be vaporized. The "gas" refers to either helium or nitrogen in the mobile phase in this separation technique. The "liquid" refers to a high–molecular-weight liquid, such as octadecane, coated on an inert solid support, such as finely ground firebrick, in the stationary phase. The stationary phase is packed into glass or metal tubing known as a column. A typical gas chromatograph is shown in Figure 6-3.

Gas chromatography is frequently used to establish the purity of a sample, identify its components, and measure the amount of each component. Gas chromatography can also be used for preparative separation of milligram quantities of reaction mixtures. A solution containing the sample to be separated and analyzed is introduced with a microliter syringe into an injector port that instantaneously vaporizes the sample. The vapor produced is partitioned between the high–molecular-weight liquid stationary phase and the helium or nitrogen mobile phase. The greater affinity a component has for the stationary phase, the longer it is retained in this phase. The larger the difference in affinity for the stationary phase of the components, the easier they are to separate. Compounds are identified on the basis of the retention time of authentic compounds, or the time from injection until a component exits the column and is detected. In addition to affinity considerations, the higher the boiling point, the longer the retention time. The detector drives a strip-chart recorder that produces triangles whose area is proportional to the amount of material passing the detector. Quantitative data can be obtained from calibration curves based on known amounts of authentic material. The free radical chlorination of cyclohexane produces a combination of unreacted cyclohexane, chlorocyclohexane, and some isomeric dichlorocyclohexanes. Each compound can be detected and its concentration determined if authentic samples are available for comparison and calibration.

Thin-layer chromatography separates small quantities of materials rapidly. These separations are used to determine the purity of a sample, identify the components of a mixture, and establish conditions for the separation and purification of larger quantities of material with a buret packed with silica gel or alumina. Thin-layer chromatography is used to prepare separations of milligram quantities of compounds, but is not generally used for quantitative analysis. The most common stationary phase is a plastic sheet coated with silica gel or alumina cut into small strips, or plates. Both silica gel and alumina are polar: they contain —O—H groups. A nonpolar solvent, such as hexane, is used as the mobile phase or mixed with a polar solvent, such as dichloromethane or diethyl ether, to adjust the polarity of the mobile phase for the best separation. A nonpolar mobile phase has minimal electrostatic interaction with the stationary phase, so compounds separate according to their polarity. The most polar compound moves the most slowly in the mobile phase, whereas the least polar compound travels most quickly. A more polar mobile phase interacts with the polar stationary phase and hastens the movement of all compounds. The stationary phase interacts with the solvent to a greater extent than the sample as a result of the greater abundance of the solvent. A few microliters of a solution of the mixture to be separated is spotted near the bottom of a thin-layer chromatography plate. The plate is placed in a covered beaker or jar containing the mobile phase. The mobile phase rises on the plate by capillary action, carrying with it components of the mixture.

Figure 6-4 shows the separation of a three-component mixture on a silica gel plate. Compound A is the most polar component, C is the least polar component, and B is of intermediate polarity. The components are identified on the basis of the ratio of the distance moved by a specific spot to the distance traveled by the solvent (i.e., mobile phase).

By definition, R_f values are equal to or less than unity. Authentic samples are often spotted on the same plate as an unknown sample to measure the R_f values under identical conditions. The basis for the separation of fluorene from fluorenone on silica gel is shown in Figure 6-5. Fluorene, a nonpolar compound, has an R_f value of nearly 1.00. The polar fluorenone has an R_f of nearly half that value, with silica gel as a stationary phase and hexane as the mobile phase. To separate large quantities of fluorene from fluorenone, a solvent or solvent mixture is selected by thin-layer chromatography. To separate fluorene and fluorenone, hexane provides two readily distinguishable separated spots. A buret is filled with a suspension of silica gel in hexane, excess hexane is drained, and the stopcock of the buret is closed. The mixture to be separated is introduced as a concentrated solution at the top of the buret, and the stopcock is opened.

Additional hexane must be added to the buret to replace the mobile phase that flows out. As the hexane moves down the buret, it carries with it the fluorene, leaving the fluorenone near the top of the silica gel. Once the nonpolar fluorene has eluted, dichloromethane is used as the mobile phase to chase out the polar fluorenone. Figure 6-6 shows this separation.

6.3.4 Distillation

Distillation is a means of purifying a liquid by vaporizing it, separating its vapor from that of impurities or other compounds, condensing the purified vapor back to a liquid, and collecting it in a separate container.

$$R_f = \frac{\text{Distance spot A moves from the origin}}{\text{Distance solvent S moves from the origin}} = A/S$$

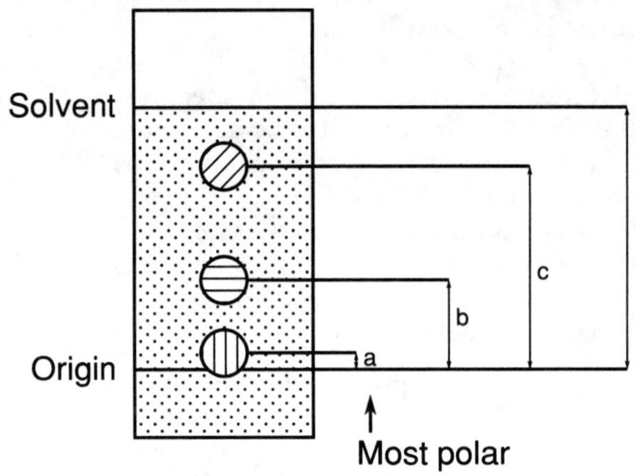

$$R_f(a) = a/S$$
$$R_f(b) = b/S$$
$$R_f(c) = c/S$$

Figure 6-4. Thin-layer chromatography separation of a three-component mixture.

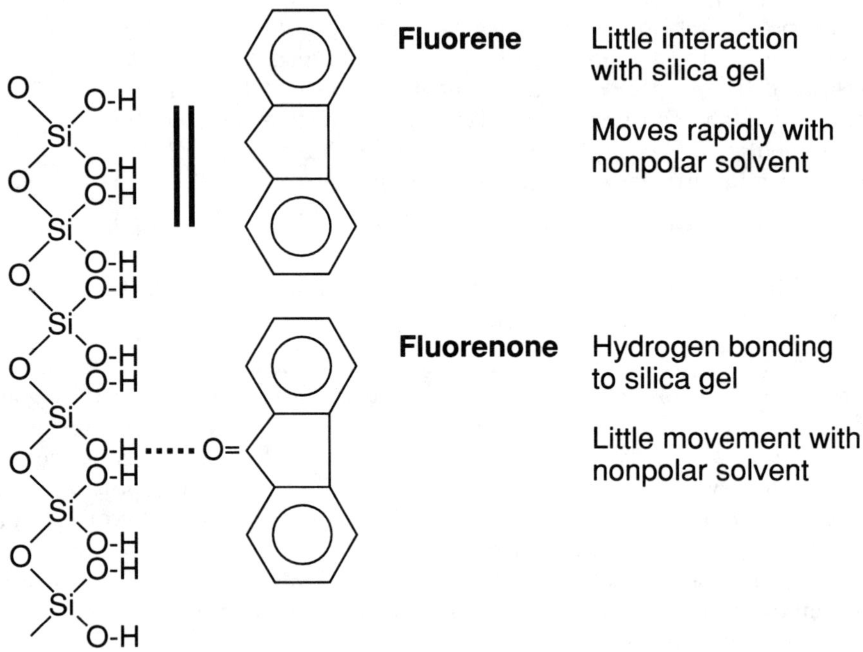

Figure 6-5. Interaction of silica gel with fluorene and fluorenone.

Every liquid has molecules above it in the vapor phase. Heating the liquid increases the kinetic energy of the molecules in the liquid state so that they are no longer attracted to other molecules of the liquid and pass into the gas or vapor phase. This change increases the partial pressure of vapor above the liquid. At the temperature at which the partial pressure of vapor above the liquid equals ambient pressure, the liquid boils. The actual temperature required to boil a liquid depends on the presence of factors that hold molecules of liquid near each other, such as van der Waals forces, dipolar electrostatic attractions, and hydrogen bonding.

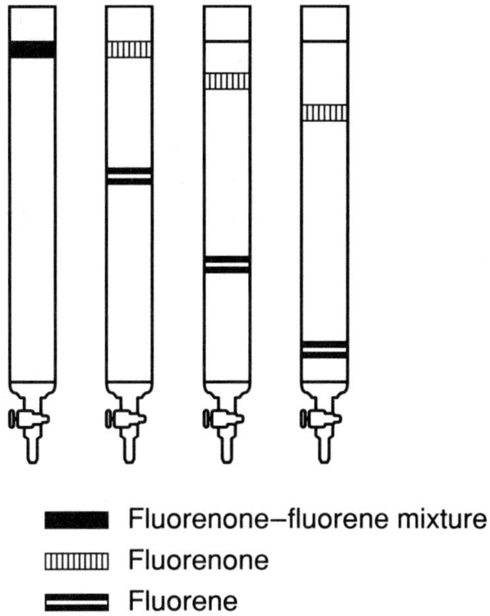

Figure 6-6. Column chromatographic separation of fluorene and fluorenone.

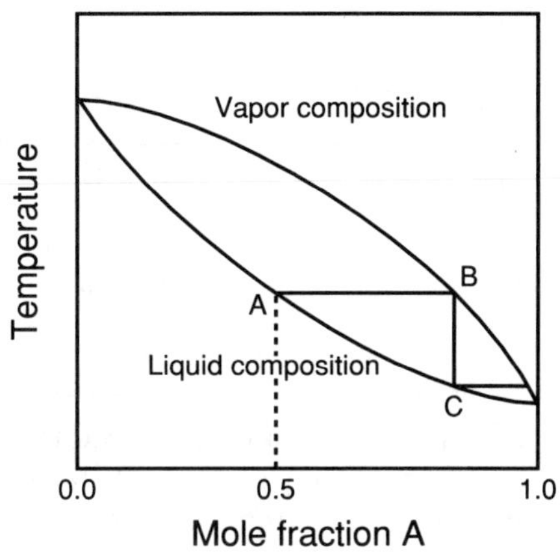

Figure 6-7. Liquid and vapor composition of an ideal two-component mixture as a function of temperature.

Distillation can be viewed as a series of vaporizations and condensations that enrich the vapor in the more volatile compound. In an equimolar mixture of two liquids A and B, if A is more volatile, the vapor above the mixture is richer in A than in B. That vapor is condensed back to a liquid, now enriched in A. The vapor above this enriched liquid is even richer in A. Each vaporization–condensation cycle is known as a theoretical plate. In research and academic laboratories, the theoretical plate has no physical being. In industrial distillations, each theoretical plate corresponds to a distinctly different heating–condensing apparatus. Liquids with widely different boiling points require few theoretical plates to achieve a vapor that is nearly pure in the low-boiling, more volatile compound. Similarly, two liquids whose boiling points are similar require several vaporization–condensation cycles to obtain a vapor that contains only one compound because less enrichment occurs at each step.

Figure 6-7 shows the vapor and liquid compositions for mixtures of A and B, where A is more volatile. Point a is the starting point of 0.5 mol fraction A in the liquid phase. Point b represents the composition of the vapor above the liquid in A at the same temperature. The vapor has a greater concentration of A than does the liquid, approximately 0.85 mol fraction A in the vapor phase. Point c represents the vapor from point b condensed to a liquid with the same 0.85 mol fraction A. The path from point a to point b to point c is one theoretical plate. Figure 6-7 shows that two theoretical plates are needed to

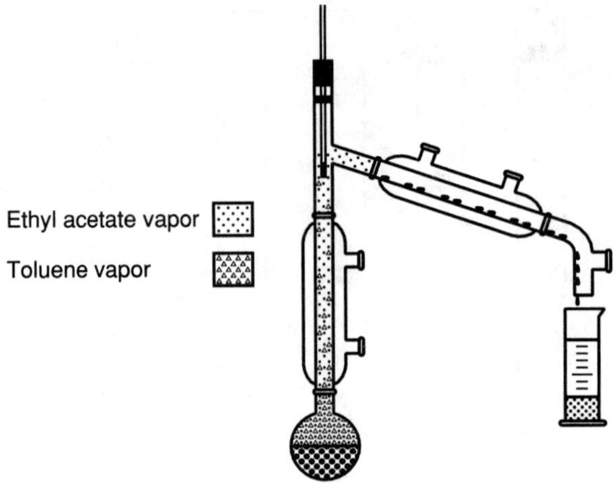

Figure 6-8. Distillation of ethyl acetate and toluene.

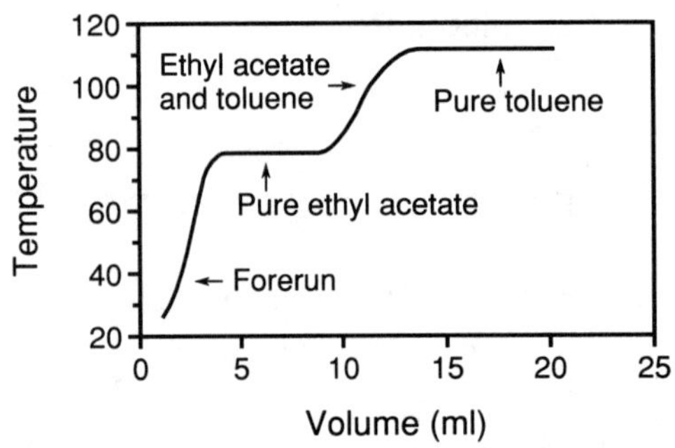

Figure 6-9. Variation of temperature with volume during the distillation of ethyl acetate and toluene.

produce a vapor of nearly pure A. A third plate would be required to complete the process. The number of theoretical plates in a research or academic laboratory distillation may be increased by increasing the surface area available for condensation. Experimentally, the fractionating column is packed with glass beads, ceramic "saddles," or copper wool.

Figure 6-8 shows the apparatus for the distillation of a mixture of ethyl acetate (boiling point = 78°C) and toluene (boiling point = 111°C). The vapor about to distill is virtually free of toluene whereas the vapor closer to the distilling flask contains increasingly higher amounts of that compound.

As each pure material is distilled, the temperature remains constant at the boiling point for the compound. An idealized graph of temperature as a function of volume for the fractional distillation of a mixture of ethyl acetate (boiling point = 78°C) and toluene (boiling point = 111°C) is shown in Figure 6-9. Four regions, or fractions, on the graph are shown. In the initial fraction, the temperature increases from room temperature (25°C) to the boiling point of ethyl acetate. The liquid collected during that region is known as forerun. Although the forerun liquid is largely ethyl acetate, it is not pure and should not be combined with the fraction that contains the pure material. Experimentally, the forerun is usually small in volume. The second fraction occurs when the temperature remains constant at 78°C, the boiling point of pure ethyl acetate. This fraction is collected in a separate container as a pure liquid. The third fraction is observed as the temperature increases from 78°C to 111°C, the boiling point of toluene. This fraction contains both ethyl acetate and toluene and should be collected in a different container. The fourth fraction boils at a constant temperature of 111°C and is pure toluene.

6.3.5 Recrystallization

Recrystallization is a technique for purifying a solid by breaking down its crystal lattice structure. The solid is dissolved in a suitable solvent, and the crystal lattice structure is allowed to form again. A saturated solution of an impure solid is prepared at an elevated temperature. When the solution cools, it becomes supersaturated with the compound, and crystals form. The more slowly the solution cools, the larger the resulting crystals. The original impurities are excluded from the crystals that form for two reasons: (1) the solution is not supersaturated with the impurities (i.e., they remain dissolved); and (2) the impurities do not easily fit into the growing crystal lattice structure. Once the solution has deposited all of the crystals that it will yield, the crystals are filtered from the solution, washed with cold solvent, and dried. If recrystallization improves the purity of the solid sample, its melting point increases over that recorded for the initial material, and the material melts over a narrower temperature range.

The choice of solvent is crucial to the success of recrystallization. The solvent must meet the following criteria: (1) it does not react chemically with the sample; (2) it dissolves the sample poorly at room temperature and well at steam bath temperature; (3) it dissolves impurities that are present, even at subambient temperatures; and (4) it is easily evaporated from the purified sample.

Water, methanol, ethyl acetate, dichloromethane, hexane, and toluene were tested as potential solvents for the recrystallization of a solid. Water was insoluble; methanol was soluble in hot solution; and ethyl acetate, dichloromethane, hexane, and toluene were soluble. Based on the second criterion for solvents, methanol is the solvent of choice to purify the solid by recrystallization if it also meets the other criteria. Ethyl acetate, dichloromethane, hexane, and toluene dissolved the sample at room temperature. To induce crystallization, the volume of solution must be substantially reduced to obtain any crystals on cooling. Because water did not dissolve the sample, it is an unacceptable recrystallizing solvent for this solute.

Fractional crystallization can be used to separate a mixture of two solids if a solvent dissolves one compound readily, even cold, and dissolves the other only when it is hot. An example is the separation of trans-cinnamic acid from urea, both of which melt at 132°C. The mixture has a melting point considerably lower than that. Typical observations on solubility are shown in Table 6-5.

These data show that a mixture of cinnamic acid and urea dissolved in hot water would yield crystals of cinnamic acid on cooling. Urea remains dissolved in the cold water. The crystals thus obtained should melt at a temperature near 132°C. Proof that the crystals are trans-cinnamic acid can be obtained by observing a mixed melting point with authentic trans-cinnamic acid.

6.3.6 Oxygen-Containing Compounds

Oxygen-containing organic compounds are classified as alcohols, aldehydes, ketones, carboxylic acids, and their derivatives, ethers and phenols. Oxygen-containing compounds have five types of general characteristics: hydrogen bonds and solubility; steric effects of substituents; electronic effects of substituents; acidity and basicity; and miscellaneous principles.

The carbon atom in alcohols bonded to the OH group is carbinol carbon. Primary and secondary alcohols have at least one H atom on the carbinol carbon. These alcohols oxidize to carbonyl compounds in the

TABLE 6-5. ***Solubility Observations***

Compound	Water	Methanol	Ethyl Acetate	Dichloromethane	Hexane	Toluene
Cinnamic acid	Soluble in hot solution	Soluble	Soluble	Soluble	Soluble	Soluble
Urea	Soluble	Soluble	Insoluble	Insoluble	Insoluble	Insoluble

presence of copper at approximately 300°C. The hydrogen atom in alcohols is weakly acidic. Thiols or mercaptans that are sulfur analogs of alcohols are represented by RSH, compared with ROH for alcohols. Hydrocarbon molecules are not associated through hydrogen bonds. As the alkane molecular chain lengthens, the solubility of alcohols in water decreases (e.g., ethyl alcohol is more soluble than decyl alcohol). Most alcohol reactions have O—H bond cleavage, which forms carboxylic acid esters, and C—O bond cleavage, which forms alkyl halides. The carbonyl oxygen atom in aldehydes and ketones forms stronger hydrogen bonds with water. Carboxylic acids, which have polar molecules, form strong hydrogen bonds with each other and also with water. The solubility of carboxylic acids in water decreases as the carbon chain lengthens. Carboxylic acids and alcohols have similar solubility characteristics. Ether molecules cannot associate with each other through hydrogen bonds, but can form hydrogen bonds with water. Like alcohols, phenols form strong hydrogen bonds.

Nucleophilic reactions are affected by steric effects, especially steric hindrance. Arrangements of atomic or functional groups cause hindrance at the reaction site, slowing the rate of S_N2 reactions. The relative rate of S_N2 reactions is affected by the molecular structure and arrangement of the alkyl halide. Molecular space may be filled by various arrangements. If the reacting part of the alkyl halide has a specific space-filling arrangement, the steric effects are dominant. Steric hindrance occurs in certain nucleophilic addition reactions (i.e., aldehydes and ketones) and in nucleophilic substitution reactions (i.e., carboxylic acid derivatives). The carbonyl carbon atom provides the reaction site or the reacting part of the molecule. Ketones with steric hindrance at the carbonyl group cannot form cyanohydrins. Aldehyde–ketone substitutions differ from carboxylic acid derivative substitutions in that nucleophilic reactions use the addition–elimination mechanism to overcome steric hindrance.

The effects of activating and deactivating substituents occur in all oxygen-containing compounds. The electronic effects include reactivity, acidity, stereoarrangements, and inductive effects in carboxylic acids. Activating substituents usually increase the reaction rate, whereas deactivating substituents decrease the reaction rate. The inductive effects are more pronounced in carboxylic acids. These effects are caused by electrostatic interaction of polarized substituent ring bonds. For example, for electronegative substituents, the ring is located at the positive end of the dipole. The acidity of phenol is linked to the resonance structures that require separation of opposite charges (i.e., energy is required to separate opposite charges). Phenol has medium resonance stabilization, whereas the phenoxide ion has greater resonance stabilization (e.g., the OH group in phenols behaves as an activating substituent). Bromination and sulfonation reactions are caused by the strong OH group. Carboxylic acid derivatives can be converted to acids, esters, amides, and ketones by substituent effects. Another important control mechanism is the enzyme-catalyzed reduction of acetaldehyde to ethanol by the reduced form of nicotinamide adenine dinucleotide, using hydride–ion transfer.

The presence of α-hydrogen in carbonyl compounds (i.e., aldehydes and ketones) makes them acidic. The α-hydrogen is attached to a carbon atom known as α-carbon. The pK_a values for α-hydrogen are approximately 20 for aldehydes and ketones. Resonance stability of the anion causes this higher acidity. Tautomers that are in reversible equilibrium are keto and enol forms of isomers, which are interconvertible. The α-, β-unsaturated carbonyls react with nucleophilic reagents by simple or conjugate addition (e.g., Michael additions, which are special conjugate additions). Delocalized carbanions are formed by the nucleophilic aromatic substitution mechanism (i.e., S_NAr).

Alcohols can be synthesized from alkenes by oxymercuration–demurcuration and hydroboration–oxidation procedures. An azeotrope is a mixture of two liquids with a boiling point that is either higher or lower than the boiling point of the ingredients. Study the permeability of biologic cell membranes and the role of crown ethers and host (i.e., crown) and guest (i.e., cation) relations. Excess acidic medium (e.g., HBr) causes dialkyl ethers to cleave and form alkyl halides. Dialkyl ethers do not react with bases. Ethers have weak basicity because of the O group. Carboxylate ions or anions, which are negatively charged, are not reactive toward nucleophilic substitution. Proton migration from α-carbon to oxygen in aldehydes and ketones with α-hydrogen forms a special isomer known as enol.

6.3.7 Reactive Intermediates and Reaction Mechanisms

The pi electrons of the double bond are available for reaction with reagents that react with a pair of electrons. Protons and carbocations (i.e., carbenium ions) are Lewis acids and electron acceptors. Carbon anions are known as carbanions. Carbocations are electron-seeking reagents. They are also known as electrophilic reagents, or electrophiles. Alkenes, which donate electrons, are Lewis bases and are nucleophilic reagents, or nucleophiles. The most important reaction of alkenes is electrophilic addition to the double bond. Figure 6-10 shows a general reaction and examples of addition reactions.

Halogenation, hydrohalogenation, and hydration of alkenes are electrophilic addition reactions. The electrophilic addition reactions of HX and HOH to asymmetrical alkenes are regioselective and follow Markovnikov's rule, which states that when HX and HOH reagents are added to asymmetrical alkenes, the hydrogen adds to the carbon of the double bond, which has more hydrogens (Figure 6-11).

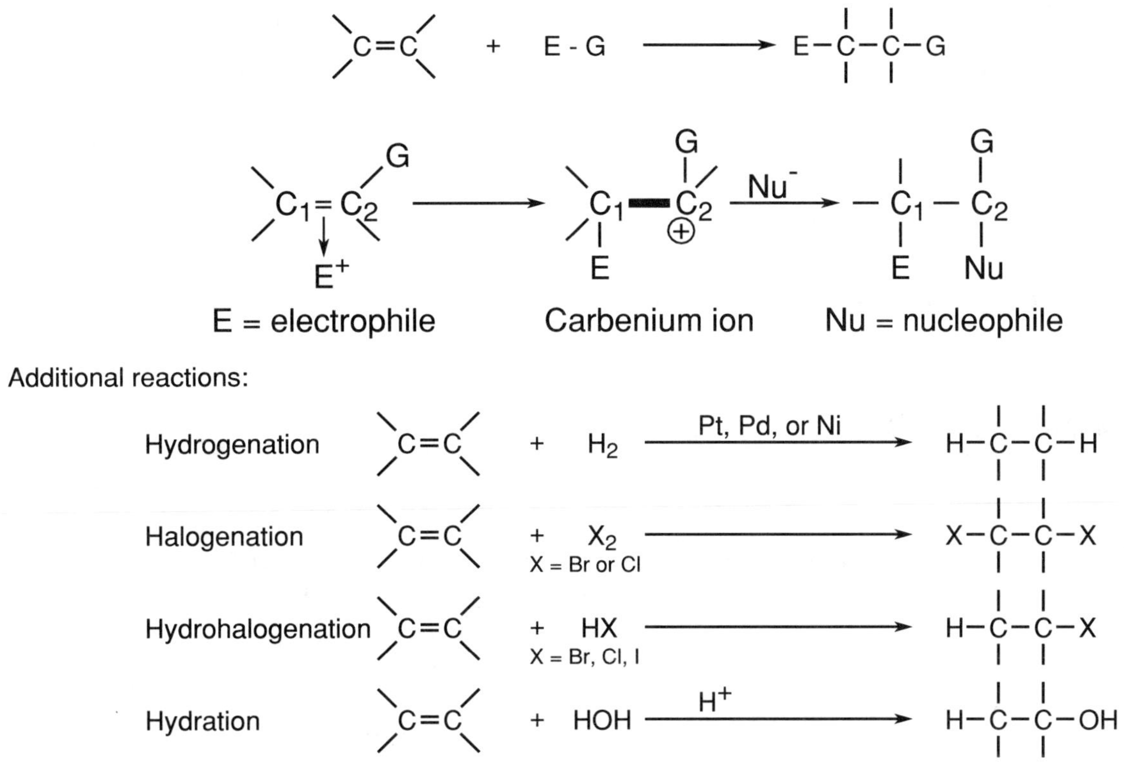

Figure 6-10. Types of addition reactions—electrophilic and nucleophilic.

Mechanism (general)

$$R-CH{=}CH_2 + H-X \longrightarrow R-\overset{+}{C}H-CH_3 + X^-$$

$$R-\overset{+}{C}H-CH_3 + X^- \longrightarrow R-\underset{\displaystyle X}{\underset{|}{C}H}-CH_3$$

Hydration

$$H_2SO_4 + HOH \longrightarrow H_3O^- + HSO_2^-$$

$$R-CH{=}CH_2 + H_3O^+ \longrightarrow R-\underset{\displaystyle OH_2^+}{\underset{|}{\overset{+}{C}H}}-CH_3 + HOH$$

$$R-\overset{+}{C}H{=}CH_3 + HOH \longrightarrow R-\underset{\displaystyle OH}{C}H-CH_3$$

$$R-\overset{\displaystyle OH_2^+}{\overset{|}{C}H}-CH_3 + HOH \longrightarrow R-\overset{\displaystyle OH}{\overset{|}{C}H}-CH_3 + H_3O^+$$

Figure 6-11. Electrophilic addition reactions using Markovnikov's rule.

Markovnikov's rule applies because the addition of the proton to the carbon that has the greater number of hydrogens yields the more stable carbocation that is formed through a lower-energy transition state. In the earlier example, a secondary carbocation (i.e., carbenium ion) is formed. The alternate mode of addition would yield the less stable primary carbocation (Figure 6-12).

The carbon skeleton of an alkene may be rearranged during electrophilic addition if the initial carbocation forms a more stable carbocation. Rearrangement may occur by methyl or hydride shift to an adjacent carbon. The rearranged structure is often the major product of the reaction (Figure 6-13).

$$R{-}CH{=}CH_2 + H^+ \longrightarrow R{-}\overset{+}{C}H{-}CH_3 \quad \text{rather than } RCH_2CH_2^+$$

$$R_2C\quad CH\quad R + H^+ \longrightarrow R_2\overset{+}{C}{-}CH_2R \quad \text{rather than } R_2CHCHR^+$$

Figure 6-12. Stability of carbocation.

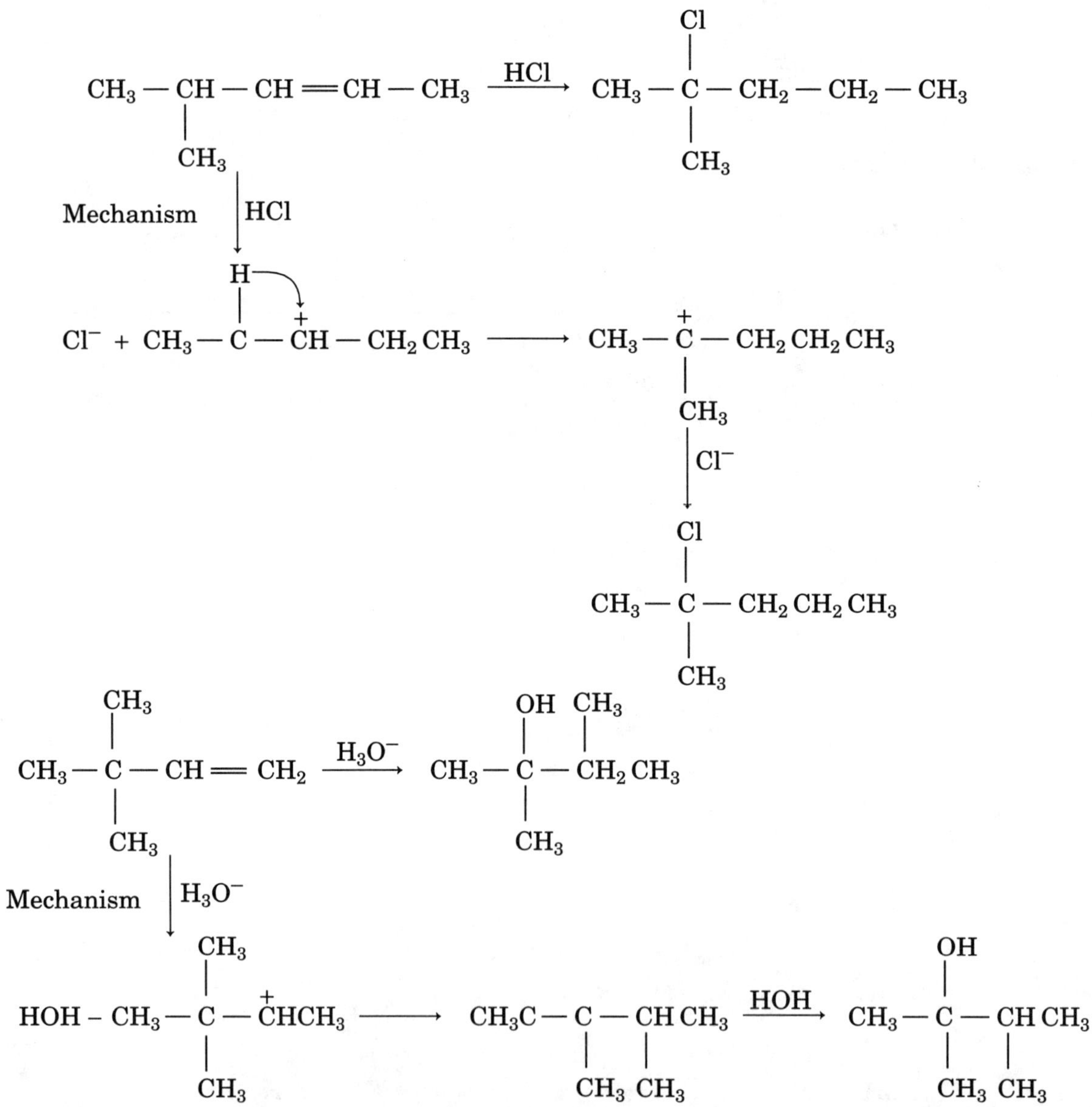

Figure 6-13. Rearrangement of electrophilic addition.

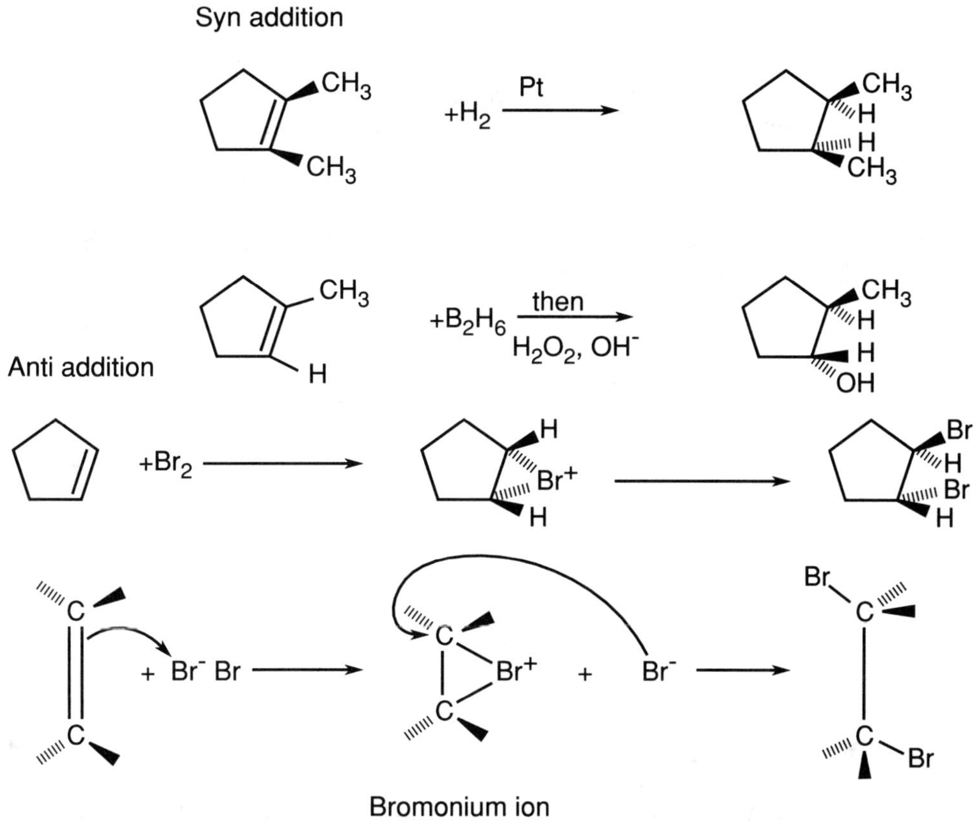

Figure 6-14. Electrophilic addition reactions: syn addition and anti addition.

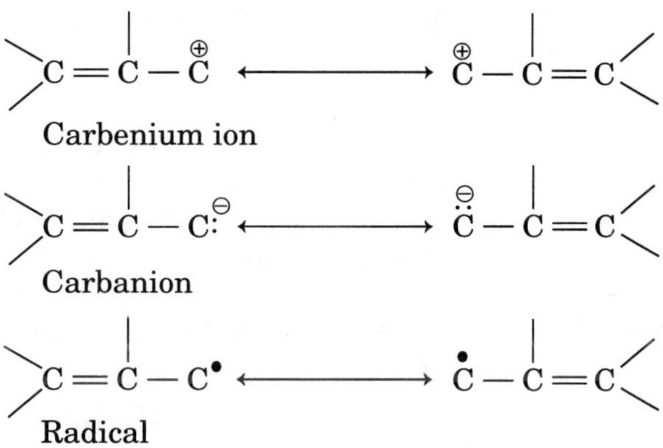

Figure 6-15. Stability of double-bond carbocations.

In some additions to a double bond, both atoms or groups of the reagent add to the same side of the double bond, resulting in syn addition. When the two atoms or groups are added on opposite sides, anti addition occurs (Figure 6-14).

The other key feature of the double bond is its ability to stabilize carbocations, or radicals on adjacent carbons (Figure 6-15). All are resonance stabilized.

The stability of the intermediate carbocation, as shown earlier (see Figure 6-10), depends on the groups attached. Groups that share electrons by pi orbital overlap (i.e., resonance) stabilize the carbenium ion. Groups that place a positive partial or total charge adjacent to the carbenium ion withdraw electrons inductively by sigma bonds to destabilize the carbocation (Figure 6-16).

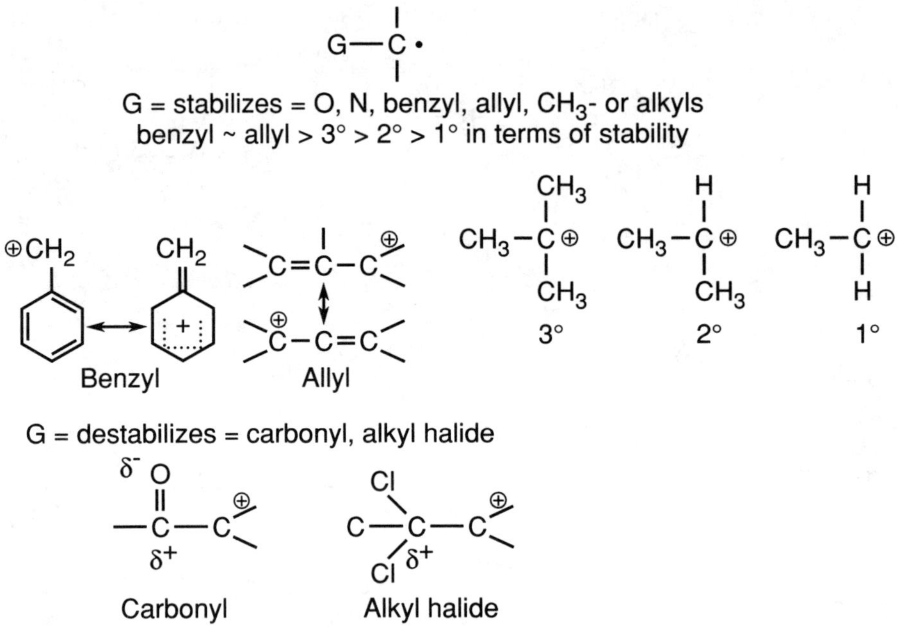

Figure 6-16. Stability of carbocations.

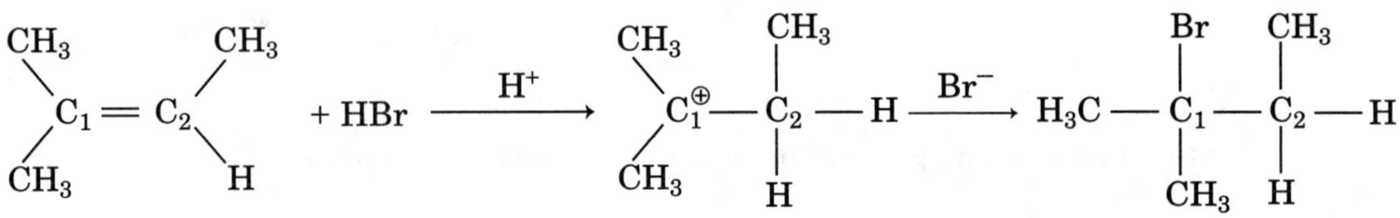

Figure 6-17. Bonding of electrophilic and nucleophilic substances.

These points are useful in predicting which carbon will become the carbenium ion and which one will bond to the electrophile and nucleophile atoms. The intermediate carbenium ion formed must be the most stable. Markovnikov's rule is a sequel to this statement: the nucleophile (i.e., a molecule with a free pair of electrons and sometimes a negative charge that seeks out partially or completely positive charge species) bonds to the most substituted carbon (i.e., the one with the fewest hydrogens attached) in the product, or equivalently, the electrophile bonds to the least substituted carbon (i.e., the one with the most hydrogens attached) in the product (Figure 6-17).

Ethene, or ethylene, is produced as fruit ripens, and it changes the color of the skin of the fruit. Fruit that is picked green for shipping often is treated with ethene to give it a ripe appearance.

6.4 NUCLEAR CHEMISTRY AND RADIOISOTOPES

6.4.1 Autoradiography

The localization and recording of a radiolabel within a solid specimen is known as autoradiography. The term does not apply to any single technique, but rather to a collection of techniques that produce an image in a photographic emulsion (Figure 6-18).

In direct autoradiography, a sample is placed on the film. Radioactive emissions produce black areas on the developed autoradiograph. This simple technique is used when spatial resolution is more important than absolute sensitivity. It produces quantitative images in which the absorbance of the film image is directly proportional to the amount of radioactivity in the sample (Figure 6-19*A* and *B*).

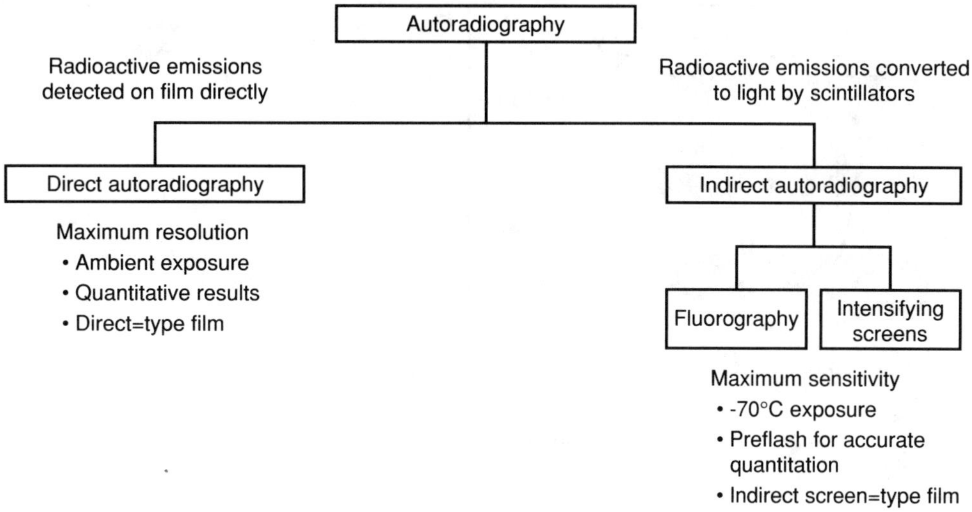

Figure 6-18. Maximizing results for sensitivity and resolution.

Figure 6-19*A* and *B*. Direct autoradiography.

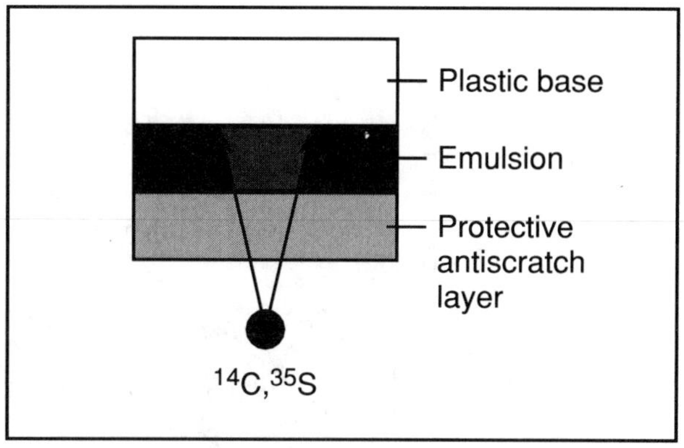

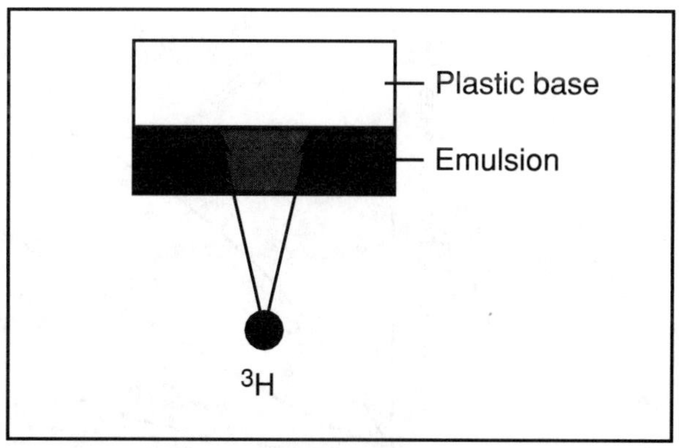

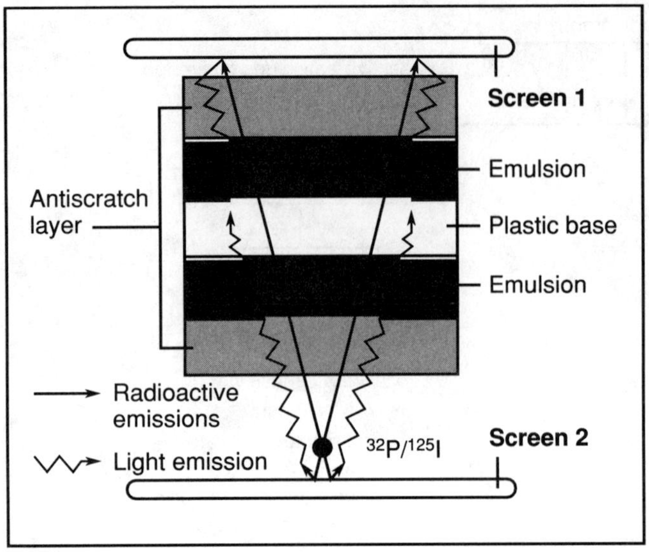

Figure 6-20. Direct or indirect autoradiography.

a

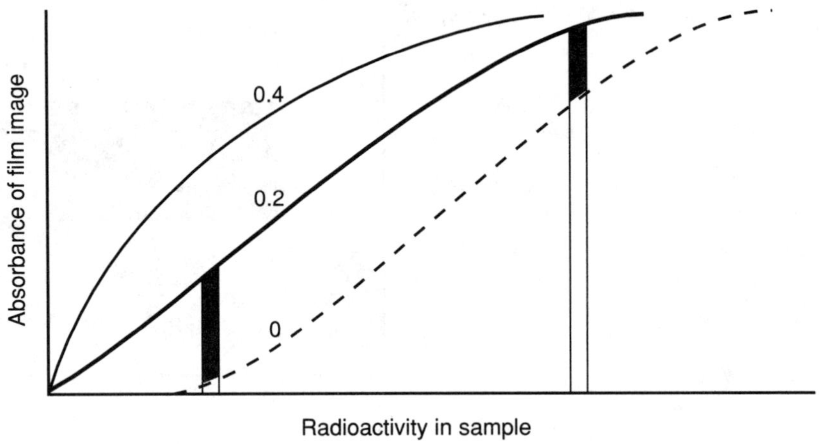

b

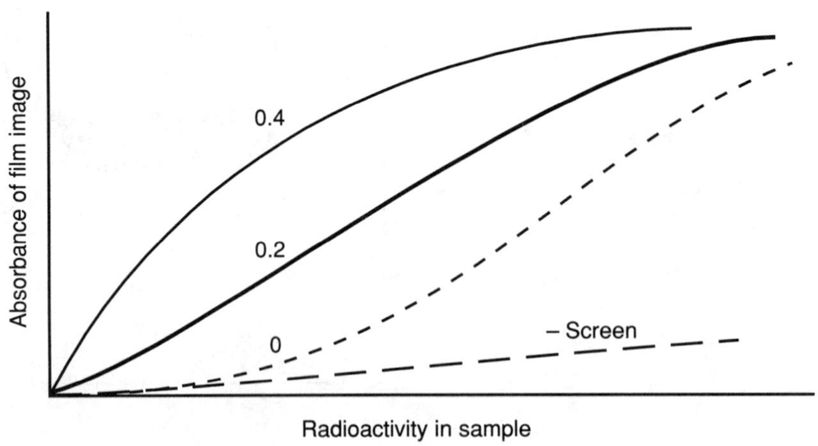

Figure 6-21*A* and *B*. Fluorography.

Direct autoradiography is best suited for use with weak to medium β-emitters if the β-particles are not absorbed within the sample before they reach the film. This problem is greatest for the weak emission of ^{3}H, but it also accounts for the decrease in efficiency of ^{35}S and ^{14}C when they are embedded in thick samples, such as agarose and polyacrylamide gels. The opposite problem limits sensitivity for high-energy β-particles, such as those from ^{32}P or for γ-rays emitted from isotopes, such as ^{125}I. These emissions pass through and beyond the film, and much of the energy is wasted (Figure 6-20). In each case, indirect autoradiography is more appropriate.

Indirect autoradiography is a technique by which emitted energy is converted to light by a scintillator that uses a fluorographic reagent or intensifying screens. Scintillators emit photons on excitation by β-particles or γ-rays. The photons are then recorded by an autoradiography film.

To a certain extent, fluorography overcomes the problem of internal absorption. The sample (e.g., a gel) can be impregnated with a scintillator. In this way, even weak β-emissions can transfer their energy to scintillator molecules, which then emit photons. If the sample is translucent, the photons travel farther than the original β-particles to form an image on the adjacent region of film. Compared with direct autoradiography, gel fluorography increases detection efficiency by more than 1000-fold for ^{3}H and by more than 10-fold for ^{35}S or ^{14}C (Figure 6-21 A, B).

For fluorography of high-energy β-particles (^{32}P) and x-rays (^{125}I), a dense, inorganic scintillator is placed behind the film. This scintillator is an intensifying screen, the most efficient of which emit blue light. Any emissions that pass through the x-ray film are absorbed by the screen and converted to light, superimposing a photographic image on the autoradiographic image. Intensifying screens are used only for isotopes that penetrate the film. If a screen is placed behind the autoradiography film, sensitivity is increased by approximately 10-fold for ^{32}P and 15-fold for ^{125}I compared with direct autoradiography.

The gain in sensitivity that is achieved by converting emissions to light is partly offset by decreased resolution and the nonlinearity of film response. The problem with nonlinearity can be overcome by pre-exposing film to an instantaneous flash of light and exposing it at $-70°C$.

6.4.2 Radioactive Isotopes

Tables 6-6, 6-7, 6-8, 6-9, and 6-10 show the characteristics of commonly used radioactive isotopes.

TABLE 6-6. *Characteristics of ^{125}I*

Characteristics	Radioactive half-life ($T_{1/2}$)	59.6 days
	Principal emission	35 keV gamma (7% emitted; 93% internally converted)
		27–32 keV x-rays (140% Te K x-rays)
Working safely with ^{125}iodine	Monitoring for contamination	Scintillation detector
	Biologic monitoring	Thyroid scans (scintillation detector)
	Annual limit on intake by inhalation	2×10^{6} Bq (≈55 β Ci)
	Dose rate from 1 GBq point source at 1 m	41 μSv/hr (4.1 mrem/hr)
	First half-value layer	0.02 mm lead
Special considerations	Volatilization of iodine is the most significant problem with this isotope. Formation of aerosols is also a hazard: simply opening a vial of sodium ^{125}I at high radioactive concentration can cause minute droplets of up to 100 Bq to become airborne. Solutions containing iodine ions should not be made acidic nor stored frozen; both lead to the formation of volatile elemental iodine.	

TABLE 6-7. ***Characteristics of ^{14}C***

Characteristics	Radioactive half-life ($T_{1/2}$)	5730 years
	Principal emission	0.156 MeV beta (maximum)
Working safely with ^{14}C	Monitoring for contamination	Thin end-window Geiger-Müller detector
	Biologic monitoring	Urine samples Breath measurements (CO_2)
	Annual limit on intake by ingestion	9×10^7 Bq (≈2.4 mCi) (labeled organic compounds)
	Maximum range in air	24 cm
	Maximum range in water	0.28 mm
	Shielding	1 cm Perspex/Plexiglas; thinner Perspex/ Plexiglas, down to 3 mm, although adequate to reduce doses, does not have good mechanical properties
Special considerations	Some organic compounds can be absorbed through gloves. Care must be taken not to generate carbon dioxide, which could be inhaled.	

TABLE 6-8. ***Characteristics of ^{35}S***

Characteristics	Radioactive half-life ($T_{1/2}$)	87.4 days
	Principal emission	0.167 MeV beta (maximum)
Working safely with ^{35}S	Monitoring for contamination	Thin end-window Geiger-Müller detector
	Biologic monitoring	Urine samples
	Annual limit on intake by inhalation	4×10^8 Bq (≈10 mCi) (inorganic compounds); 2×10^8 Bq (≈5 mCi) (elemental sulfur)
	Maximum range in air	26 cm
	Maximum range in water	0.32 mm
	Shielding	1 cm Perspex/Plexiglas; thinner Perspex/Plexiglas; down to 3 mm. although adequate to reduce doses, does not have good mechanical properties
Special considerations	Organic compounds are often strongly retained, and no limits of exposure have been set for them. Care must be taken not to generate sulfur dioxide or hydrogen sulfide, which could be inhaled. Radiolysis of ^{35}S amino acids during storage and use may lead to the release of ^{35}S-labeled volatile impurities.	

TABLE 6-9. ***Characteristics of ^{51}Cr***

Characteristics	Radioactive half-life ($T_{1/2}$)	27.7 days
	Principal emission	0.32 MeV gamma (9.8%); 5 keV x-ray (22% V 51 K x-rays)
Working safely with ^{51}Cr	Monitoring for contamination	Scintillation detector
	Biologic monitoring	Whole body
	Annual limit on intake by inhalation	7×10^8 Bq (≈20 mCi)
	Dose rate from 1 GBq point source at 1 m	4.7 μSv/hr (0.47 mrem/hr)
	First half-value layer	≈3 mm lead
Special considerations	In general, ^{51}Cr requires no special precautions beyond those necessary for any radionuclide of this emission energy. ^{51}Cr in the form of chromate is not selectively absorbed by any organ.	

TABLE 6-10. ***Characteristics of*** ^{32}***P***

Characteristics	Radioactive half-life ($T_{1/2}$)	14.3 days
	Principal emission	0.709 MeV beta (maximum)
Working safely with 32p	Monitoring for contamination	Geiger-Müller detector
	Biologic monitoring	Urine samples
	Annual limit on intake by inhalation	3×10^7 Bq (≈1 mCi*) (class D)
	Maximum range in air	790 cm
	Maximum range in water	0.8 mm
	Shielding	1 cm Perspex/Plexiglas cuts out betas and minimizes production of Bremsstrahlung
Special considerations	^{32}P is the highest-energy radionuclide commonly found in life science research laboratories; it requires special care. Exposure should be avoided (e.g., tubes containing even small quantities of ^{32}P should be held no longer than necessary; a stand or holder should be used). If more than ≈1 mCi is used, wrist and finger dosimeters should be worn.	

* Based on occupational effective dose equivalent limit of 50 mSv for stochastic risks.

6.5 SAMPLE TEST

1. What chemical compound has the formula PCl_3?
   A. Phosphorus trichlorite
   B. Phosphorus trichloride
   C. Phosphorus trichlorate
   D. Phosphorus trichlorine

2. What is the formula for the chemical compound barium oxide?
   A. BaO
   B. BaO_2
   C. Ba_2O
   D. Ba_2O_3

3. Which compound contains the lowest percentage of carbon by mass?
   A. CH_4
   B. CH_3CO_2H
   C. $Na_2C_2O_2$
   D. $C_6H_{12}O_6$

4. A compound has the empirical formula CH_2Cl and a molecular mass of 198 g $mole^{-1}$. Using the atomic weights C = 12, H = 1, and Cl = 35.5, what is the molecular formula?
   A. CH_2Cl
   B. $C_2H_4Cl_2$
   C. $C_3H_6Cl_3$
   D. $C_4H_8Cl_4$

5. Balance the following hypothetical equation with the minimum integral coefficients.
   $CrPO_4 + Bi_2(SiO_4)_3 \rightarrow BiPO_4 + Cr_2(SiO_4)_3$
   What is the correct coefficient for $BiPO_4$?
   A. 1
   B. 2
   C. 3
   D. 4

6. A chemist who is attempting to identify the main component in a commercial record cleaner finds that 25 ml of the substance has a mass of 20 g. Which compound is the most likely choice?
   A. Chloroform, which has a density of 1.5 g/cm^3
   B. Diethyl ether, which has a density of 0.7 g/cm^3
   C. Isopropyl alcohol,which has a density of 0.8 g/cm^3
   D. Toluene, which has a density of 0.9 g/cm^3

7. How many grams of HCl are required to react completely with 1 mol Zn?
   $HCl_{(aq)} + Zn_{(s)} \rightarrow ZnCl_{2(aq)} + H_{2(g)}$
   A. 18
   B. 36
   C. 54
   D. 72

8. The total pressure of a mixture of gases is:
   A. obtained by multiplying the individual pressures by the number of moles and averaging the product.

B. the sum of the partial pressures of the components.
C. dependent only on the pressure of the gas that is present in the greatest quantity.
D. the product of the partial pressures of the components.

9. What volume is occupied by 2.00 mol methane (CH_4) at 273 K and 2.00 atm?
A. 22.4 L
B. 11.2 L
C. 10.00 L
D. 44.8 L

10. Four identical 1.0-L flasks contain different gases at 0°C and 1 atm pressure. Which gas has the lowest density?
A. He
B. Cl_2
C. CH_4
D. C_3H_6

11. A technician forces 1 L nitrogen and 1 L carbon dioxide initially at 1 atm into a single 500-ml vessel. What is the new nitrogen pressure if the temperature remains unchanged?
A. 1 atm
B. 2 atm
C. 3 atm
D. 4 atm

12. Given the unbalanced reaction $N_{2(g)} + Br_{2(g)} \rightarrow NBr_{3(g)}$, how many liters of gaseous bromine are needed to react with 2 L nitrogen?
A. 1
B. 3
C. 4
D. 6

13. The boiling point for ethylene glycol is 198°C; for water, 100°C; for formamide, 111°C; for ethanol, 79°C; and for methanol, 65°C. Which compound has the highest vapor pressure at room temperature?
A. Ethylene glycol
B. Water
C. Ethanol
D. Methanol

Questions 14 and 15 refer to the following phase diagram:

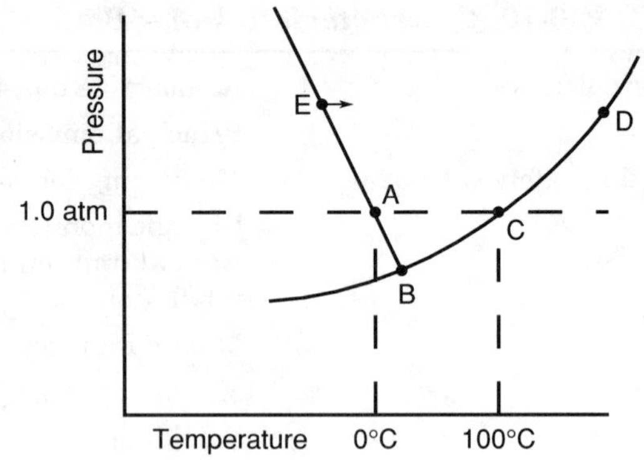

14. The triple point of water is located at the temperature and pressure represented by point:
A. A.
B. B.
C. C.
D. D.

15. What physical change is represented by arrow E?
A. Sublimation
B. Condensation
C. Melting
D. Deposition

16. Adding a nonvolatile solute to a solvent:
A. decreases the freezing point and increases the boiling point.
B. increases the freezing point and decreases the boiling point.
C. increases both the freezing and boiling points.
D. decreases both the freezing and boiling points.

17. In any cubic lattice, an atom lying at the corner of a unit cell is shared equally by how many unit cells?
A. 1
B. 2
C. 8
D. 16

18. What are electrolytes?
A. Solutions that contain solvated electrons
B. Solutions that conduct an electric current
C. Solutions that contain soluble salts, strong acids, or strong bases
D. Both B and C

19. What volume of 2.0 M HCl must be used to prepare 10.0 L 0.50 M HCl solution?
A. 25 L
B. 2.5 L
C. 0.25 L
D. 250 L

20. A student has 500 L 4×10^{-3} M solution of NaOH. How many atoms of sodium are contained in this sample?
A. 6.02×10^{23}
B. 3.01×10^{23}
C. 1.2×10^{24}
D. 4.50×10^{22}

21. Which pair of liquids would be infinitely miscible?
A. Ethanol and water
B. Benzene and water
C. Ether and water
D. Chloroform and water

22. Which compound is nonpolar?
A. NH_3
B. BCl_3
C. H_2O
D. CO

23. What is the conjugate acid of NH_3?
A. OH^-
B. NH_2^-
C. H_3O^+
D. NH

24. When $NaC_2H_3O_2$ is dissolved in water, the resulting solution is:
A. acidic.
B. basic.
C. neutral.
D. colligative.

25. Which system is a buffer?
A. 10 ml 0.1 M NH_4Cl and 10 ml 0.1 M HCl
B. 10 ml 0.1 M NH_4Cl and 10 ml 0.1 M NaCl
C. 10 ml 0.1 M NH_4Cl and 10 ml 0.1 M NH_3
D. 10 ml 0.1 M NH_4Cl and 10 ml 0.1 M NaOH

26. Given the reaction $HCl + Ba(OH)_2 \rightarrow BaCl_2 + H_2O$, what volume of 1 N HCl is required to react completely with 10 ml 1 N $Ba(OH)_2$?
A. 5 ml
B. 10 ml
C. 15 ml
D. 20 ml

27. In the reaction, $B_2H_6 + 2N(CH_2CH_3)_3 \rightarrow 2H_3B - N(CH_2CH_3)_3$, what is the role of $N(CH_2CH_3)_3$?
A. Lewis acid
B. Lewis base
C. Brønsted-Lowry acid
D. Brønsted-Lowry base

28. In the equilibrium $4\ NH_{3(g)} + 3\ O_{2(g)} \rightleftharpoons 2\ N_{2(g)} + 6\ H_2O_{(l)}$, $\Delta H = -303$ kcal, which change will cause the equilibrium to shift to the right?
A. Increase the temperature
B. Selectively absorb the water
C. Add a catalyst
D. Selectively absorb the O_2

29. In the reaction $2\ XY_{(g)} \rightleftharpoons X_{2(g)} + Y_{2(g)}$, K = 0.9 at 243 K, 1 mol XY was injected into a 1-L container at 243 K. What is the equilibrium expression?
A. $0.9 = \dfrac{(1 - 2x)^2}{x^2}$
B. $0.9 = \dfrac{x^2}{(1 - 2x)^2}$
C. $0.9 = \dfrac{x^2}{(1 - 2x)}$
D. $0.9 = \dfrac{(1 - 2x)}{x^2}$

30. Which compound is the most soluble in water?
A. $CaSO_4$, $K_{sp} = 10^{-5}$
B. CuI, $K_{sp} = 10^{-12}$
C. AgI, $K_{sp} = 10^{-16}$
D. CuS, $K_{sp} = 10^{-45}$

31. What is the concentration of silver in a saturated silver iodide solution?
A. 10^{-16} M
B. 10^{-32} M
C. 10^{-4} M
D. 10^{-8} M

32. The K_{sp} of $Fe(OH)_2$ is 10^{-15}. A system at equilibrium is a brown solution, $Fe(OH)_{2(aq)}$, and a brown solid, $Fe(OH)_{2(s)}$. If 50 ml NaOH is added, what will occur?
A. Additional solid forms; solution color pales
B. Some solid dissolves; solution color deepens

C. Gas evolves; solution color changes to green
D. No change

33. The heat of formation of an element in its standard state is:
A. the ΔH of its reaction with hydrogen.
B. the ΔH of its reaction with oxygen.
C. zero.
D. determined with the molecular mass.

34. When a sample is burned in a bomb calorimeter containing 1.00 kg water, the temperature of the water increases by 1°C. If the heat capacity of the system is 0 kJ/K and the specific heat of water is 4.18 J/K g, how much heat is evolved?
A. 2.09 kJ
B. 8.36 kJ
C. 1.00 kJ
D. 4.18 kJ

35. Calculate the heat of formation of ethanol, C_2H_5OH, with the following information:

$C_2H_5OH_{(l)} + 3\ O_{2(g)} \rightarrow 2\ CO_{2(g)} + 3\ H_2O_{(l)}$ $\quad \Delta H = -1300 kJ$
$C_{(s)} + O_{2(g)} \rightarrow CO_{2(g)}$ $\quad \Delta H = -400\ kJ$
$H_{2(g)} + 0.5\ O_{2(g)} \rightarrow H_2O_{(l)}$ $\quad \Delta H = -300\ kJ$

A. −2000 kJ
B. +2000 kJ
C. −400 kJ
D. +400 kJ

36. When must a reaction be spontaneous, independent of T?
A. $\Delta H = 0, \Delta S > 0$
B. $\Delta H = 0, \Delta S < 0$
C. $\Delta S = 0, \Delta H > 0$
D. $\Delta H < 0, \Delta S > 0$

37. What is the rate of a unimolecular reaction?
A. k[A]
B. $k[A]^2$
C. k[A][B]
D. $k[A][B]^2$

38. The rate constant for a first-order reaction is 0.40 min^{-1}. What is the initial rate if the initial concentration of the compound is 0.50 M?
A. 0.90 mol L^{-1} min^{-1}
B. 0.10 mol L^{-1} min^{-1}
C. 0.20 mol L^{-1} min^{-1}
D. 0.40 mol L^{-1} min^{-1}

39. Which event is necessary for a reaction to occur between two molecules?
A. A collision between two molecules has an energy greater than the E_a.
B. A collision between two molecules has an energy less than the ΔH of the reaction.
C. The activated complex has sufficient vibrational energy to break bonds.
D. The activated complex has less potential energy than the reaction products.

Questions 40 and 41 refer to the following diagram:

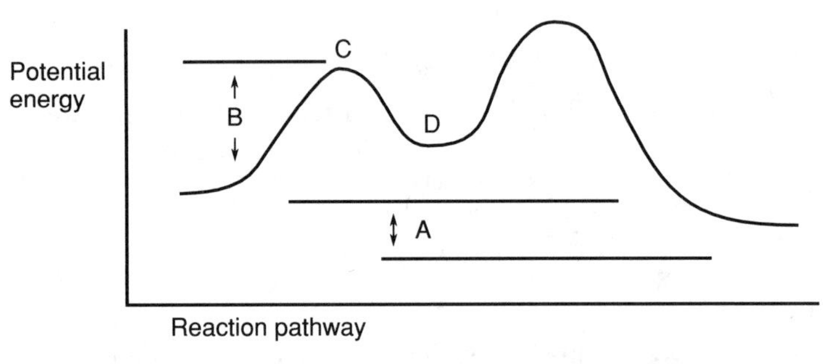

40. What point on the reaction diagram is a reaction intermediate?
A. A
B. B
C. C
D. D

41. What point on the reaction diagram is a transition state?
A. A
B. B
C. C
D. D

Questions 42 and 43 refer to the following information and cell diagram:

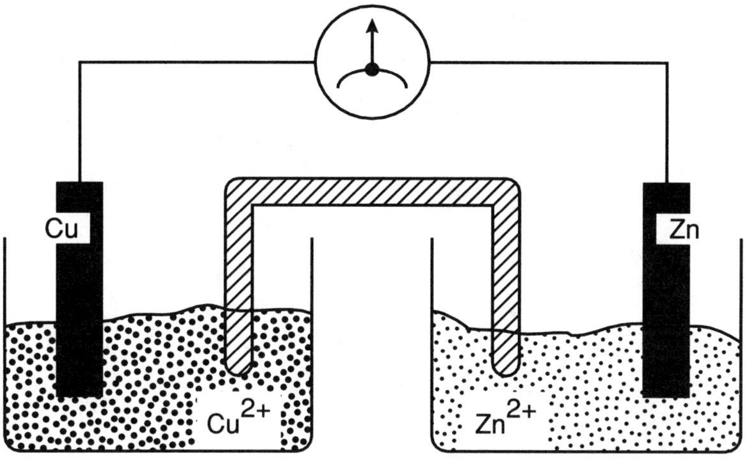

$Zn^{2+} + 2\,e^- \rightarrow Zn \quad E° = -0.76\ V$

$Cu^{2+} + 2\,e^- \rightarrow Cu \quad E° = +0.34\ V$

42. Which reactions will produce a spontaneous reaction ($\Delta G < 0$) for the cell?
A. $Cu^{2+} + Zn \rightarrow Cu + Zn^{2+}$
B. $Cu + Zn^{2+} \rightarrow Cu^{2+} + Zn$
C. $Cu^{2+} + Zn^{2+} \rightarrow Cu + Zn + 4\,e^-$
D. $Cu + Zn + 4\,e^- \rightarrow Cu^{2+} + Zn^{2+}$

43. If the cell contains 1.0 M $CuSO_4$ and 1.0 M $ZnSO_4$, what is the potential, E, of the cell?
A. −1.10 V
B. +1.10 V
C. +2.20 V
D. −2.20 V

44. What is the oxidation state of nitrogen in NO_3^-?
A. −3
B. 0
C. +3
D. +5

45. Based on the following information, which metal is the strongest reducing agent?
(i) $Zn^{2+} + Fe \rightarrow$ No reaction
(ii) $Fe^{2+} + Zn \rightarrow Zn^{2+} + Fe$
(iii) $Mg^{2+} + Zn \rightarrow$ No reaction
(iv) $Zn^{2+} + Mg \rightarrow Mg^{2+} + Zn$
(v) $Cu^{2+} + Zn \rightarrow Cu + Zn^{2+}$
A. Cu
B. Fe
C. Mg
D. Zn

46. Oxygen has six valence electrons. Which electron arrangement is the ground state for oxygen?

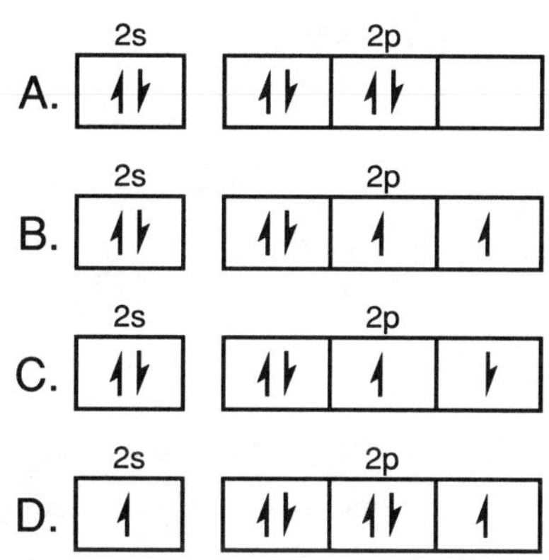

47. Which ion is isoelectronic with Ar?
A. Ca^+
B. S^-
C. K^+
D. P^{2-}

48. Which of the following best describes the bonding in HCN?
A. Ionic only
B. Two sigma bonds and two pi bonds
C. Three sigma bonds and one pi bond
D. Four sigma bonds

49. How many electrons can occupy a shell with $n = 3$?
A. 2
B. 8

C. 18
D. 42

50. How many electrons can occupy a subshell with $l = 2$?
A. 2
B. 6
C. 10
D. 14

51. Which element does not obey the octet rule?
A. C
B. Ne
C. P
D. H

52. What element has the electron configuration [Kr] $4d^5 5s^2$?
A. Mn
B. Tc
C. Re
D. Uns (#107)

53. Which element is classified as a semimetal or metalloid?
A. Carbon
B. Sulfur
C. Arsenic
D. Lead

54. Which element is liquid at room temperature?
A. F_2
B. Cl_2
C. Br_2
D. I_2

55. Which elements are known collectively as the noble gases?
A. He, Ne, Ar, Kr, Xe
B. F, Cl, Br, I, At
C. Be, Mg, Ca, Sr, Ba, Ra
D. Li, Na, K, Rb, Cs, Fr

56. How many electrons can be contained in all of the orbitals with $n = 3$?
A. 2
B. 8
C. 18
D. 32

57. Which atoms are listed in increasing size?
I. Al, Si, P, S
II. S, P, Si, Al
III. I, Br, Cl, F
IV. F, Cl, Br, I
A. I and III
B. II and IV
C. I and IV
D. II and III

58. What is the value of 1 for a 3d orbital?
A. 0
B. 1
C. 2
D. 3

59. Which atom requires the most energy to remove a valence electron?
A. Li
B. Na
C. K
D. Rb

60. Which metal yields an oxide with the formula MO when reacted with oxygen?
A. Sodium
B. Potassium
C. Aluminum
D. Magnesium

61. Which compound is caustic soda?
A. NaOH
B. Na_2CO_3
C. NaCl
D. Na_2SO_4

62. Which radioactive decay process does not involve a change in atomic number?
A. Electron capture
B. Gamma emission
C. Positron emission
D. Beta emission

63. The half-life of ^{131}I is 8.0 days. How many grams of ^{131}I remain after 16.0 days in a sample that initially contained 1.00 g ^{131}I?
A. 0.50
B. 0.25
C. 0.13
D. 0.05

64. What is the missing product of the reaction $^{43}_{19}K \rightarrow ^{43}_{20}Ca + ?$
A. $^{4}_{2}He$
B. $^{0}_{-1}e$
C. $^{0}_{1}e$
D. γ

65. What is the missing product of the reaction $Ni^* \rightarrow Ni + ?$
A. $^{4}_{2}He$
B. $^{0}_{-1}e$
C. $^{0}_{1}e$
D. γ

66. What is the best description of the bonding in CO_2?
   A. One sigma bond and three pi bonds
   B. Three sigma bonds and one pi bond
   C. No sigma bonds and four pi bonds
   D. Two sigma bonds and two pi bonds

67. Which molecule violates the octet rule?
   A. BH_3
   B. CH_4
   C. NH_3
   D. H_2O

68. Which molecule represents molecule 1 in a Fisher projection?

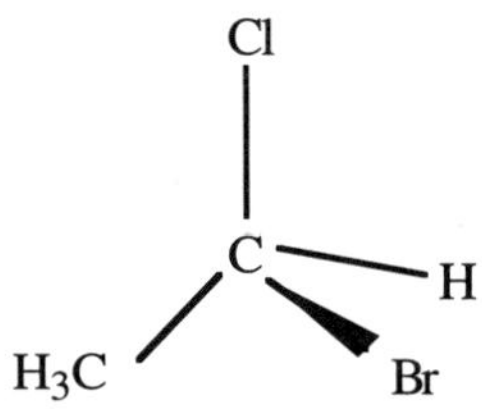

Molecule 1

A. 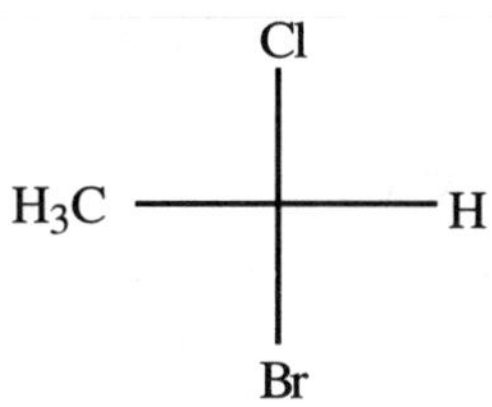

B. 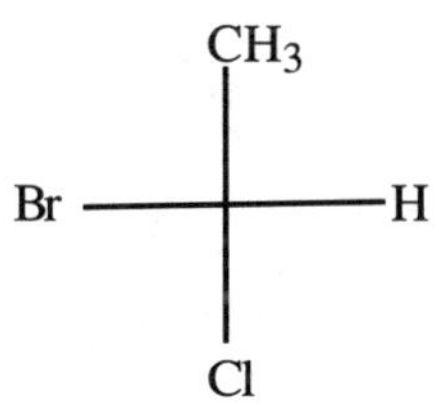

C. 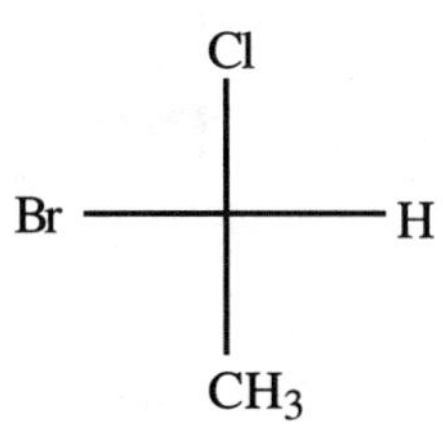

D. 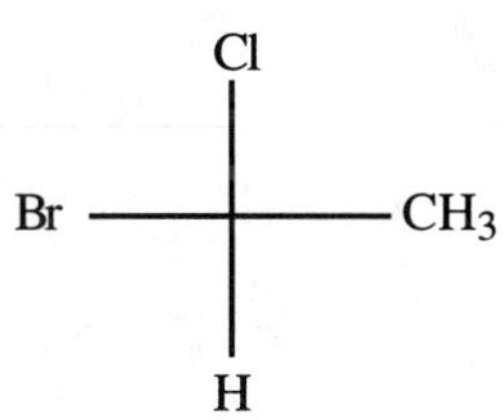

69. Which molecule is in the S configuration?

A. 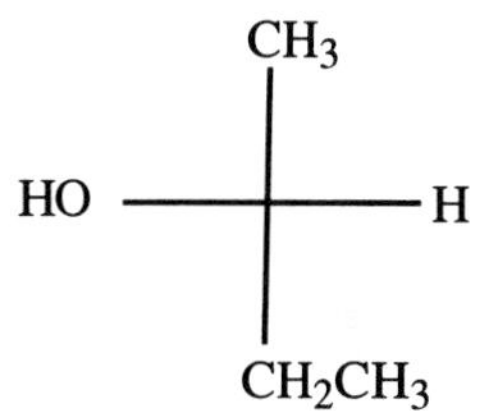

B. 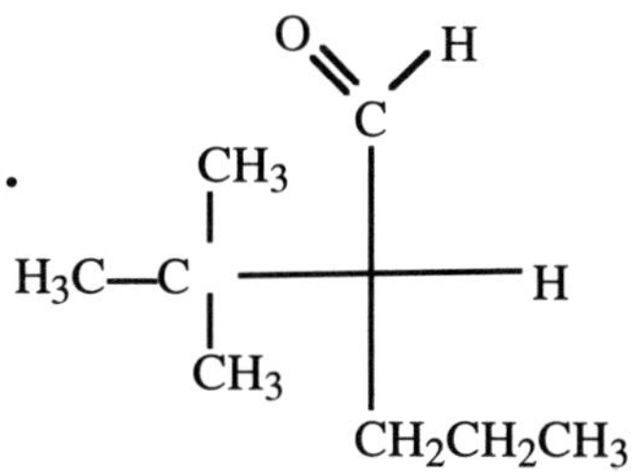

C. 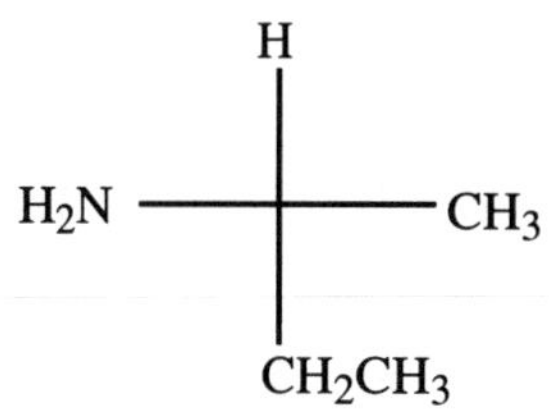

D. 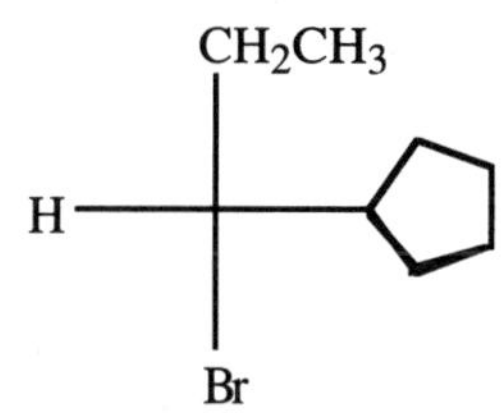

70. Which molecule is an enantiomer of molecule 2?

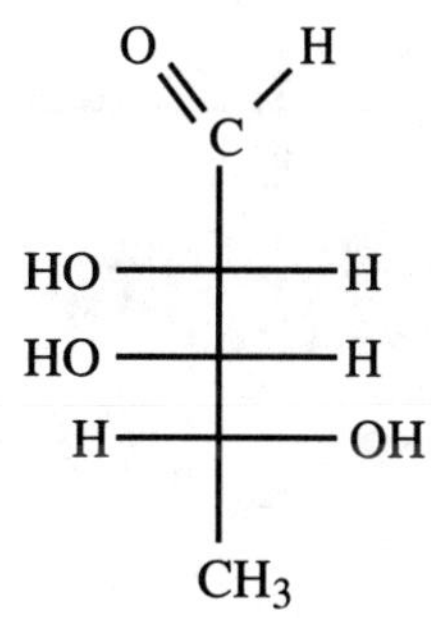

Molecule 2

A.

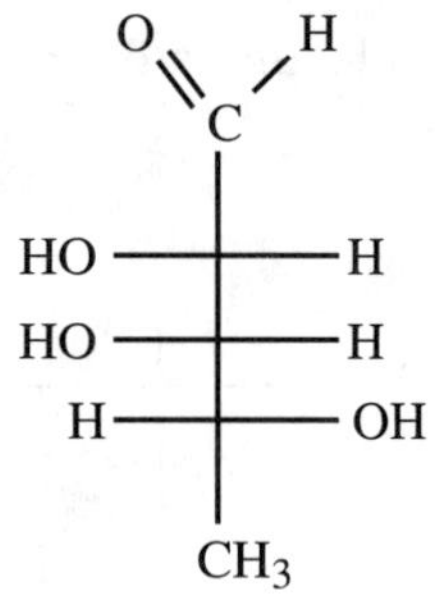

B.

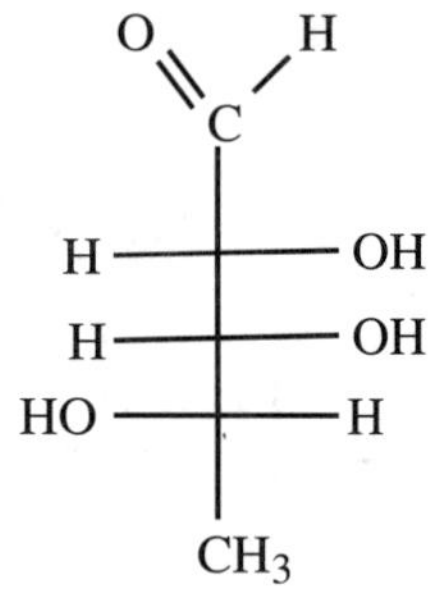

C.

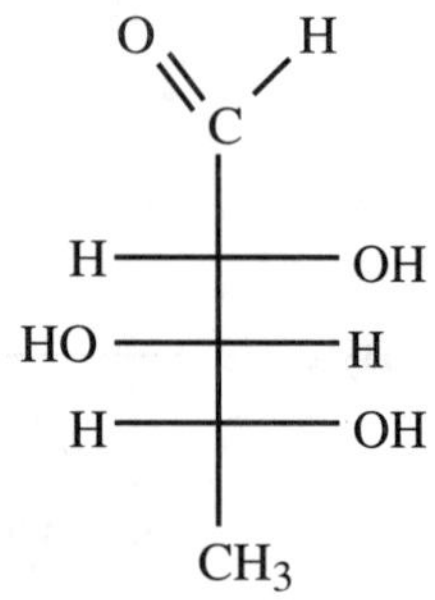

D.

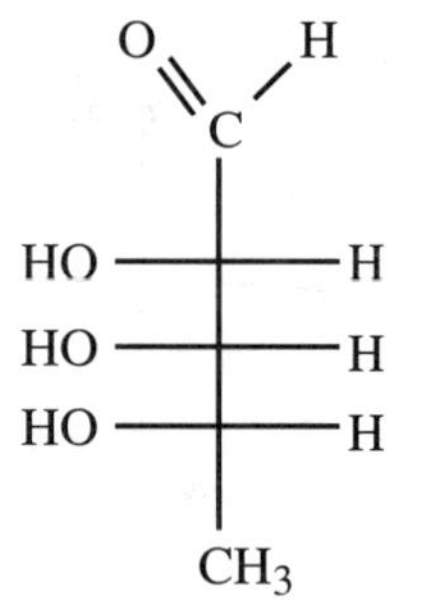

71. How many stereoisomers of molecule 3 exist?

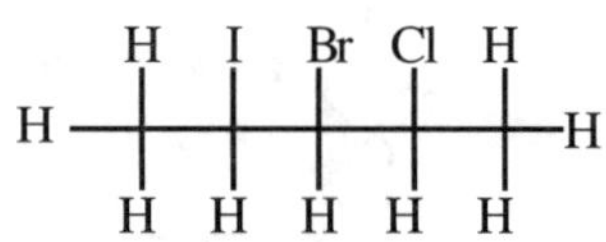

Molecule 3

A. 4
B. 8
C. 16
D. 32

72. Of the labeled carbons in molecule 4, which is a tertiary carbon?

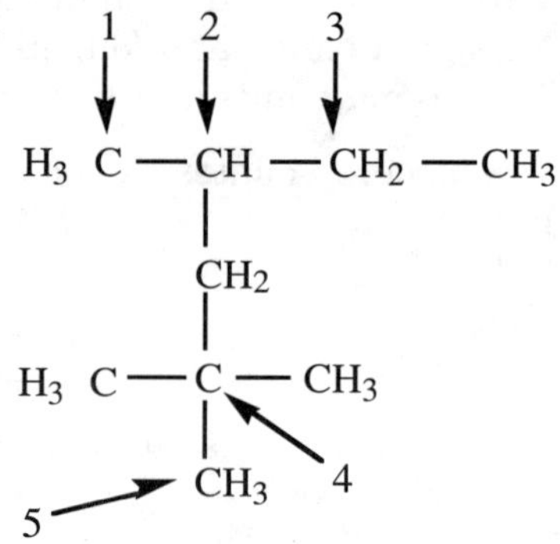

Molecule 4

A. 1
B. 2
C. 3
D. 4

73. The compound with the highest boiling point is:
A. n-hexane.
B. 2-methylpentane.
C. 2,3-dimethylbutane.
D. cyclohexane.

74. Which Newman projection represents the highest energy configuration?

A.

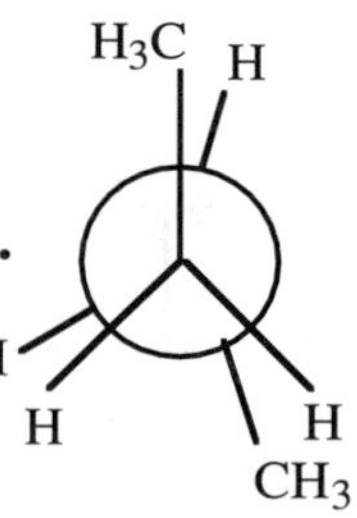

B.

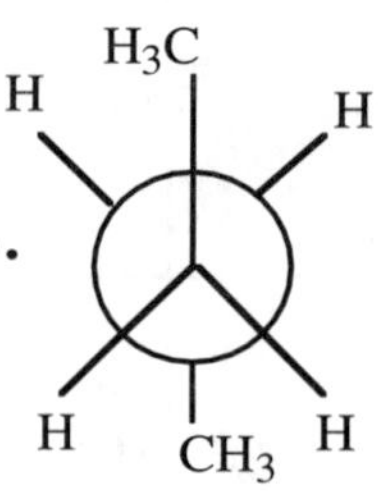

C.

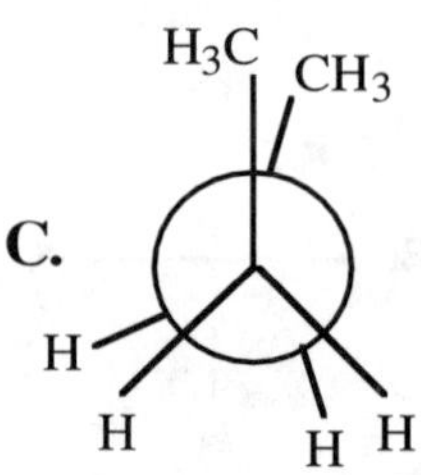

D. 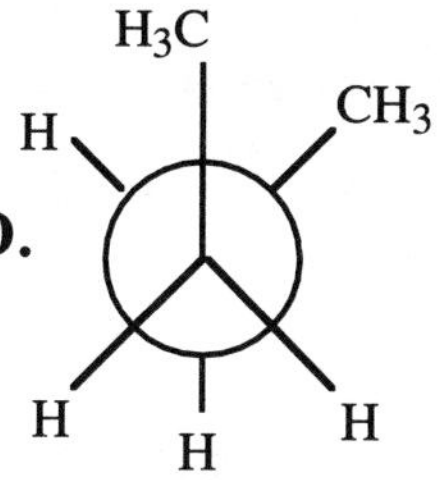

75. What is the product of the following reaction?

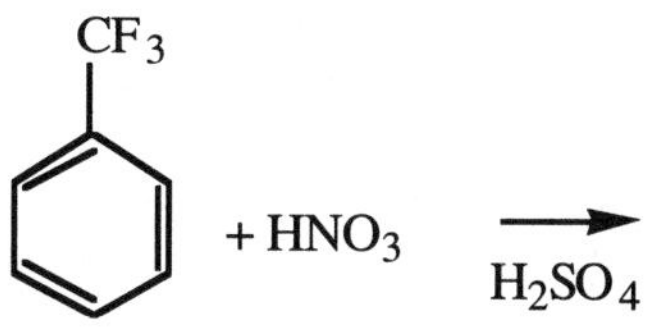

A. 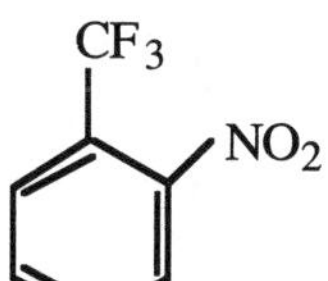

B. 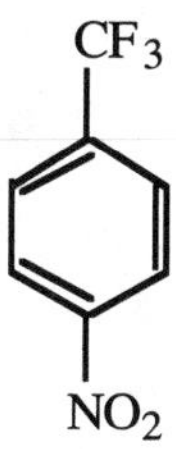

C. 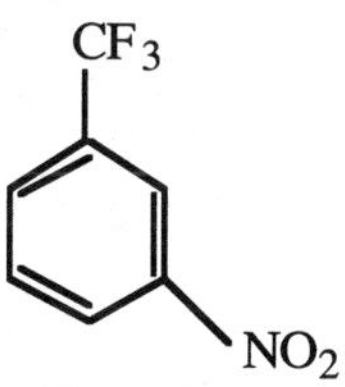

D. 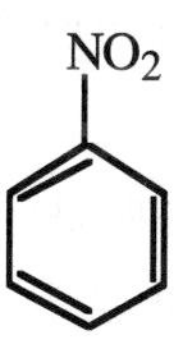

76. Which compound is not aromatic?

A. 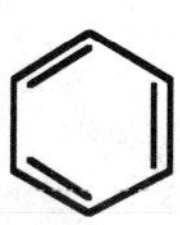

B. 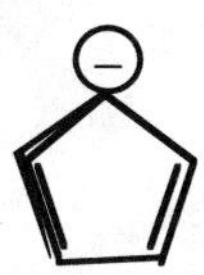

C. 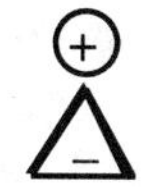

D. 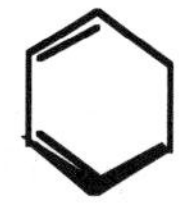

77. What is the product of the following reaction?

$$H_3CCH{=}CH_2 + HBr \longrightarrow ?$$

A. 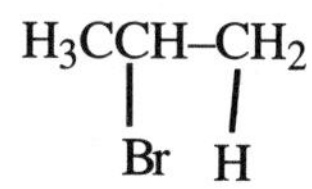

B. 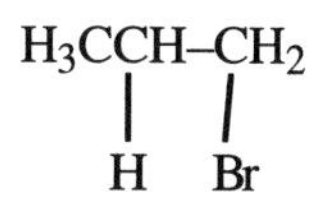

C. 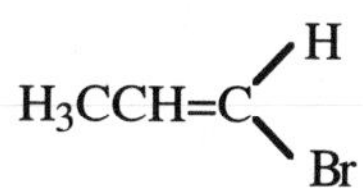

D. $H_3CC(Br){=}CH_2$

78. The reaction of a primary alcohol with CrO_3 yields:
A. an aldehyde.
B. a carboxylic acid.
C. a ketone.
D. an ether.

79. The Williamson ether synthesis is the reaction of:
A. ROH and R'X
B. RCOOH and R'X
C. RONa and R'X
D. ROH and R'Na

80. What is the name of the following compound?

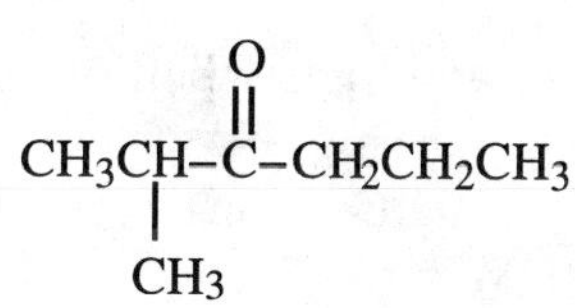

A. 2-methyl-3-hexanal
B. 1-methyl-3-hexanal

C. 2-methyl-3-hexanone
D. 1-methyl-3-hexanone

81. Which species is a ketal?

A. 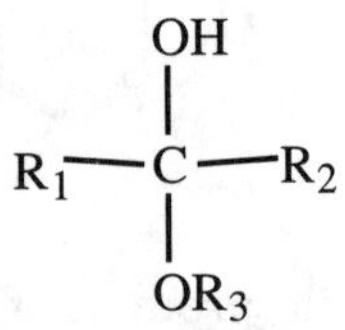

B. 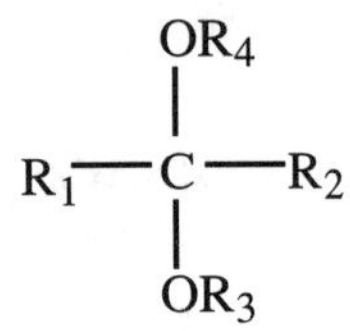

C. 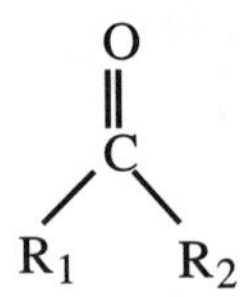

D. 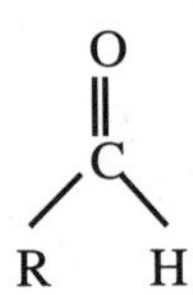

82. What is the major product in the following reaction?

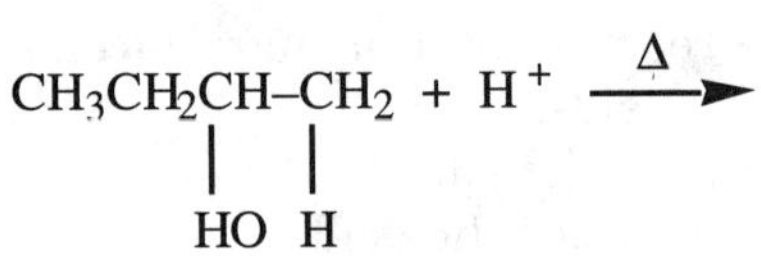

A. $CH_3CH_2CH{=}CH_2$

B. $CH_3CH{=}CH{-}CH_3$

C. 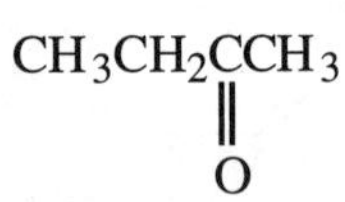

D. $CH_3CH_2CH_2CH_3$

83. Alcohols have higher boiling points than the corresponding alkanes (e.g., methane boils at $-164°C$, whereas methanol boils at 65°C). Why?
A. Higher molecular mass
B. Hydrogen bonding
C. London dispersion forces
D. Higher density

84. Which carboxylic acid is the strongest?

A. 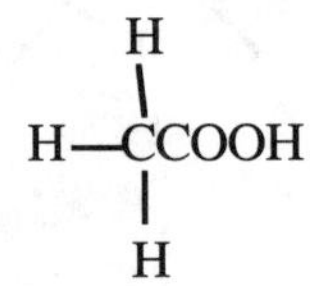

B. 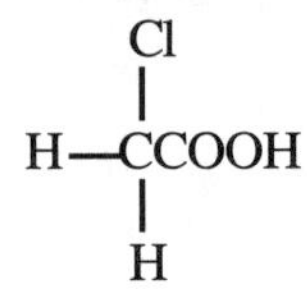

C. 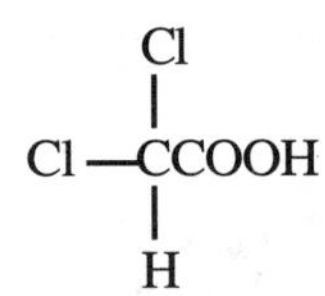

D. 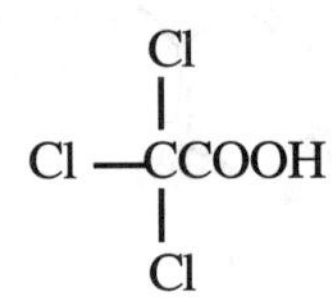

85. The reaction of a carboxylic acid and an alcohol produces:
A. an anhydride.
B. an ether.
C. an ester.
D. an acid with a longer carbon chain.

86. What is the name of the following compound?

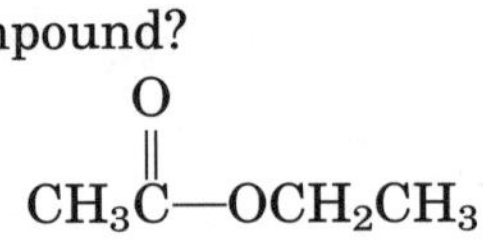

A. Ethanoic acid
B. Ethanoic anhydride
C. Ethyl ethanoate
D. Ethanamide

87. A general reagent for the conversion of an acyl chloride to an ester is:
A. excess ammonia.
B. an alcohol in the presence of pyridine.
C. a dialkyl cadmium compound.
D. hydrogen in the presence of palladium.

88. Which compound has the lowest melting point?

A. Ethanamide
B. N-ethylethanamide
C. N, N-diethylethanamide
D. Ethene

89. Which compound is the strongest base in the gas phase?
A. Trimethylamine
B. Dimethylamine
C. Methylamine
D. Ammonia

90. What is the product of the following reaction?

$RC(=O)NH_2 + LiAlH_4 \longrightarrow$

A. $R\text{–}C\equiv N$

B. RCH_2NH_2

C. $RC(=O)H$

D. $RC(=O)NH_3^+$

91. What is the product of the following reaction?
$CH_2{=}CHC{\equiv}N + H_2/Pt \rightarrow ?$
A. $CH_3CH_2C{\equiv}N$
B. $CH_2{=}CHNH_2$
C. $CH_3CH_2CH_2NH_2$
D. $CH_3CH_2CH{=}NH$

92. Which compound is aniline?

A.
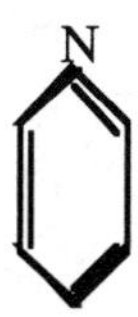

B.
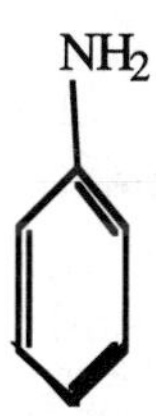

C.
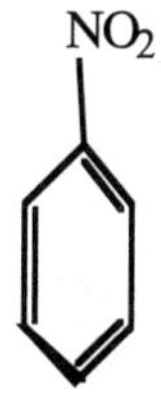

D.
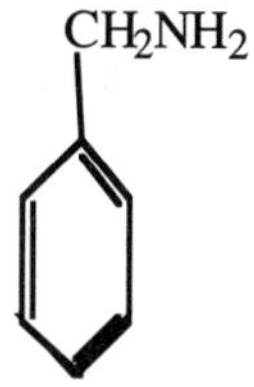

93. A peptide linkage between two amino acids is best described by:
A. the condensation of two carboxylic acids groups on amino acids.
B. the interaction between amine and carboxyl groups of amino acids.
C. a hydrogen bond formed between the —COOH group and —NH_2 groups of amino acids.
D. a new carbon–carbon interaction between amino acids.

94. The isoelectric point of amino acids is defined as occurring when:
A. all —COOH sites are protonated.
B. all —NH_2 sites are deprotonated.
C. the amino acid present as a zwitterion is at a minimum.
D. the amino acid present as a zwitterion is at a maximum.

95. One useful method for determining the N-terminal amino acid residue is the Sanger method. In this reaction, using 2,4-dinitrofluorobenzene, the terminal amino acid contains:
A. a nitro group.
B. a fluorophenyl group.
C. a 2,4-dinitrophenyl group.
D. a fluoro group.

96. Which functional group is not commonly found in amino acids?
A. Thiol, —SH
B. Nitrosyl, —NO
C. Hydroxyl, —OH
D. Amino, —NH_2

97. How many amino acids occur naturally in proteins?
A. 10
B. 12

C. 18
D. 20

98. What is the product of the reaction of glycine with benzoyl chloride and $NaOH_{(aq)}$?

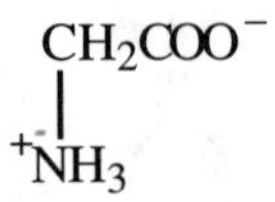

Glycine

A. $Ph\overset{O}{\overset{\|}{C}}NHCH_2COOH$
B. $(Cl^-)(^+H_3NCH_2COOH)$
C. H_2NCH_2COOCl
D. $H_2NCH_2COOCH_2C_6H_5$

99. Which characteristic does NOT describe globular proteins?
A. Insoluble in water
B. Intramolecular hydrogen bonding
C. Folded into compact units
D. Functions usually related to the regulation of life processes

100. Stereochemical studies of naturally occurring amino acids show that they all have the same configurations around the carbon bonded to the alpha-amino group as:
A. D-gylceraldehyde.
B. L-glyceraldehyde.
C. D-tartaric acid.
D. L-tartaric acid.

101. Which labeled carbon is the anomeric carbon?

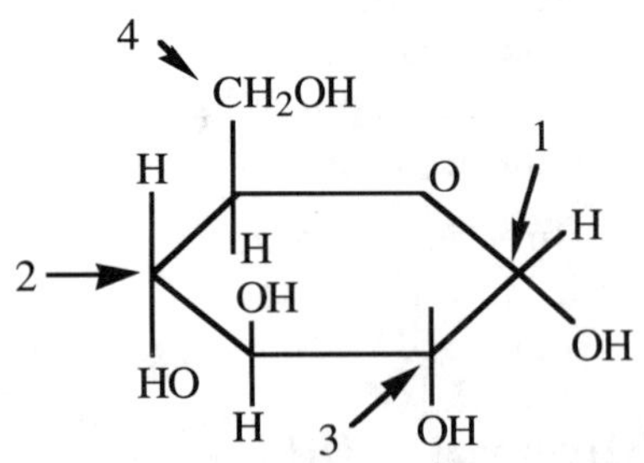

A. 1
B. 2
C. 3
D. 4

102. Which straight-chain aldose provides the following cyclic structure?

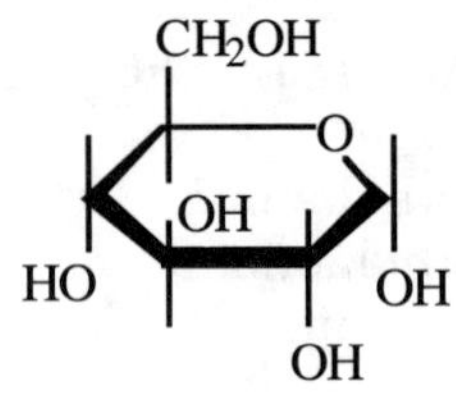

A.

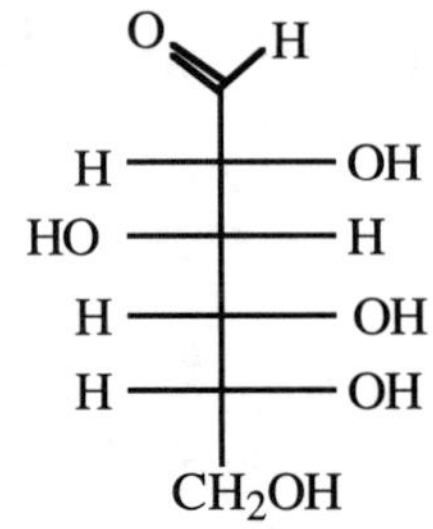

B.

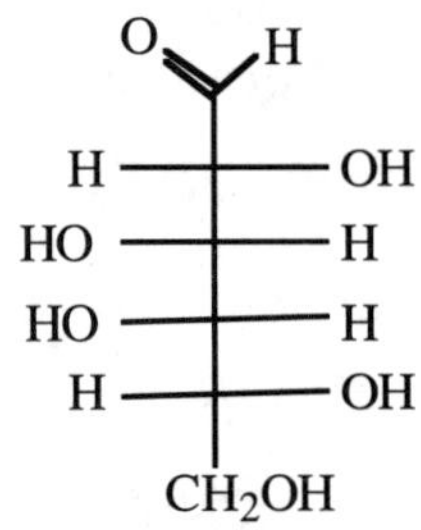

C.

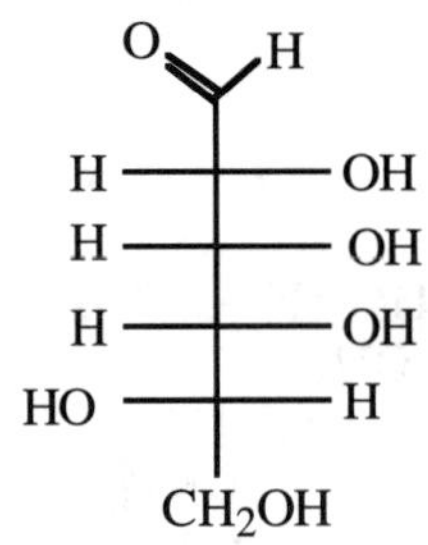

D.

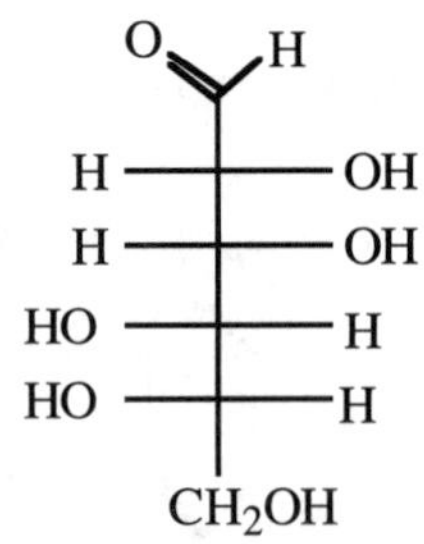

103. Which procedure is used in the Kiliani-Fischer synthesis to lengthen the carbon chain of aldoses?
A. Reaction with H_2CO_3 followed by hydrolysis

B. Reaction with $H_2C{=}O$ followed by hydrolysis
C. Reaction with H_3COH followed by hydrolysis
D. Reaction with HCN followed by hydrolysis

104. What is the product of a Ruff degradation that starts with:

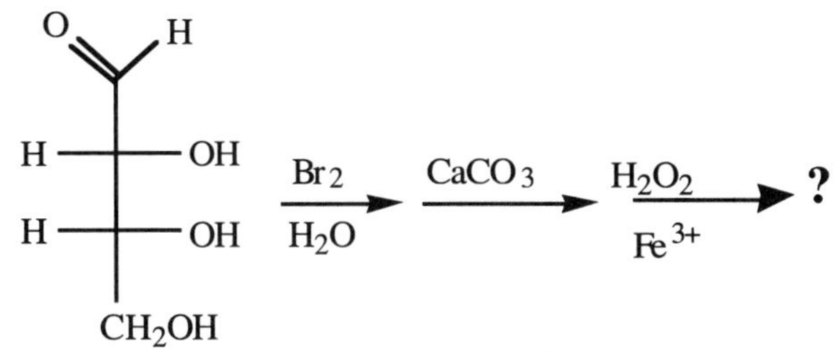

A.
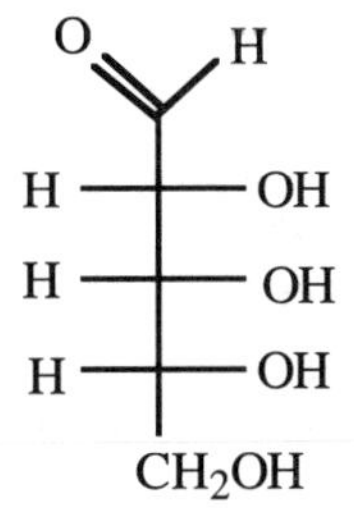

B.
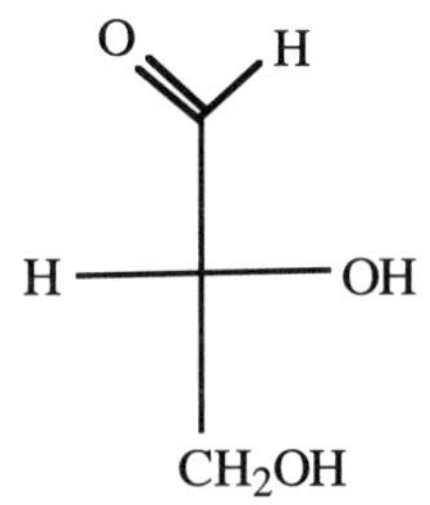

C.
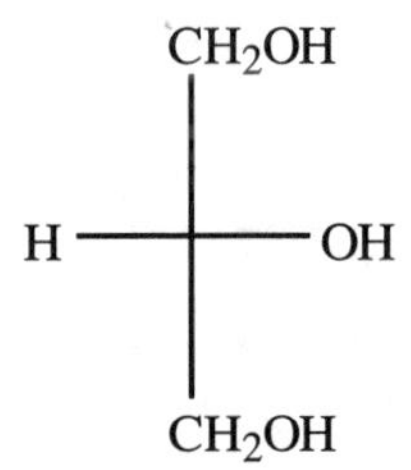

D.
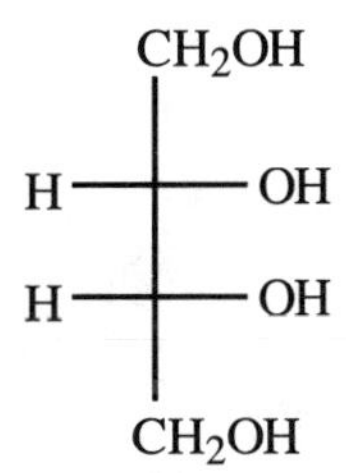

105. Which reagent tests can be used to differentiate between aldoses and ketoses?
A. Fehling's reagent
B. Tollen's reagent
C. Bromine water
D. Benedict's solution

106. High-resolution mass spectrometric analysis of compound A gave a molecular formula of $C_9H_{10}O_2$. The infrared spectrum showed strong absorption at 1715 cm^{-1} as well as many other medium-intensity bands. The nuclear magnetic resonance spectrum consisted of three sharp peaks at ∂ = 5.00 ppm (area 2) and ∂ = 1.96 ppm (area 3). What is the structure of compound A?

A.
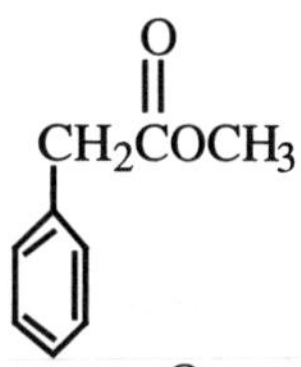

B.
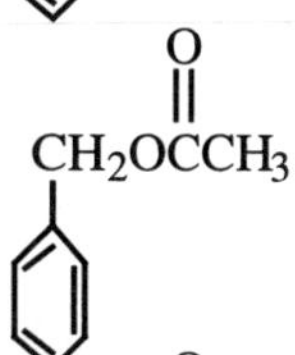

C.
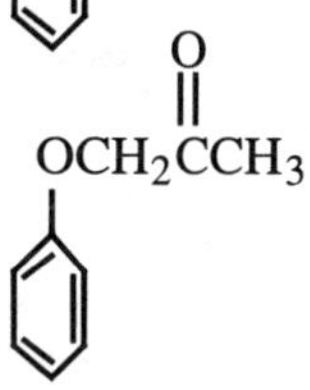

D.
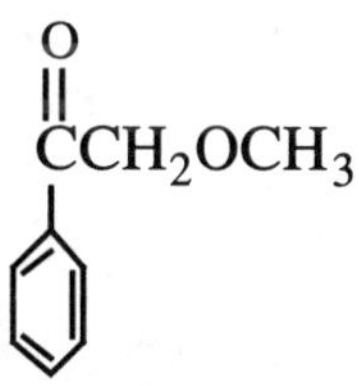

107. From a high-resolution mass spectrum of compound B, a molecular formula of $C_6H_{14}O$ was assigned. In the infrared spectrum, the strongest absorption greater than 1400 cm^{-1} occurred at 2900 cm^{-1}. In nuclear magnetic resonance, compound B showed a septet at ∂ = 3.62 ppm (area 1), J = 7 Hz, and a doublet at ∂ = 1.10 (area 6), J = 7 Hz. What is the structure of compound B?

A. 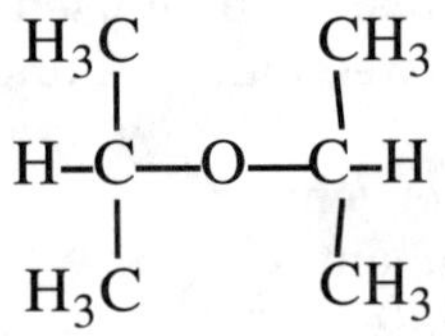

B. 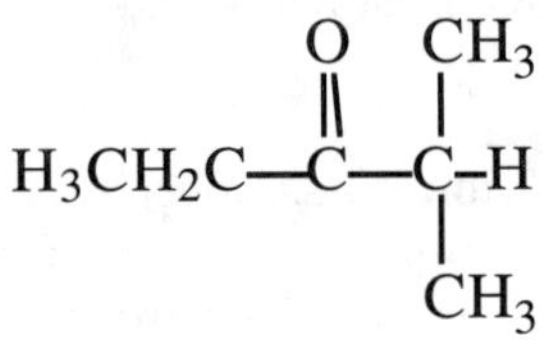

C. $H_3CH_2CH_2C–O–CH_2CH_2CH$

D. 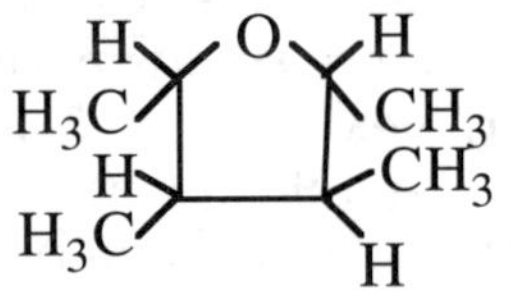

108. For two compounds to be separated by $NaHCO_3$ extraction, they must have different:
- **A.** dipole moments.
- **B.** acid–base properties.
- **C.** boiling points.
- **D.** molecular weights.

109. Which pair of compounds could be separated most readily by solvent extraction?
- **A.** Aminocyclohexane and chlorocyclohexane
- **B.** Cyclohexanol and cyclohexanone
- **C.** Phenol and p-cresol
- **D.** Butanoic acid and 2-methylpropanoic acid

110. Carboxylic acids are generally separated as their methyl esters in gas chromatography. Why are they difficult to separate by this technique?
- **A.** Carboxylic acids all have the same nominal polarity
- **B.** Carboxylic acids are insoluble in most organic solvents, whereas their methyl esters are soluble
- **C.** Carboxylic acids decompose readily in a gas chromatographic column
- **D.** Carboxylic acids do not vaporize readily, but their methyl esters do so easily

111. Which pair of compounds would be separated most readily on silica gel by thin-layer chromatography?

A. 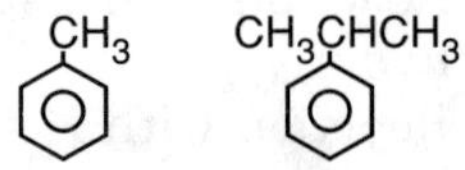

B. $CH_3CH_2CH_2CH_2CH_2Cl$
$CH_3CH_2CH_2CH_2CH_2Br$

C. $CH_3CH_2CH_2CH_2\overset{O}{\overset{\|}{C}}CH_3$
$CH_3CH_2CH_2\overset{O}{\overset{\|}{C}}CH_2CH_3$

D. 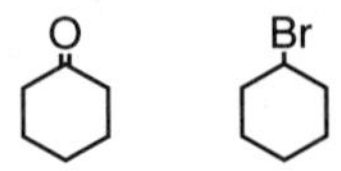

112. Fractionating columns in distillations are frequently packed with glass beads, ceramic saddles, or copper wool to:
- **A.** increase the condensation of vapor in the fractionating column.
- **B.** decrease the rate at which pure liquid distills.
- **C.** maintain a constant temperature in the fractionating column.
- **D.** provide a surface on which impurities may be absorbed and removed.

113. According to the following temperature versus volume graph of distillation, how many compounds were present in the initial mixture?

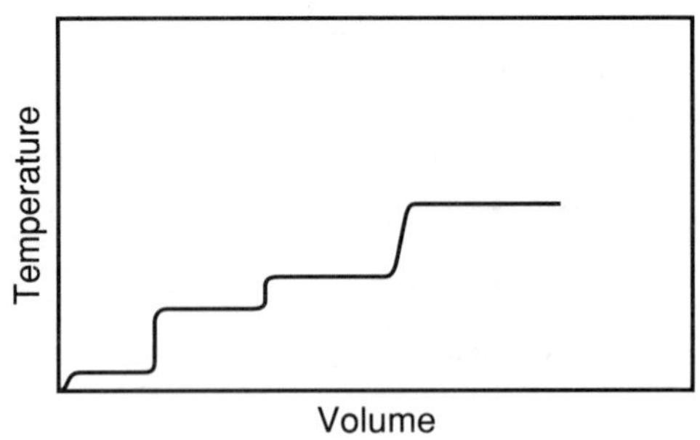

- **A.** 1
- **B.** 2
- **C.** 3
- **D.** 4

114. An impure solid has the following solubility test results: water, insoluble;

methanol, insoluble; hexane, soluble in hot solution; and dichloromethane, soluble. Which solvent would be most appropriate for the recrystallization of this impure solid?

A. Water
B. Methanol
C. Hexane
D. Dichloromethane

115. Impurities are removed during recrystallization because:

I. Impurities do not "fit" into a growing crystal lattice.
II. Impurities decrease the melting point of the compound.
III. Impurities remain dissolved in the solvent.

A. I only
B. I and II
C. I and III
D. I, II, and III

116. A double bond can stabilize an adjacent carbenium ion by __________ the positive charge with its __________ bond.

A. neutralizing, pi
B. neutralizing, sigma
C. delocalizing, pi
D. delocalizing, sigma

117. The reaction of H^+ with the following compound forms which carbenium ion:

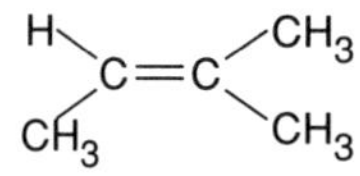

A. 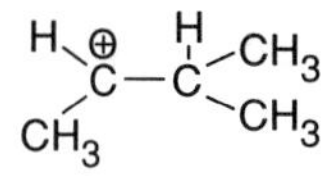

B. 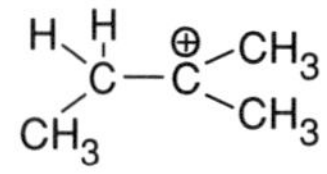

C. 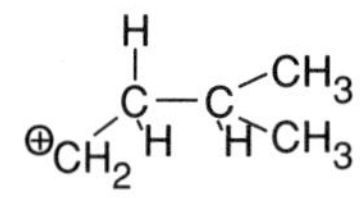

D. None of the above

118. A sample of ^{32}P disintegrates at a rate of 30,000 disintegrations per minute (dpm). Determine the radioactivity in microcuries [1 Ci $= 3.7 \times 10^{10}$ disintegrations per second (dps)].

A. 3.7×10^{6} mCi
B. 32×10^{-4} mCi
C. 3.7×10^{-2} mCi
D. 1.5×10^{-2} mCi

6.6 ANSWERS AND EXPLANATIONS

1. [B] Topic: nomenclature. When naming small inorganic compounds, the more electropositive element is listed first. The other element is named as an anion. Anion endings are -ide for elemental anions and -ite and -ate for oxygen-containing polyatomic anions. The ending -ine is used for elements.
2. [A] Topic: nomenclature. Barium is a +2 cation, and oxide is a −2 anion. The correct formula would contain 1 barium and 1 oxide.
3. [C] Topic: percent composition. Determine the molecular weight of each species: 1 = 16 g/mol; 2 = 61 g/mol; 3 = 102 g/mol; 4 = 192 g/mol; 5 = 28 g/mol. Next, divide the mass of carbon by the molecular weight: 1 = 12/16 = 0.75; 2 = 24/61 = 0.40; 3 = 24/102 = 0.24; 4 = 72/196 = 0.37; 5 = 24/28 = 0.86.
4. [D] Topic: empirical/molecular formula. Determine the mass of the empirical formula unit (49 g). Divide the result into molecular mass (= 4). The molecule contains four empirical units.
5. [B] Topic: balancing equations. Start with the most complicated molecule, $Bi_2(SiO_4)_3$. Balance Bi with 2 on the product side and $CrPO_4$ with 2.
6. [C] Topic: density. Divide the mass of the sample by the volume.
7. [D] Topic: stoichiometry. Balance the equation by placing 2 with HCl. The mole ratio calculation gives 2 mol HCl/1 mol Zn. The molecular weight of HCl is 36 g/mol.
8. [B] Topic: Dalton's law of partial pressure.
9. [A] Topic: ideal gas law and Avogadro's gas law. At standard temperature and pressure, 1 mol ideal gas occupies 22.4 L. Avogadro's gas law states that the amount of gas present is directly proportional to the pressure. If both the number of moles and the pressure double, the volume and temperature are constant.

10. [A] Topic: ideal gas law. Substitute mass/molecular weight for n in the ideal gas law. Solve for density with mass/volume. The density is proportional to the molecular weight.

11. [B] Topic: Boyle's law. To halve the volume, double the pressure.

12. [D] Topic: law of combining volumes. The law of combining volumes allows substitution of volumes of gas for moles in stoichiometric calculations in gas-phase reactions.

13. [D] Topic: vapor pressure. The boiling point is the point at which the vapor pressure of the liquid equals the atmospheric pressure. The lower the boiling temperature, the closer the vapor pressure is to the atmospheric pressure.

14. [B] Topic: phase diagrams. A is the normal freezing point; C is the normal boiling point; and D is the critical point.

15. [C] Topic: phase changes. The change is from solid to liquid.

16. [A] Topic: colligative properties. The addition of an impurity to a material increases the boiling point according to $\Delta T_b = k_b m$, where ΔT_b is the change in boiling point, k_b is a constant, and m is the molality of the solution. The addition of an impurity decreases the freezing point according to $\Delta T_f = k_f m$. For this reason, salt is used to melt ice.

17. [B] Topic: cubes. Any atom on the corner of a cube is one-eighth within the cube; therefore, any corner atom is shared by eight atoms.

18. [D] Topic: solutions. Electrolytes are solutions that conduct electrons and are either soluble salts, acids, or bases. Any compound that ionizes in solution is an electrolyte.

19. [B] Topic: concentration units. Using the formula $C_1V_1 = C_2V_2$ for this dilution problem, solve for V_1.

20. [C] Topic: concentration units. Molarity is moles per liter. Multiply the concentration by the volume to obtain the value in moles. According to Avogadro's number, there are 6.02×10^{23} molecules per mole; therefore, there are 2 mol NaOH, and in solution, this quantity ionizes to 2 mol Na^+.

21. [A] Topic: polarity. Water is polar, so only another polar compound is completely miscible.

22. [A] Topic: polarity. Draw the molecule in a three-dimensional view, and look for a permanent dipole moment.

23. [D] Topic: conjugates. When ammonia ionizes in aqueous solution, the reaction is $NH_3 + H_2O \leftrightarrow NH_4^+ + OH^-$. A base is a proton acceptor.

24. [B] Topic: salt hydrolysis. Acetate, $C_2H_3O_2^-$, is the conjugate base of a weak acid, acetic acid. The resulting conjugate base of a weak acid is a strong conjugate base that reacts with water.

25. [C] Topic: buffers. A buffer includes a weak base (i.e., acid) and the salt of its conjugate acid (i.e., base). See question 23. A has a strong acid, B has two salts, and D has a strong base.

26. [B] Topic: neutralization reaction. The unit of concentration is N, or normality, which is defined as the gram-equivalent weight of a substance dissolved in 1 L solution. HCl has one reactive H per molecule, giving a gram-equivalent weight that is equal to the molecular weight. $Ba(OH)_2$ has two reactive hydroxyl ions, each equivalent to a proton. Therefore, the gram-equivalent weight is one-half the molecular weight. Equal volumes of solutions of equal normality are needed for a complete reaction.

27. [B] Topic: acid definition. A Lewis acid is an electron pair acceptor. A Lewis base is an electron pair donor. A Brønsted-Lowry acid is a proton donor. A Brønsted-Lowry base is a proton acceptor. In the course of the reaction, no proton is exchanged. Because N has a lone pair of electrons [$:N(CH_2CH_3)_3$], it is an electron donor.

28. [B] Topic: equilibrium. Removing a product causes the shift to the right.

29. [B] Topic: equilibrium calculations. To solve any similar problem (e.g., gas phase, acid–base, or solubility equilibrium), consider the problem in three phases:

$$2\,XY_{(g)} \leftrightarrow X_{2(g)} + Y_{2(g)}$$

t_o	1M	0	0
Δ	$-2x$	$+x$	$+x$
t_{eq}	$1-2x$	x	x

(1) t_o = concentration at the start; (2) Δ = concentration change; and (3) t_{eq} = equilibrium concentration. Place the information into the equilibrium expression for the reaction. The general form of an equilibrium expression is: for $xA + yB \leftrightarrow aX + bY$.

$$K = \frac{\text{Concentration of products}}{\text{Concentration of reactants}} = \frac{[X]^a\,[Y]^b}{[A]^x\,[B]^y}$$

where a, b, x, and y are the coefficients from the balanced chemical equation.

30. [A] Topic: equilibrium. All of the salts form the same number of ions in solution, so the K_{sp} values can be compared. If the salts form different numbers of ions in solution, the molar solubility must be calculated.

31. [C] Topic: solubility equilibrium. The expression for K_{sp} for this equilibrium is $K_{sp} = [Ag^+][I^-]$. Substitute x for the concentration, and solve for x. The K_{sp} value was given previously.

$$AgI_{(s)} \leftrightarrow Ag^+_{(aq)} + I^-_{(aq)}$$
$$\qquad\quad x \qquad\quad x$$

$x^2 = 10^{-16}$

Therefore: $x = 10^{-4}$

32. [A] Topic: common ion effect (Le Chatelier principle). The chemical equation describing the equilibrium is $Fe(OH)_{2(s)} \leftrightarrow Fe^{2+}_{(aq)} + 2\ OH^-_{(aq)}$. The question states that NaOH, a strong base, has been added. Strong bases ionize completely in water, $NaOH_{(aq)} \rightarrow Na^+_{(aq)} + OH^-_{(aq)}$. Both equations have hydroxide as a product. Adding the product of the equilibrium causes reactants to form.

33. [C] Topic: heat of formation. The heat of formation is the heat needed to form a compound from its components. Elements do not need to be formed.

34. [D] Topic: calorimetry. Heat q, evolved in a calorimeter, is $q = C\Delta T$. C = heat capacity = specific heat × mass; ΔT = change in room temperature. C = (4.18 J/Kg)(1.00 kg) = 4.18 kJ/K. Then q = (4.18 kJ/K)(1K) = 4.18 kJ.

35. [C] Topic: Hess's law. The three given reactions can be added to obtain the desired reaction. Heat of formation is the formation of the compound from the component elements; in this case, $2\ C + 3\ H_2 + 1/2\ O_2 \rightarrow C_2H_5OH$. The first given reaction contains information on ethanol, but as a reactant. Reversing the reaction is equivalent to multiplying by −1, which changes the sign of the heat ΔH. To remove unwanted species, the other reaction is used to cancel. Two carbon dioxides are removed as reactants. To cancel out, two carbon dioxides are needed as products. Similar reasoning can be used to remove the water. The solution is as follows:

$$-1[C_2H_5OH + 3\ O_2 \rightarrow 2\ CO_2 + 3\ H_2O\ \Delta H = -1300\ kJ] = \cancel{2\ CO_2} + \cancel{3\ H_2O} \rightarrow C_2H_5OH + \cancel{6/2\ O_2}\ \Delta H = +1300\ kJ$$
$$2[C_{(s)} = O_{2(g)} \rightarrow CO_{2(g)}\ \Delta H = -400\ kJ] = 2C_{(s)} + \cancel{4/2\ O_{2(g)}} \rightarrow \cancel{2\ CO_{2(g)}}\ \Delta H = -800\ kJ$$
$$3[H_{2(g)} = 1/2\ O_{2(g)} \rightarrow H_2O_{(l)}\ \Delta H = -300\ kJ] = 3H_{2(g)} + (1/2)\cancel{3/2}\ O_{2(g)} \rightarrow \cancel{3\ H_2O_{(l)}}\ \Delta H = -900\ kJ$$

$$2\ C + 3\ H_2 = 1/2\ O_2 \rightarrow C_2H_5OH,\ \Delta H = -400\ kJ$$

---

36. [D] Topic: spontaneity and Gibbs' free energy theory. Free energy is the relation between enthalpy (ΔH, heat that seeks a minimum value) and entropy (ΔS, which seeks a maximum value). The relation is $\Delta G = \Delta H - T\Delta S$, resulting in the following:

ΔH	ΔS	ΔG	
>0	>0	>0 <0	at low temperatures (nonspontaneous) at high temperatures (spontaneous)
>0	<0	>0	at all temperatures (never spontaneous)
<0	>0	<0	at all temperatures (always spontaneous)
<0	<0	>0 <0	at high temperatures (nonspontaneous) at low temperatures (spontaneous)

37. [A] Topic: rate laws. Unimolecular refers to one molecule. Bimolecular refers to two molecules and does not distinguish between two different molecules or two of the same type. The order of the reaction is the sum of the coefficients in the rate law and refers to the number of molecules participating in the rate-determining step.

38. [C] Topic: reaction rates. See solution for question 37. Substitute 0.4 for k and 0.5 for the concentration, and multiply. A unimolecular reaction is first order.

39. [A] Topic: activation energies. In a successful reaction, the molecules collide in the correct orientation and with sufficient energy to overcome the activation energy barrier.

40. [D] Topic: reaction diagrams. In a reaction diagram, A is the change in enthalpy; ΔH is the energy difference between the reactants and the products; B is the energy of activation; E_a is the energy required for the reactants to react; C is the transition state, an energy maximum; and D is an intermediate, an energy minimum located between the reactants and the products.

41. [C] Topic: reaction diagram.

42. [A] Topic: spontaneity. For the reaction to occur spontaneously, the potential (E°) for the cell must be greater than 0. In thermodynamics, $\Delta G° < 0$ for a spontaneous reaction and $\Delta G° = -nFE°$, where n = number of electrons transferred and F = Faraday's constant.

43. [B] Topic: Nernst equation. Because the concentrations of the ions are equal, $\log Q = 0$, so $E = E°$.

44. [D] Topic: oxidation states. Because $O = -2$ and $3O = -6$, what positive charge is needed to give a value of -1? Nitrogen has a charge of $+5$.

45. [C] Topic: redox reactions. A reducing agent in a redox reaction is the species that is oxidized. Simply stated for metals, it prefers to be a cation, not the neutral element. By comparing the given reactions, Mg always reacts and Mg^{2+} never does.

46. [B] Topic: electron configurations. The Aufbau principle states that the orbitals of lowest energy must fill first. Hund's rule states that the lowest electron configuration has the maximum number of unpaired spins. The unpaired spins must be in the same direction.

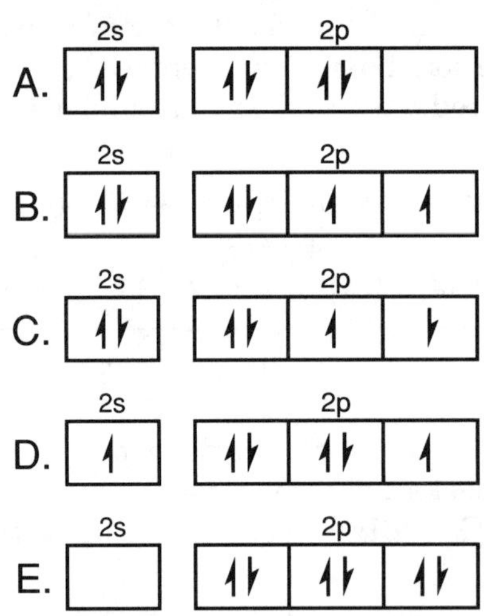

47. [C] Topic: electron configurations. The electron configuration of argon is $[Ne]3s^23p^6$.

48. [B] Topic: bonding. Ionic bonding usually occurs in compounds consisting of metals and nonmetals; HCN contains only nonmetals. To answer this question, draw the Lewis dot structure of HCN. In general, H forms one bond, O forms two bonds, N forms three, and C forms four. The result is H—C≡N. The first bond between atoms is a sigma bond, and if multiple bonds are present, all bonds after the first are pi bonds. Two sigma bonds and two pi bonds are present.

49. [C] Topic: quantum numbers. For the principle quantum number 3, s, p, and d orbitals are allowed. The 3s orbital can contain two electrons, the 3p orbital can contain six electrons, and the 3d orbital can contain ten electrons, for a total of eighteen allowed electrons.

50. [C] Topic: quantum numbers. The azimuthal quantum number refers to the shape of an orbital. $l = 0$ means s, $l = 1$ means p, $l = 2$ means d, and $l = 3$ means f. The question refers to a d orbital that can hold 10 electrons.

51. [C] Topic: octet rule. The elements C, N, O, F, Ne, and H always obey the octet rule. To violate the octet rule, most elements use d orbitals, which for these elements are not allowed by quantum mechanics. Their principle quantum number is 2 or less, which allows for l, with allowed values of $0 \rightarrow n - 1$, 0, and 1, only s and p orbitals. These orbitals can hold a maximum of eight electrons.

52. [B] Topic: electron configurations.

53. [C] Topic: metalloids. Most periodic tables have a red zigzag line through the p block. Elements shown along this line are metalloids.

54. [C] Topic: halogens. Fluorine and chlorine are gases, bromine is one of two liquid elements (mercury is the other), and iodine is a solid. In general, the greater the molecular weight for a series of related compounds, the higher the melting and boiling points.

55. [A] Topic: group names. The groups are: (1) noble gases, (2) halogens, (3) alkaline earths, (4) alkali metals, and (5) group V elements.

56. [C] Topic: electron shells. The electron shells refer to the principle quantum number and increase +1 for each horizontal row of the periodic table. Row 1 ($n = 1$) contains only the s orbital (two electrons); row 2 ($n = 2$) contains s and p orbitals (eight electrons); and row 3 ($n = 3$) has s, p, and d orbitals available (eighteen electrons, but the d orbitals are not used yet).

57. [B] Topic: periodic trends. Size increases from the top to the bottom and from the right to the left of the periodic table.

58. [C] Topic: quantum numbers. The values of 1 are: $0 \rightarrow$ s, $1 \rightarrow$ p, $2 \rightarrow$ d, and $3 \rightarrow$ f.

59. [A] Topic: ionization energy trends. Ionization energies increase from the top to the bottom and from the left to the right of the periodic table.

60. [D] Topic: ionic compounds. O is a -2 anion and needs a $+2$ cation to form a 1:1 ionic compound.

61. [A] Topic: descriptive chemistry. Sodium hydroxide is known generically as caustic soda; NaCl is known as salt.

62. [B] Topic: decay process. Gamma radiation is only release of energy. Electron capture and positron emission decrease the atomic number by 1; beta emission increases the atomic number by 1.

63. [B] Topic: half-life. Sixteen days includes two half-life periods. In the first half-life period, 50% of the sample decayed (1 g $\rightarrow$ 0.5 g); in the second, 50% of the sample decayed (0.5 g $\rightarrow$ 0.25 g).

64. [B] Topic: nuclear reactions. The atomic mass is unchanged, but the atomic number is increased by 1 (i.e., beta emission).

65. [D] Topic: nuclear reactions. The atomic mass and atomic number are unchanged, but energy is released (i.e., gamma emission).

66. [D] Topic: covalent bonding. Draw a Lewis dot structure: O=C=O. In forming covalent bonds, the first bond between atom pairs is a sigma bond. Further bonds are pi bonds.

67. [A] Topic: octet rule.

68. [C] Topic: stereoview. In a Fisher projection, the horizontal bonds point out of the page and vertical bonds are behind, or pointing into the page. Rotating the molecule to the right by approximately 60° gives the correct orientation.

69. [C] Topic: Cahn-Ingold-Prelog rules. To assign an absolute configuration, the four atoms or groups attached to the chiral carbon are ranked by mass. The largest mass is the highest range, 1. An arrow is drawn from 1 to 2 to 3 to 4. If the arrow is clockwise, R, for rectus, is assigned. If the arrow is counterclockwise, S, for sinister, is assigned. However, if group 4 is horizontal, the arrow is reversed.

70. [B] Topic: enantiomers. An enantiomer is a nonsuperimposable mirror image. Enantiomers have similar chemical and physical properties, except for rotation of light and reactions with chiral reagents. Diastereomers are stereoisomers that are not mirror images. They have similar chemical properties, but different physical properties.

71. [B] Topic: stereoisomers. The number of stereoisomers is 2^n, where n is the number of chiral carbons present.

72. [B] Topic: carbon types. Carbon atoms are typed by the number of C—C bonds formed. A primary carbon forms one bond, a secondary carbon forms two bonds, a tertiary carbon forms three bonds, and a quaternary carbon forms four bonds.

73. [D] Topic: physical properties of alkanes. Cyclic hydrocarbons have a higher boiling point than straight-chain analogs because of London dispersion forces.

74. [C] Topic: conformation of alkenes. The highest-energy form has the most steric interactions.

75. [C] Topic: directors in aromatic electrophilic substitution reactions. The group $—CF_3$ is a meta director. Some other groups and their influences are the following:

Activators: Ortho & para directors	$—NH_2, -O\overset{\overset{O}{\Vert}}{C}R, -R, -OH, —NH\overset{\overset{O}{\Vert}}{C}R, —Ph$
Deactivators: Meta directors	$—NO_2, —\overset{\overset{O}{\Vert}}{C}—R, —NH_3{}^+, —\overset{\overset{O}{\Vert}}{C}—OR$
Deactivators: Ortho & para directors	Halogens

76. [D] Topic: aromaticity. This compound is not planar, and all of the carbons in the ring are not sp^2 or sp hybrids.

77. [A] Topic: addition reactions. This example is an addition across a C—C double bond. This class of reaction follows Markovnikov's rule.

78. [A] Topic: oxidation reactions of alcohols. CrO_3 is an average oxidizing agent and oxidizes 1° alcohols to aldehydes. To produce a carboxylic acid, a stronger oxidizing agent, such as $KMnO_4$, is needed. Oxidizing agents react with 2° alcohols to form ketones and do not react with 3° alcohols. For a reaction to occur, the alcohol carbon must possess an H.

79. [C] Topic: name reactions. The Williamson ether synthesis is the reaction of an alkoxide and alkyl halide.

80. [C] Topic: nomenclature. The compound is a ketone, so the suffix is -one. The longest carbon chain is six (hexane). Use the lowest number combination from an end.

81. [B] Topic: reaction products. A ketal is produced in the reaction of a ketone with two alcohols under acidic conditions.

82. [B] Topic: reaction products. The reaction is a dehydration, which results in a C═C bond. The major product is the most substituted double bond because of a rearrangement.

83. [B] Topic: physical properties. Alcohols meet the criteria for hydrogen bonding (i.e., electronegative element, N, O, or F, with an H attached and a lone pair of electrons). The intermolecular force is strong and causes a high boiling point.

84. [D] Topic: acid strength. Cl is an electron-withdrawing group. The inductive effect results in a withdrawing of electrons from the O—H bond, weakening the bond and producing a stronger acid. The higher the degree of substitution, the greater the effect.

85. [C] Topic: reaction products. Anhydrides are formed by the removal of water from two carboxylic groups. Ethers would form from alcohols in the Williamson ether synthesis.

86. [C] Topic: nomenclature. The compound is an ester, named by changing the acid ending with -ioc to -ate and naming the organic group attached to the oxygen. The others are as follows:

A. CH_3COOH (common name = acetic acid) B. $CH_3\overset{\overset{O}{\Vert}}{C}O\overset{\overset{O}{\Vert}}{C}CH_3$ D. $CH_3\overset{\overset{O}{\Vert}}{C}NH_2$

87. [B] Topic: reaction reagents. Acylchlorides, PhC(═O)Cl, react with excess ammonia to form amides; with an alcohol to form esters; with a dialkyl cadium compound, R_2Cd, to form ketones; and with H_2/Pd to form aldehydes.

88. [C] Topic: physical properties. The trisubstituted N does not possess a bond for use in hydrogen bonding. The result is a lower melting point.

89. [A] Topic: physical properties. In the gas phase, the inductive effect of the donor group, Me, increases the electron density on the central N. The higher the degree of substitution, the greater the effect. This question is similar to question 84.

90. [B] Topic: reaction products. $LiAlH_4$ is a reducing agent. The product usually contains more Hs along a unit of unsaturation. This example reduces a C═O group to a CH_2 group. This reaction is typical with $LiAlH_4$.

91. [C] Topic: reaction products. H_2/M is also a reducing agent. The product usually contains hydrogens along a unit of unsaturation. In this example, there are two units of unsaturation, C═C and C≡N. Both units are reduced by this strong reducing agent.

92. [B] Topic: nomenclature. The correct names are as follows:

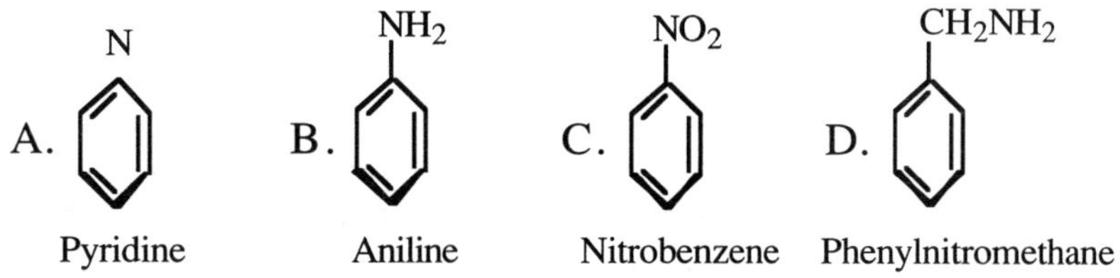

93. [B] Topic: peptides. A peptide linkage is formed by the loss of water from the —COOH and —NH_2 groups on amino acids. The formation and the correct way to draw the peptide are shown. For example:

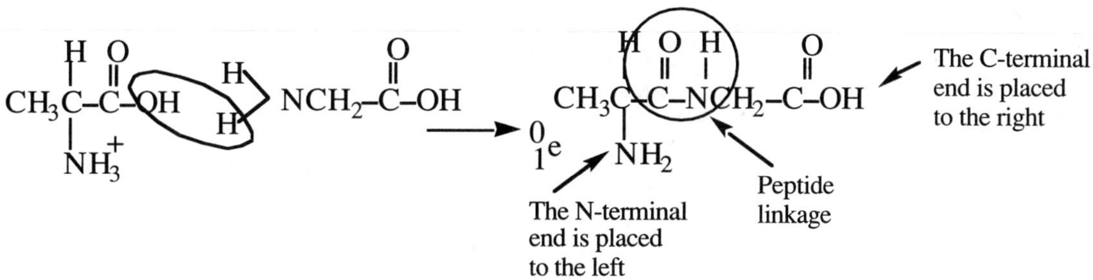

94. [C] Topic: properties. The isoelectric point occurs when the rate of reaction 1 is equal to the rate of reaction 2 and the concentration of the zwitterion is maximized.

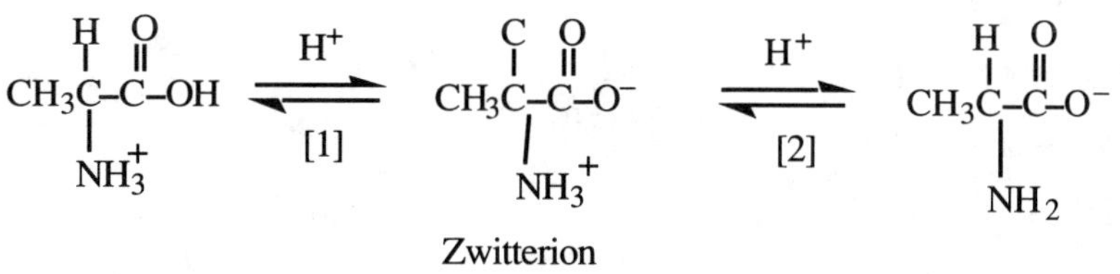

95. [C] Topic: reaction types. The Sanger method labels the N-terminal end with a 2,4-dinitrophenyl group. The dinitrofluorobenzene reacts with any free amino group, but only an α-amino group is at the N-terminal end.

96. [B] Topic: amino acids. Nitrosyl groups are usually found bonded to transition metals.

97. [D] Topic: amino acids. Twenty amino acids occur naturally.

98. [A] Topic: reactions. Amino acids exhibit the reactions that the functional groups possess. Amines react with acid chlorides, and —Cl is replaced by the —NHR group, yielding the observed product.

99. [A] Topic: globular proteins. Hemoglobin and lysozyme are globular proteins that are soluble in water. Globular proteins have low molecular weights (e.g., lysozyme is an enzyme with a molecular weight of 14,600).

100. [B] Topic: configuration of amino acids. All naturally occurring amino acids have the same configuration as L-glyceraldehyde.

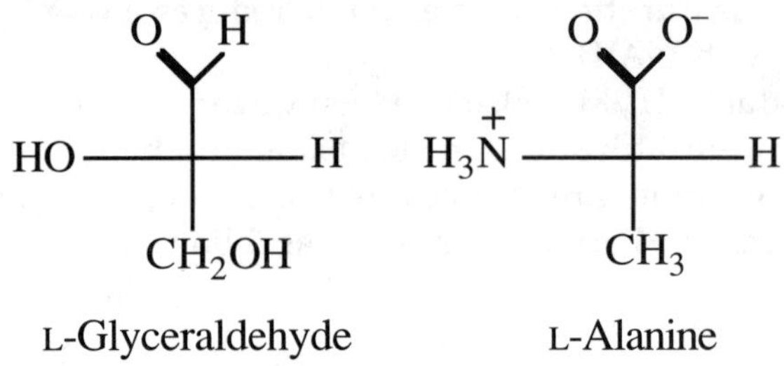

101. [A] Topic: diastereomeric forms. In a cyclic representation of the structure, carbon 1 is known as the anomeric carbon. The forms are designated as the α-anomer or the β-anomer, depending on the orientation of the OH group. In the α-anomer, the —OH is in the down orientation; in the β-anomer, the —OH is in the up orientation.

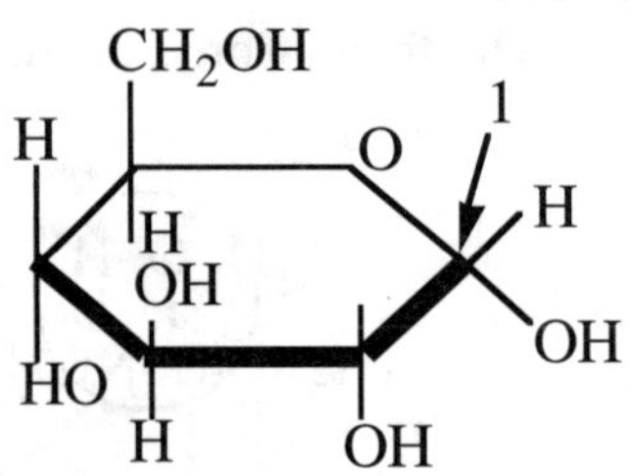

102. [A] Topic: sugar structures. To relate a linear structure to a cyclic structure, follow this procedure:

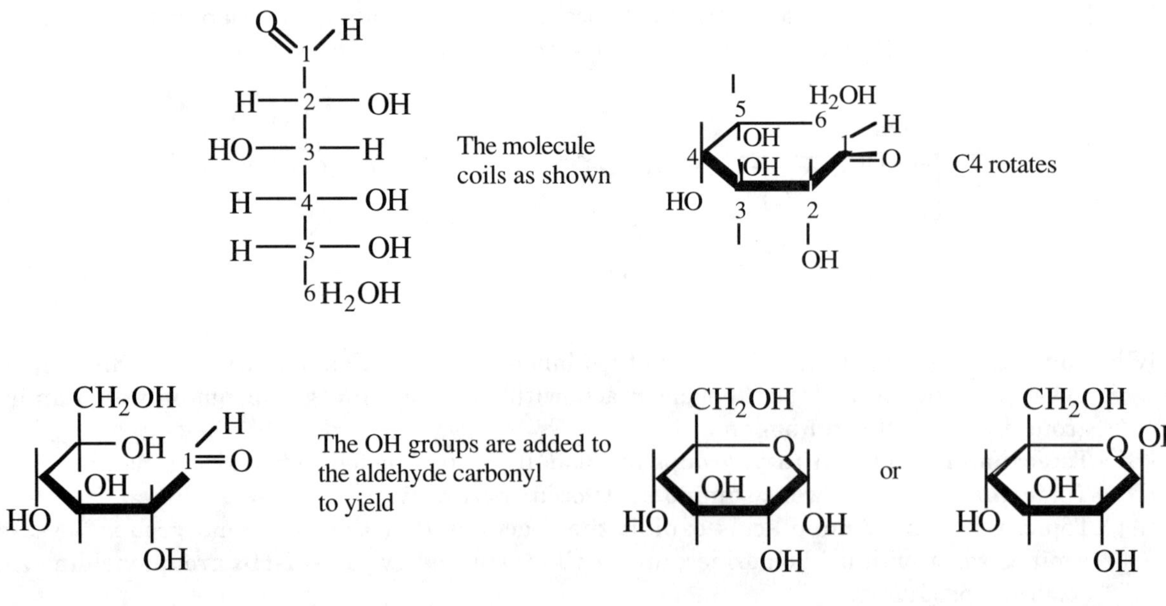

103. [D] Topic: name reactions. The Kiliani-Fischer synthesis uses HCN followed by hydrolysis to lengthen the carbon chain by one unit.

104. [B] Topic: name reactions. The Ruff degradation shortens the carbon chain by one H—C—OH unit. It is the reverse reaction of Kiliani-Fischer synthesis.

105. [C] Topic: chemical tests. Fehling's reagent, Tollen's reagent, and Benedict's solution are all tests for sugars. They do not differentiate between aldoses and ketoses. Bromine water reacts only with aldoses. It converts aldoses to an aldonic acid.

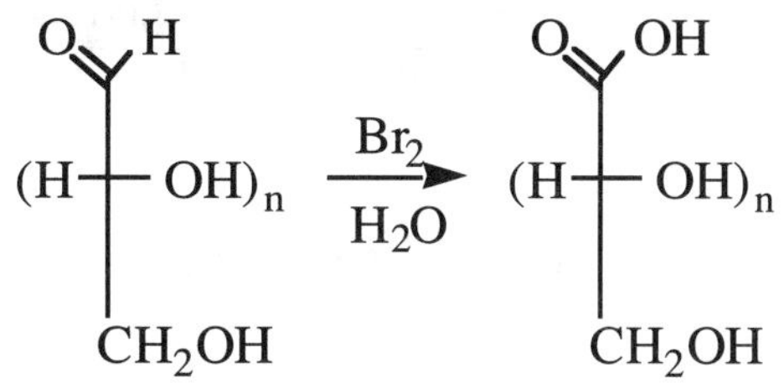

Aldose Aldonic acid

106. [C] Topic: spectroscopy. The IR signal at 1715 cm^{-1} indicates a ketone. The nuclear magnetic resonance signal at 7.22 indicates C_6H_5; the other signals are not coupled. A peak of area 2 suggests CH_2, and a peak of area 3 suggests CH_3. A group neighboring an O is in the range of 3–5.

107. [A] Topic: spectroscopy. The IR information suggests that there is no carbonyl, C═O, in this molecule. The formula shows that there are only six carbons. The nuclear magnetic resonance data of a doublet at 1.10 ppm suggest a group next to a carbon with one hydrogen, and the septet suggests a group next to carbons with six hydrogens.

108. [B] Topic: Separations and purifications. Separation by solvent extraction requires different acidity and basicity. Sodium bicarbonate is a weak base. To serve as the basis of a separation, one compound must react with $NaHCO_3$, whereas the other does not.

109. [A] Topic: Separations and purifications. This question is an application of the same principle as question 66 using HCl. An amine can be protonated and therefore water solubilized, leaving behind the alkyl halide. The remaining pairs of compounds are not readily distinguishable by their acid–base properties.

110. [D] Topic: Separations and purifications. Compounds to be separated by gas chromatography must be capable of being vaporized. Carboxylic acids form hydrogen-bonded dimers that maintain low vapor pressure. Hydrogen-bonded dimers do not form from methyl esters.

111. [D] Topic: Separations and purifications. Thin-layer chromatography separates compounds on the basis of polarity. A ketone and an alkyl halide have different polarities, whereas those of the other compounds are similar.

112. [A] Topic: Separations and purifications. Distillation is a series of vaporizations and condensations. The efficiency of distillation improves if more condensations occur in the fractionating column.

113. [D] Topic: Separations and purifications. A pure compound distills at a constant temperature. Temperature remains constant in four regions, so four compounds were initially present.

114. [C] Topic: Separations and purifications. The best solvent for recrystallization on the basis of solubility tests is the one that must be heated for the solute to dissolve. Pure crystals are easily obtained by cooling the solution to less than room temperature.

115. [C] Topic: Separations and purifications. Crystals grow in highly ordered patterns into which impurities do not fit unless the impurities closely resemble the compound. With an appropriate solvent, the impurities remain in solution as the pure crystals form.

116. [C] Topic: hydrocarbons.

117. [B] Topic: hydrocarbons. The only possible cations from this double bond are 2° and 3°. Tertiary cations are more stable than secondary cations.

118. [D]

$$1 \text{ dpm} = \frac{1 \text{ disintegration}}{1 \text{ min}} = \frac{1 \text{ disintegration}}{60 \text{ sec}}$$

$$60 \text{ dpm} = \frac{1 \text{ disintegration}}{1 \text{ sec}} = 1 \text{ disintegrations per second (dps)}$$

$$30{,}000 \text{ dpm} = \frac{30{,}000}{60} = 500 \text{ dps}$$

$$1 \text{ mCi} = \frac{3.7 \times 10^{10}}{10^6} = 3.7 \times 10^4 \text{ dps}$$

$$\text{The } ^{32}\text{P activity} = 500 \text{ dps} \times \frac{1 \text{ mCi}}{3.7 \times 10^4 \text{ dps}} = \frac{500}{3.7 \times 10^4} \text{ mCi}$$

$$\text{Using estimation: } \frac{5}{3.7} \cong \frac{6}{4} \cong 1.5$$

$$\text{The best estimate is } 1.5 \times \frac{10^2}{10^4} = 1.5 \times 10^{-2} \text{ mCi}$$

6.7 REFERENCES

Burkett A, Sedenair J: *Test Bank for Chemistry,* 2nd ed. Boston, Allyn and Baker, 1989.

Jacob SW, Francone CA: *Structure and Function in Man,* 5th ed. Philadelphia, WB Saunders, 1982.

Masterson W: *Test Bank for Chemistry.* Philadelphia, WB Saunders, 1989.

7 CHAPTER

Test-Taking Skills

7.0 INTRODUCTION TO THE VCAT

The Veterinary College Admission Test (VCAT) requires a half-day for administration. The test takes approximately 4 hours. The VCAT is administered three times a year, usually in October, November, and January. Candidates report at 8:00 A.M. The test usually begins at 8:45 A.M. and ends at 12:30 P.M. A 15-minute break, but no lunch break, is scheduled. Any other breaks are determined by the proctor and vary among test centers.

The test has approximately 230 multiple-choice questions. The time allowed per item may vary depending on the length of the section and the difficulty of the questions. Each multiple-choice question has four answer choices, only one of which is correct. The VCAT is divided into five sections, each of which is timed separately (Table 7-1). You may work on only one section at a time. You may not return to earlier sections or turn to later sections. Six scores are reported on the VCAT: Verbal Ability, Biology, Chemistry, Quantitative Ability, Reading Comprehension, and Composite. Books, papers, reference materials, food and drink, and calculators, including watch calculators, are not allowed in the testing room.

7.1 GRE GENERAL TEST

By 1997, a completely modular computer-delivered test is expected to replace the traditional paper-and-pencil version of the Graduate Record Examination (GRE) General Test. The new General Test will likely consist of revised versions of the current verbal, quantitative, and analytical measures as well as a mathematical reasoning measure and a writing measure.

Table 7-2 shows a typical GRE Computer-Adaptive Test (GRE-CAT) schedule. Table 7-3 shows a typical paper-and-pencil GRE schedule. Individual GRE sections may vary by a few questions. The total amount of time allowed to complete each section is adjusted so that the average time per question is approximately the same, regardless of the number of questions in that section.

7.2 GRE CHEMISTRY TEST

The chemistry test consists of approximately 150 multiple-choice questions to be answered in approximately 170 minutes. Some of the questions are grouped in sets and based on information such as a

TABLE 7-1. ***VCAT Schedule***

Section	Number of Questions	Time Allotted	Average Time per Item
Verbal Ability	50	35 minutes	42 seconds
Quantitative Ability	40	35 minutes	53 seconds
Chemistry	50	35 minutes	42 seconds
Break	. . .	10 minutes	. . .
Biology	50	35 minutes	42 seconds
Reading Comprehension	40	35 minutes	53 seconds

TABLE 7-2. ***GRE-CAT Schedule***

Subtest	Number of Questions	Time	Minimum Number of Answers Required for a Score
Verbal	30	30 minutes	24
Quantitative	28	45 minutes	23
Analytical	35	60 minutes	28

descriptive paragraph or experimental results. From the five answer choices provided for each question, students choose the one that is correct or most nearly correct. A periodic table is printed in the test booklet. Test questions are constructed to simplify mathematical manipulations. As a result, calculators, tables, and logarithms are not needed. If the solution of a problem requires the use of logarithms, the necessary values are included with the questions.

The content of the test emphasizes the four traditional divisions of chemistry and some interrelations among these fields. Because of these interrelations, it is impossible to categorize all questions as testing only one field of knowledge. The distribution of test items is: analytical chemistry, 15%; inorganic chemistry, 25%; organic chemistry, 30%; and physical chemistry, 30%.

7.3 GRE BIOLOGY TEST

The GRE Biology Test contains approximately 210 five-choice questions, some of which are grouped in sets and based on descriptions of laboratory and field situations, diagrams, or experimental results. The total time allotted for this test is usually 170 minutes.

TABLE 7-3. ***Paper-and-Pencil GRE Schedule***

Subtest	Number of Questions	Time
Sentence completion, reading comprehension, analogies, and antonyms	38	30 minutes
Quantitative problems and comparisons	30	30 minutes
Analytical and logical reasoning	25	30 minutes
Verbal	38	30 minutes
Quantitative problems and comparisons	30	30 minutes
Analytical and logical reasoning	25	30 minutes

To cover the broad field of the biological sciences, the material is organized into three major areas: cellular and molecular biology; organismal biology; and ecology, evolution, and population biology. Approximately equal weight is given to these three areas.

7.4 MCAT

The Medical College Admission Test (MCAT) requires 5 hours and 45 minutes. Two sections are administered in the morning. The remaining two are administered after a lunch break. Table 7-4 shows the MCAT schedule.

7.5 SELF-ASSESSMENT

If you have not spent adequate time developing speed and accuracy, you may consider postponing the test until the next administration. Doing poorly on the test is demoralizing and does not enhance your standing with application committees. However, if you have prepared adequately for the VETs, you are now ready to develop your test-taking strategies.

7.6 SPEED

Managing time well on the VETs is important. No extra points are awarded for finishing a subtest. Speed is important, but it is always a tradeoff with accuracy. Under actual testing conditions, your goal is to obtain the highest possible score. Speed varies from section to section. In addition, within each subtest, some questions are designed to take longer than others. Most students do not spend an equal amount of time on each item within a subtest.

A good test-taking strategy is to complete the relatively easy questions quickly, thereby earning certain points and saving time for more difficult questions. No extra points are awarded for answering the single most difficult question. A better strategy would be to spend the same amount of time answering three easier questions.

Subscores are given for each topic. A natural tendency is to spend more time on the science topics that you like and to avoid those areas that you dislike. The suggestions in this book encourage a disciplined approach. However, the pressure of the testing situation has a tendency to make everyone revert to past behaviors.

Approximately 6 weeks before the test, concentrate on increasing speed. Work with a clock in view. Take approximately 10 items at a time, work for accuracy, and note how long it takes to achieve accuracy. On the next set of practice items, work slightly faster. If your accuracy level is the same, work faster on the next set. When your accuracy level begins to suffer, work at that speed to increase your accuracy. Increase your speed only when your accuracy level is high. Work in this way on all of the subtests.

TABLE 7-4. ***MCAT Schedule***

Section	Number of Questions	Time
Verbal Reasoning	65	85 minutes
Break	. . .	10 minutes
Physical Sciences	77	100 minutes
Lunch	. . .	10 minutes
Writing Sample	2	60 minutes
Break	. . .	10 minutes
Biological Sciences	77	100 minutes

As you work to build speed, look for shortcuts. For example: Would a quick estimate have allowed you to eliminate several answer choices quickly? Were there other, faster ways to answer a question? Did you become stubborn about answering a question that simply required too much time?

7.7 THREE WEEKS BEFORE THE TEST

1. Take a full simulated test 3 or 4 weeks before the actual test. The results will help you to decide whether you are ready to take the test and how you can spend your last few weeks of study most profitably. The model test in Chapter 8 can also help you to identify your weaknesses. Some students participate in a simulation together. The more closely the simulation resembles the actual test, the more benefit it provides. For example, if you take the simulated test at home, do not play the radio or accept telephone calls during the test, and follow the time limits carefully.
2. After you complete the model test, score one point for each correct answer. No points are deducted for incorrect or unanswered items. To discover your raw score, determine the percentage of correct answers. For example, if you answered 35 of 50 questions correctly, your raw score is 70%. The scaled score varies from test to test, depending on test difficulty, item analysis, and other variables. There is no advantage in taking the VETs just to discover that you were not ready. You can take the VETs as many times as you want, but all of your scores are forwarded to the schools where you apply.
3. Establish and maintain a daily test-taking schedule that includes the time you get up, your morning routine, your diet (e.g., eating a healthful, filling breakfast), and the time you go to sleep. You cannot perform your best on a morning test if you maintain a night study schedule until the test day.

7.8 ONE WEEK BEFORE THE TEST

1. If possible, on the Saturday before the test, travel to the testing location at the same time as you will on the day the test is given. Note the route, amount of traffic, available parking, and other variables. Locate the testing room, nearest fire exit, restroom, snack bar, and nearest telephone. Preparation is a good antidote to anxiety.
2. Schedule review sessions that emphasize short-term memory tasks. The rest of your study time should be spent completing test items from each section under timed conditions. During these final sessions, simulate actual test situations as closely as possible. For example, do not spend too much time solving one problem. In a good simulation, you feel stress, but not anxiety.
3. During the final practice sessions, use the strategies that you have developed and practiced. For example, consider each choice carefully, mark the answer clues in the question, and cross out obviously wrong answers. Work with the watch that you will bring to the test. It should have a large, clear face and a minute hand. Before the test, you should know what speed produces the highest level of accuracy on each subtest.

7.9 THE DAY BEFORE THE TEST

1. Assemble the items that you will take to the test site. Take a watch; three or four well-sharpened No. 2, or HB, pencils with erasers; juice or water; and a nutritious snack.
2. The night before the test, eat a high-carbohydrate dinner. This practice, known as carbohydrate packing, is common among competitive athletes because the carbohydrates convert to energy by morning.

7.10 THE TEST DAY

1. Eat a high-protein breakfast. Research at Johns Hopkins shows that eating protein at breakfast is particularly important for problem-solving activities. Allow time to eat your breakfast calmly.
2. Arrive at the testing site early. Standby candidates who have been instructed to report at 8:00 A.M. should be there by 7:45 A.M.

3. If you are not familiar with the test site, locate important areas, such as restrooms, the snack bar, and telephones.
4. As soon as the test starts, write out short-term memory items.
5. If your mind goes blank when you read the first question, go on to the next. Continue until you find a question that you can answer. Then go back to the skipped questions. Once you start, maintain the pace that you know gives you the highest level of accuracy.
6. Follow your strategies throughout the test. Do not be distracted by what others are doing. Periodically make sure that your mark on the answer sheet corresponds to the number of the question that you are answering.
7. Do not omit any questions. If you do not know an answer, simply fill in your predetermined guess answer. There is no penalty for wrong answers.
8. During breaks, do not talk to other test takers. Keep your energies focused on the test.
9. Do not engage in any activity that diverts your attention from the test or distracts others (e.g., reading books or newspapers).
10. Focus only on the test section in front of you. Do not attempt to remember earlier sections of this test or other tests.
11. During the break, stretch and take 10 to 20 short, deep breaths.

7.11 RULES FOR THE TEST

1. The testing room must be well lighted, ventilated, and accessible to individuals with impaired mobility.
2. Seating suitable for left-handed examinees is usually available on request.
3. Exact timing is essential for test results to be usable. Two timepieces should be used to ensure accurate timing in case one of them fails. Each part of the test should be timed with a stopwatch; if none is available, a wristwatch may be substituted. Note the beginning time of the test according to a wall clock so that if the stopwatch malfunctions, there will be an alternate means of timing the test.
4. The use of books; scratch paper; slide rules; calculators, including watch calculators; or any other aids is prohibited. Only your pencils, admission ticket, test booklet, and answer sheet may be on the desk during the examination.
5. Examinees must mark their answer sheets with a No. 2 pencil. The use of any other writing instrument can affect machine scoring and produce inaccurate scores.
6. Examinees are not permitted to smoke or talk during the test.

7.12 AFTER THE TEST

1. If you feel sick during the test or you realize that you are not adequately prepared, you can void your test. The proctor will void the test in front of you. You will not receive a score for the voided test.
2. Do not compare what you remember answering with what someone else remembers answering. This practice is unreliable.
3. Both preparation and luck have a part in any event. If you are not happy with your performance, you can take the test again.

7.13 REFERENCES

Association of American Medical Colleges: *MCAT Student Manual.* Washington, DC, AAMC, 1993.
Association of American Medical Colleges: *MCAT Student Application and Booklet.*
Educational Testing Service: *GRE General Test #9*. Princeton, NJ, ETS, 1994.
Educational Testing Service: *GRE Candidate Booklet.* Princeton, NJ, ETS, 1995.
The Psychological Corporation: *Veterinary College Admission Test* candidate information booklet. San Antonio, TX, The Psychological Corporation, 1995.

8

CHAPTER

Model Test

8.0 INTRODUCTION

The model test contains five subtests: Biology, Chemistry, Reading Comprehension, Quantitative Reasoning, and Verbal Ability. The model test is designed in accordance with the Psychological Corporation's Veterinary College Admission Testing Program in conformity with sample items and course outlines. The model test is not a copy of the actual test, which is guarded closely and may not be duplicated.

The time allotted for each subtest in the model test is based on a careful analysis of the Psychological Corporation test schedule. The model test may not contain the same number of questions as the actual test. It may be helpful to record your time for each subtest. Because the subtests are timed uniformly, if you follow all of the directions, your scores will be comparable. If your speed increases, you may assume that you are making progress.

The official Veterinary College Admission Test (VCAT) schedule differs from the model test schedule (Table 8-1).

8.1 BIOLOGY

For each question, read all of the choices carefully. Select the answer that is correct or most nearly correct. Blacken the answer space that corresponds to your choice. This section contains 53 items.

Time limit: 35 minutes

1. Which organelle is INCORRECTLY matched with its function?
   A. Mitochondria: fermentation
   B. Chloroplast: fixation of CO_2
   C. Lysosome: storage of hydrolytic enzymes
   D. Golgi apparatus: packaging and secretion of glycoprotein

2. The corpus luteum secretes:
   A. LH.
   B. progesterone.
   C. FSH.
   D. HCG.

TABLE 8-1. ***Model Test Schedule***

Subtest	Number of Questions	Time Allotted
Biology	53	35 minutes
Chemistry	60	35 minutes
Reading Comprehension	47	35 minutes
Quantitative Reasoning	40	35 minutes
Verbal Ability	60	35 minutes

3. When members of two species benefit from living in close association, the relation is called:
- **A.** mutualism.
- **B.** commensalism.
- **C.** parasitism.
- **D.** predation.

4. Which substance has the highest energy content per gram?
- **A.** Proteins
- **B.** Fats
- **C.** Carbohydrates
- **D.** Phospholipids

5. Cyanide blocks cellular production of energy at which stage?
- **A.** Glycolysis
- **B.** Citric acid cycle
- **C.** Electron transport system
- **D.** Oxidative phosphorylation

6. Lysosomes:
- **A.** are the site of protein synthesis.
- **B.** form the rough endoplasmic reticulum.
- **C.** contain digestive enzymes.
- **D.** contain the enzymes for oxidative phosphorylation.

7. Which condition causes a gene frequency to depart from the equilibrium expected from the Hardy-Weinberg law?
- **A.** Random assortment
- **B.** Nonrandom mating
- **C.** Large population
- **D.** No mutation

8. Which substance is NOT secreted into the human digestive tract?
- **A.** Bile
- **B.** Insulin
- **C.** Ptyalin
- **D.** Pepsinogen

9. Which ability is shared by both eukaryotic animal cells and animal viruses?
- **A.** The ability to undergo mutation
- **B.** The ability to reproduce through mitosis
- **C.** The ability to produce proteins
- **D.** The ability to enter other cells and cause lysis

10. A major difference between fungi and bacteria is that only fungi:
- **A.** are photosynthetic.
- **B.** can produce spores.
- **C.** are always diploid.
- **D.** can undergo meiosis and mitosis.

11. Blood that is pumped from the left ventricle of the heart:
- **A.** is highly oxygenated.
- **B.** flows into the aorta.
- **C.** is under high pressure.
- **D.** all of the above.

12. Muscles are bound to joints by:
- **A.** cartilage.
- **B.** tendons.
- **C.** ligaments.
- **D.** myosin fibers.

13. The development of the ovarian follicle is initiated by:
- **A.** FSH.
- **B.** LH.
- **C.** estrogen.
- **D.** progesterone.

14. In the immune system, B cells:
- **A.** are lymphocytes that release antibodies.
- **B.** are special phagocytic neutrophils.
- **C.** are transformed into macrophages at the site of inflammation.
- **D.** are lymphocytes that destroy foreign cells.

15. A relation in which one species benefits and the other is harmed is called:
- **A.** mutualism.
- **B.** socialism.
- **C.** commensalism.
- **D.** parasitism.

16. Translation of the genetic code does NOT directly require:
- **A.** activated tRNA–AA.
- **B.** ribosomes.
- **C.** mRNA.
- **D.** DNA.

17. What is the correct hierarchy (i.e., from highest to lowest) of taxonomy?
A. Class, order, family, genus
B. Order, family, genus, class
C. Family, genus, class, order
D. Family, class, order, genus

18. Who said, "Under certain conditions gene frequencies and genotypic frequencies remain constant from generation to generation in sexually reproducing populations"?
A. Dalton
B. Hardy-Weinberg
C. Mendel
D. Mendeleyev

19. In the following pedigree, a blackened symbol indicates that a specific trait is present. What is the most likely pattern of inheritance?

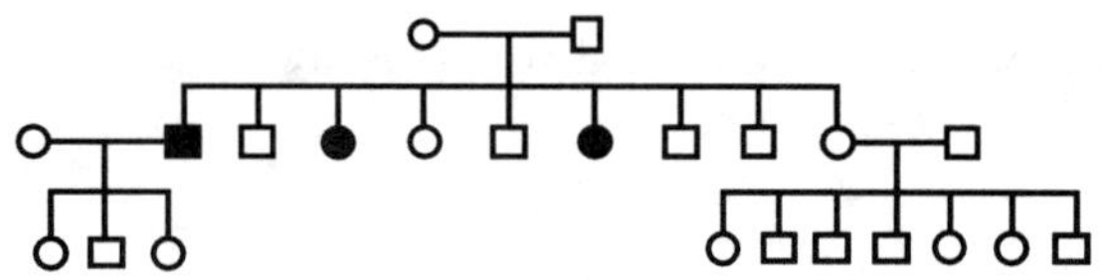

A. Autosomal dominant inheritance
B. Autosomal recessive inheritance
C. Sex-linked inheritance
D. Triglyceride inheritance

20. Which substance is NOT generally absorbed into the blood capillaries of the intestinal villi?
A. Water
B. Glucose
C. Amino acids
D. Triglycerides

21. Which of the following is required to convert fructose-6-phosphate to fructose 1, 6-diphosphate during glycolysis?
A. Oxygen
B. An excess of fructose-6-phosphate
C. A kinase enzyme that is specific for fructose-6-phosphate
D. Any enzyme that catalyzes the reactions of glycolysis

22. A membrane is found on all of the following structures EXCEPT:
A. lysosomes.
B. endoplasmic reticulum.
C. mitochondria.
D. centrioles.

23. During facilitated diffusion:
A. carrier substances carry molecules across the membrane.
B. molecules can go against the concentration gradient.
C. molecules require energy.
D. saturation kinetics is not observed.

24. If red blood cells are placed in a hypertonic solution, they:
A. remain the same.
B. hemolyze.
C. crenate.
D. swell.

25. The bronchi are prevented from collapsing by the:
A. cartilage rings.
B. alveolus.
C. bony rings.
D. epiglottis.

26. The greatest resistance to blood flow is in the:
A. capillaries.
B. veins.
C. arteries.
D. arterioles.

27. Bacteriophages:
A. cause disease in humans.
B. contain both DNA and RNA.
C. are viruses.
D. are bacteria.

28. Which structure protects a bacterium from phagocytosis by white blood cells?
A. Mesosome
B. Cilia
C. Capsule
D. Nucleoid

29. The chromosomes coil and become visible and the nuclear membrane disintegrates during what phase of mitosis?
A. Anaphase
B. Telophase
C. Prophase
D. Metaphase

30. The genetic code is composed of sequences of:
A. three nucleotides.
B. three nucleosides.
C. three amino acids.
D. two amino acids.

31. The following is one strand of a double helix of DNA, showing only nitrogen bases. What is the structure of its complementary strand? (A = adenine, G = guanine, T = thymine, C = cytosine, U = uracil)

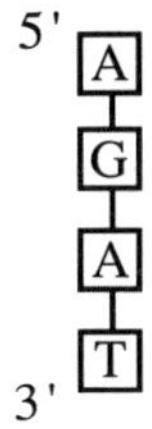

A.
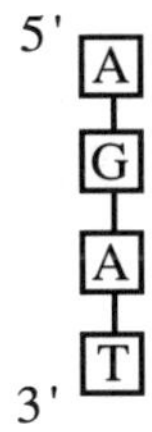

B.
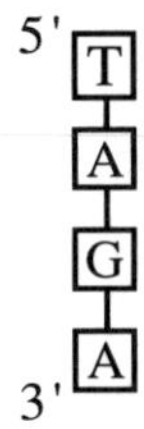

C.
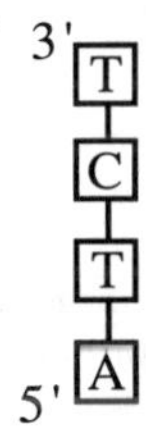

D.
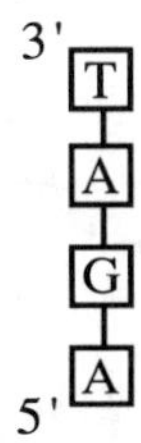

32. Which of the following are involved in the immune system?
A. Neutrophils
B. Platelets
C. Lymphocytes
D. Basophils

33. All of the following are part of the kidney EXCEPT:
A. glomerulus.
B. loop of Henle.
C. Bowman's capsule.
D. malpighian tubules.

34. Where does reabsorption of most water, glucose, amino acids, sodium, and other nutrients occur?
A. In the small intestines
B. In the collecting duct
C. In the distal convoluted tubules
D. In the proximal convoluted tubules

35. Control of body temperature is localized in the:
A. skin.
B. heart.
C. cerebrum.
D. hypothalamus.

36. Which of the following is NOT a feature of the unit membrane model of the cell membrane?
A. Continuous lipid bilayer
B. Globular proteins floating in lipids
C. Hydrophobic ends of lipids in contact with water
D. Continuous protein bilayers outside the lipid layer

37. If a cell is placed in a solution that causes it to shrink because of water loss, that solution is:
A. hypotonic.
B. isotonic.
C. hypertonic.
D. homeostatic.

38. Glycolysis, which is the first series of reactions in the oxidative breakdown of glucose, is sometimes used as a synonym for the:
A. Krebs cycle.
B. Calvin cycle.
C. Embden-Meyerhof pathway.
D. electron transport system.

39. Fertilization of an ovum by sperm normally occurs in the:
A. uterus.
B. vagina.
C. oviduct.
D. fallopian tube.

40. Which of the following is NOT a function of the liver?
- **A.** Synthesis of insulin
- **B.** Synthesis of carbohydrates, proteins, and fats
- **C.** Detoxification of drugs
- **D.** Synthesis of bile

41. Which statement about gene mapping is correct?
- **A.** Only three-factor crosses may be used to sequence gene loci
- **B.** The recombination frequencies are always representative of the recombination rates of the gene loci
- **C.** The recombination frequency is equal to the map units
- **D.** Viral DNAs are used for gene mapping

42. Which statement about cytoplasmic inheritance is correct?
- **A.** It does not follow mendelian laws
- **B.** The maternal cytoplasm plays the dominant role
- **C.** Replication of mitochondria is an example
- **D.** All of the above

43. Homozygous refers to:
- **A.** similar types of chromosomes.
- **B.** similar functions on an evolutionary basis.
- **C.** particles in a solution that are not separable microscopically.
- **D.** identical alleles for a given trait.

44. Which statement about X and Y chromosomes is INCORRECT?
- **A.** X is larger than Y
- **B.** They are not homologous
- **C.** XY is a genotypic male
- **D.** Traits that appear on X, but not on Y, are called sex-linked traits

45. Which statement is INCORRECT?
- **A.** Genotype is the alleles for a given trait in an individual
- **B.** Phenotype is the expression of the genotype
- **C.** A given genotype will produce different phenotypes
- **D.** Different genotypes may produce the same phenotype

46. Diseases such as blights, wilts, and galls are caused by:
- **A.** fungi.
- **B.** viroids.
- **C.** rickettsiae.
- **D.** bacteria.

47. Which disease is fungal?
- **A.** Influenza
- **B.** Pneumonia
- **C.** Both A and B
- **D.** Ringworm

48. Which is not a family in suborder Eubacteriineae?
- **A.** Rhizobiaceae
- **B.** Chlamydobacteriales
- **C.** Achromobacteriaceae
- **D.** Parvobacteriaceae

49. A vaccine usually causes:
- **A.** passive immunity.
- **B.** active immunity.
- **C.** the production of antibodies.
- **D.** both B and C.

50. Which disease is viral?
- **A.** Anthrax
- **B.** Syphilis
- **C.** Polio
- **D.** Tuberculosis

51. All of the following are infections EXCEPT:
- **A.** typhoid.
- **B.** botulism.
- **C.** common flu.
- **D.** strep throat.

52. All of the following are types of bacteria EXCEPT:
- **A.** metatrophic.
- **B.** parasitic.
- **C.** autotrophic.
- **D.** eucalyptic.

53. Infectious diseases are:
- **A.** inherited.
- **B.** caused by pathogens.
- **C.** caused by rickettsiae.
- **D.** caused by bacterial respiration.

8.2 CHEMISTRY

For each question, read all of the choices carefully. Select the answer that is correct or most nearly correct. Blacken the answer space that corresponds to your choice. This section contains 60 items.

Time limit: 35 minutes

1. A neutral atom that has 53 electrons and an atomic mass of 111 has:
A. no other isotopes.
B. an atomic number of 58.
C. a nucleus that contains 58 neutrons.
D. a nucleus that contains 53 neutrons.

2. Which measurement or technique can be used to find the atomic, or molecular, weight of a substance?
A. Heat of combustion
B. Boiling point elevation
C. Boiling point of the pure substance
D. Electrical conductivity

3. How many grams of HCl are required to react completely with 32.5 g Zn, producing zinc chloride and hydrogen?
A. 9
B. 18
C. 36
D. 72

4. What is the sum of the coefficients of all species in the following balanced equation?
$Pb(NO_3)_2 \rightarrow NO_2 + PbO + O_2$
A. 18
B. 15
C. 12
D. 9

5. The boiling point of acetic acid is 118°C. Estimate the boiling point of a solution of a nonelectrolyte in acetic acid.
A. 115°C
B. 118°C
C. 120°C
D. 100°C

6. If the standard heats of formation of SO_2 and SO_3 are -70 and -95 kcal/mol, respectively, what is the heat of reaction for the following?
$SO_2 + 1/2\ O_2 \rightarrow SO_3$
A. -25 kcal
B. -165 kcal
C. 25 kcal
D. 165 kcal

7. If 50 ml 2.0 M NaOH is mixed with 50 ml 4.0 M nitric acid, what is the pH of the final solution?
A. 1.00
B. 7.00
C. 14.00
D. 10.00

8. What volume is occupied by 0.50 mol ideal gas at 760 torr and 0°C?
A. 2.24 L
B. 11.2 L
C. 22.4 L
D. 44.8 L

9. What volume of HI is produced if 14.2 L hydrogen and 23.5 L iodine react at standard temperature and pressure?
$H_2 + I_2 \rightarrow 2\ HI$
A. 14.2 L
B. 23.5 L
C. 28.4 L
D. 47.0 L

10. A gas mixture contains equal numbers of CO molecules and CO_2 molecules, and no others. Assuming ideal gas behavior, which statement is true?
A. The total mass of CO_2 and CO is the same
B. The partial pressure of CO_2 and CO is the same
C. Because carbon dioxide molecules have more mass, they have more inertia and contribute more to the total pressure
D. The density of CO_2 and CO is the same

11. Which compound is INCORRECTLY named?
A. $V(ClO_3)_3$, vanadium (III) chlorate
B. $Na_2C_2O_4$, sodium oxalate
C. $AlPO_4$, aluminum phosphate
D. $KHSO_4$, krypton bisulfate

12. Fe metal adopts a body-center cube structure. How many Fe atoms are present in the unit cell?
A. 1
B. 2
C. 4
D. 6

13. Which combination(s) of quantum numbers CANNOT be used to solve the Schrödinger wave equation for the hydrogen atom?

	n	l	m	s
I.	9	0	0	−5/2
II.	2	1	0	−1/2
III.	1	3	3	1/2

A. I
B. III
C. I and II
D. I and III

14. Atom A has three valence electrons, and atom B has seven valence electrons. The formula expected for an ionic compound of A and B is:
A. AB.
B. AB_3.
C. AB_2.
D. A_2B.

15. Which trend in first ionization potential is NOT correct?
A. Rb < Sb < Cl < Ne
B. Na < Mg < P < Cl
C. Be < Sb < P < N
D. F < N < B < Li

16. In which molecule is the octet rule violated?
A. $SnCl_2$
B. $PbCl_4$
C. F_2
D. All of the above

17. Which oxidation state would NOT be expected?
A. Ar(0)
B. Pb(IV)
C. Nb(V)
D. N(VI)

18. Which molecule(s) would be expected to be polar?
I. NO
II. $GaCl_3$
III. HF
IV. $COCl_2$

A. I
B. II and IV
C. I, III, and IV
D. I, II, and III

19. What is the pH of a 0.0100 molar HNO_3 aqueous solution?
A. 7.00
B. 12.00
C. 2.00
D. 2.76

20. In the following hypothetical half-reactions, which statement is true?
$M^{2+} + e^- \rightarrow M^+ \quad E^\circ = -0.579\ V$
$M^{3+} + e^- \rightarrow M^{2+} \quad E^\circ = 0.735\ V$
A. M^{2+} is reduced
B. M^{3+} is reduced
C. This reaction is never spontaneous
D. More information is needed

21. If 75% of a radioactive isotope decays in 300 days, what is its half-life?
A. 100 days
B. 150 days
C. 200 days
D. 300 days

22. Which arrangement of atoms is most likely?

A. O—C—O—O

B. 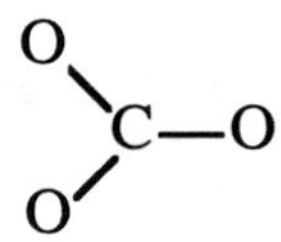

C. 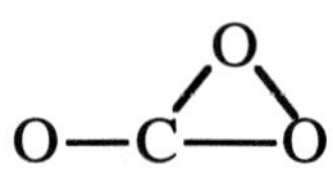

D. 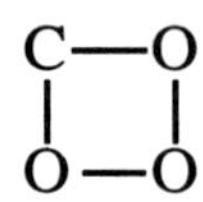

23. What is the molecular formula for a compound with an empirical formula of NO and a molecular mass of 90 g/mol?
A. NO
B. N_2O_2
C. N_3O_3
D. N_4O_4

24. Which ion is formed by an element with the electron configuration $1s^22s^22p^4$?
A. +2
B. +4
C. −2
D. −4

25. Element A has three isotopic forms with masses of 21.0, 25.0, and 26.0 AMU, respectively. Element B also has three isotopic forms with masses of 22.0, 24.0, and 26.0 AMU, respectively. Which statement is true?
  A. Element A has a higher atomic mass than element B
  B. Element B has a higher atomic mass than element A
  C. Elements A and B have identical atomic masses because the sums of their isotopic masses are equal
  D. More information is needed to predict which atomic mass is greater

26. Which oxidation state would NOT be expected?
  A. Ar(0)
  B. Ag(I)
  C. S (VII)
  D. Na(III)

27. Which gives the correct hybridization for the central atom in the following molecule?
$AlCl_3$ N_3^- CS_2
  A. sp^3 sp^2 sp^2
  B. sp^3 sp sp^2
  C. sp sp^3 sp^2
  D. sp^2 sp sp^2

28. The biologic effect of radiation is measured in units of:
  A. geigers.
  B. electron volts.
  C. curies.
  D. rems.

29. When sulfuric acid is added to sodium chloride, the gas emitted has the formula:
  A. Cl_2.
  B. HCl.
  C. H_2S.
  D. SO_3.

30. Which species CANNOT behave as a reducing agent?
  A. ClO^-
  B. ClO_2^-
  C. ClO_3^-
  D. ClO_4^-

31. Which carbon backbone forms the structure of 2,3,6-trimethyloctane?

A. 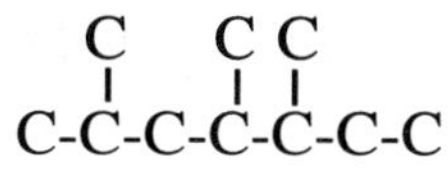

B. 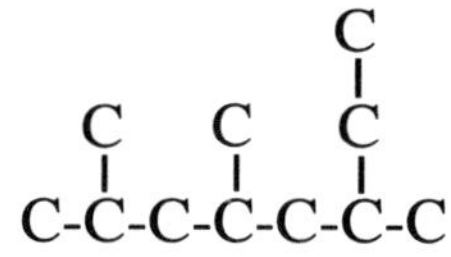

C. 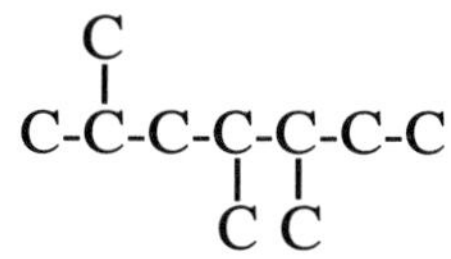

D. 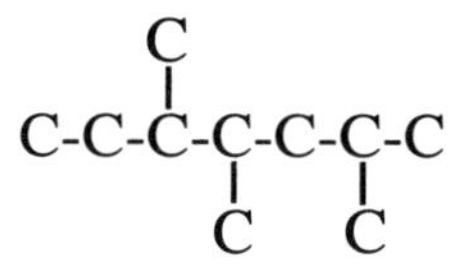

32. Which compound has the highest dipole moment?

A. 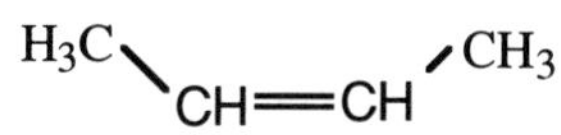

B. 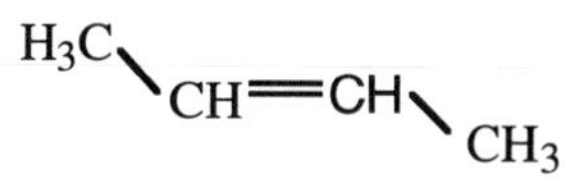

C. $H_3C-C\equiv C-CH_3$

D. 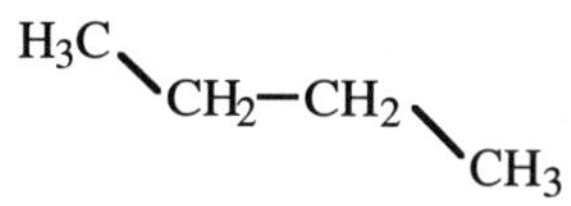

33. What is the product of the reaction between 1,1,1-tribromo-2-butene and HBr?

A. 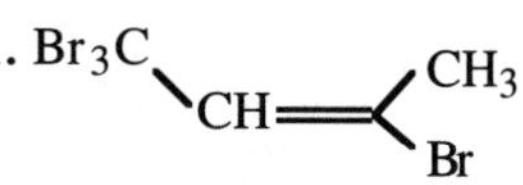

B. 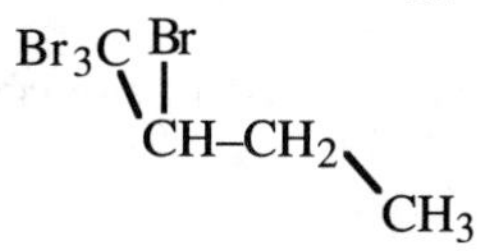

C. $Br_3C-C\equiv C-CH_3$

D. 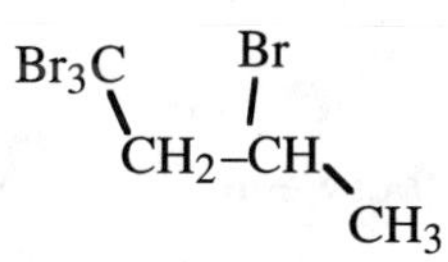

34. What is the product of the reaction between Br^+ and anisole?

A. 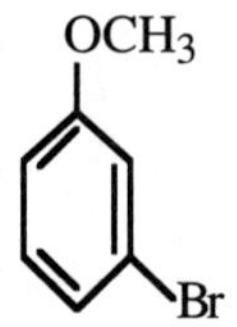

B. 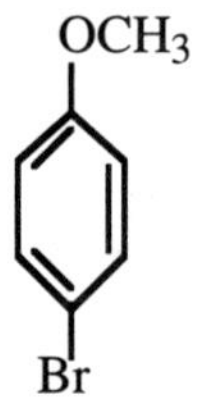

C. 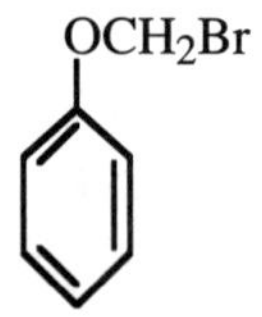

D. 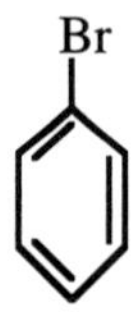

35. Which acid is strongest?
A. Isopropanol
B. Sec-butanol
C. Tert-butanol
D. Propanol

36. Which substance is the least soluble in water?
A. Ethanol
B. Propanol
C. Butanol
D. Pentanol

37. Which alcohol is most likely to undergo S_N2 substitutions?
A. CH_3OH
B. CH_3CH_3OH
C. $(CH_3)_2CHOH$
D. $(CH_3)_3COH$

38. What is the relation between these straight-chain aldoses?

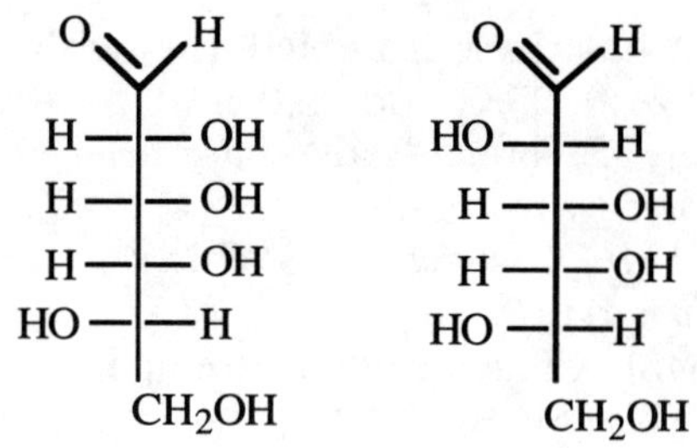

A. Anomers
B. Enantiomers
C. Epimers
D. Racemers

39. Which of the following is NOT a product of the following reaction?

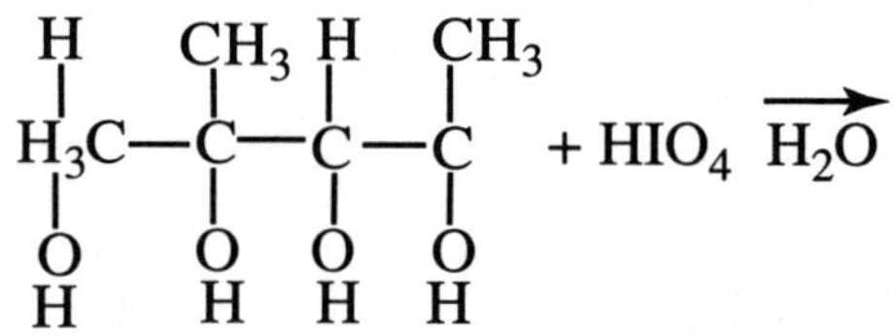

A. $H_3C\overset{O}{\overset{\|}{C}}H$

B. $H_2C{=}O$

C. $(CH_3)_2C{=}O$

D. $(CH_3)_3COH$

40. Name the following compound.

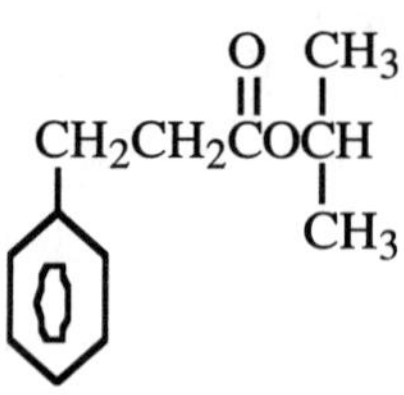

A. Isopropyl benzoate
B. Benzyl isopropyl ester
C. Isopropyl-3-phenylproponate
D. Isoalkyl chloride

41. What is the product of the following reaction?
$(CH_3)_3CCH_2CH_2OH + KMnO_4 \rightarrow$

A. $(CH_3)_3CCH_2\overset{\overset{O}{\|}}{C}H$

B. $(CH_3)_3CCH{=}CH_2$

C. $(CH_3)_3C\overset{\overset{O}{\|}}{C}CH_3$

D. CH_3COOH

42. Which is NOT a property of phenols?

A. They are more acidic than alcohols, but less acidic than carboxylic acids

B. Most reactions involve breaking the O—H bond

C. They cannot be dehydrated

D. They are easily oxidized to ketones

43. Which reagent is used in a Fridel-Crafts acylation?

A. CuX

B. RX and $AlCl_3$

C. $KMnO_4$

D. RC(=O)X and $AlCl_3$

44. Which sugar is a furanose?

A.

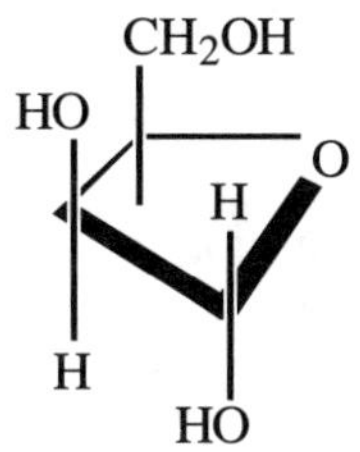

B.

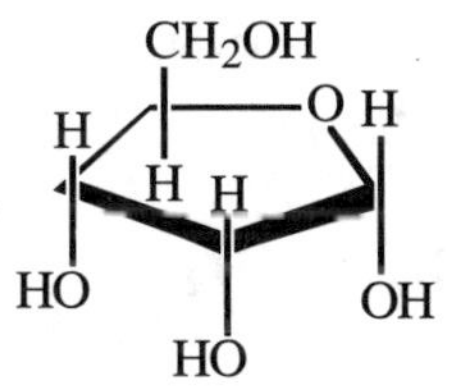

C.

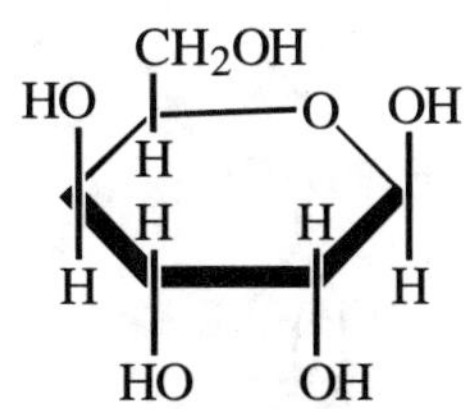

D.

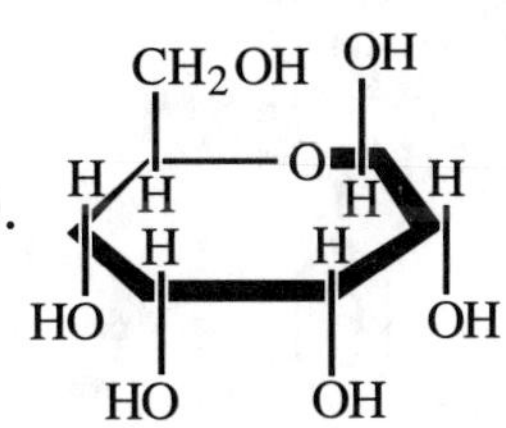

45. Which structure is consistent with these infrared (IR) and ^{1}H nuclear magnetic resonance (NMR) data?

IR: 3620 cm^{-1}, broad peak	NMR: 1:1 doublet, mass S, area 6
2980 cm^{-1}, strong peak	2:6 broad, area 1
No other strong peaks	3:9 septet, area 1

A.

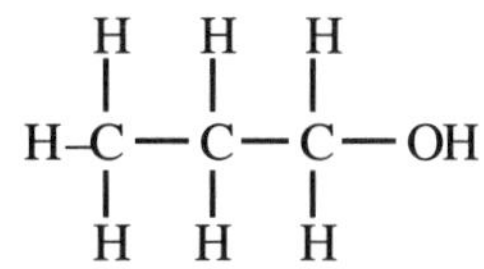

B.

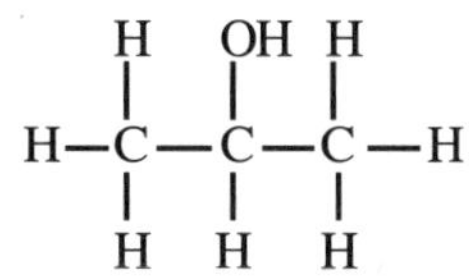

C.

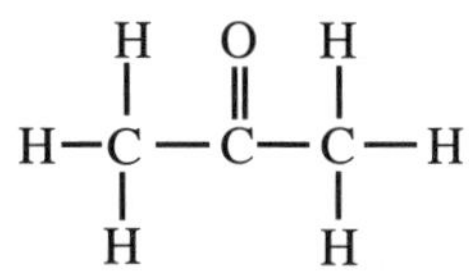

D.

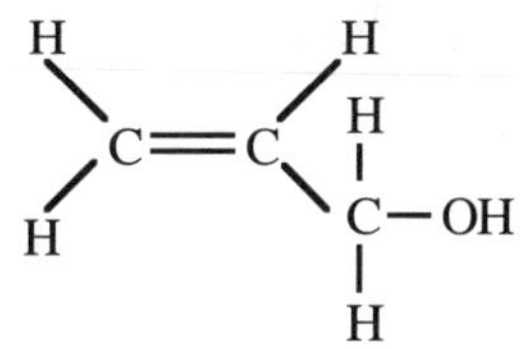

46. Aldehydes and ketones react with secondary amines to form compounds known as:

A. amides.

B. enamines.

C. lipids.

D. barbiturates.

47. Which of the following best describes a transesterification reaction?

A. High-boiling ester + high-boiling alcohol → Higher-boiling ester + low-boiling alcohol

B. High-boiling ester + low-boiling alcohol → Higher-boiling ester + high-boiling alcohol

C. Low-boiling ester + high-boiling alcohol → High-boiling ester + low-boiling alcohol

D. Low-boiling ester + low-boiling alcohol → High-boiling ester + high-boiling alcohol

48. What is the product of the following reaction?

$$H_2C{=}CH\overset{O}{\overset{\|}{C}}OCH_3 + CH_3CH_2CH_2CH_2OH \xrightarrow{H^+}$$

A. $H_2C{=}CH\overset{O}{\overset{\|}{C}}OCH_2\,(CH_2)_2CH_3$

B. 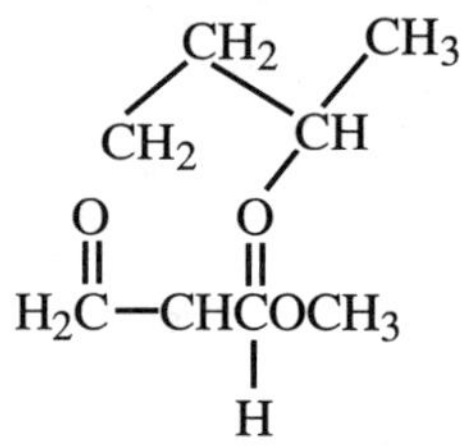

C. 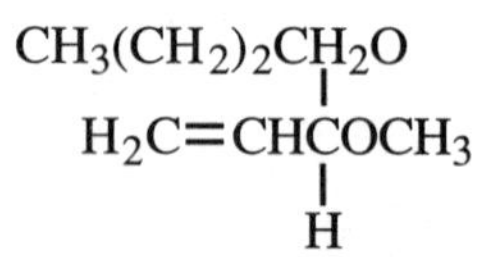

D. 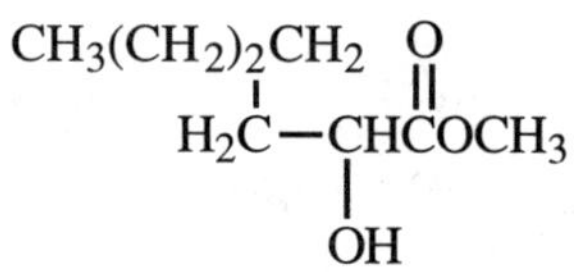

49. Which step is NOT a chain-propagating step for a radical reaction?

A. $(C_6H_5)_3C\cdot + O_2 \rightarrow (C_6H_5)_3C{-}O{-}O\cdot$

B. $(C_6H_5)_3C{-}O{-}O\cdot + (C_6H_5)_3CH \rightarrow (C_6H_5)_3C\cdot + (C_6H_5)_3C{-}O{-}OH$

C. $(C_6H_5)_3C\cdot + (C_6H_5)_3C{-}O{-}OH \rightarrow (C_6H_5)_3C{-}O{-}O\cdot + (C_6H_5)_3CH$

D. $(C_6H_5)_3C\cdot + (C_6H_5)_3C\cdot \rightarrow (C_6H_5)_3C{-}C(C_6H_5)_3$

50. Reduction of an organic compound usually entails:

A. a decrease in its oxygen content.
B. an increase in its oxygen content.
C. a decrease in the length of the longest carbon chain.
D. an increase in the length of the longest carbon chain.

51. A compound with an empirical formula of $C_5H_{10}O$ showed the following spectral characteristics: IR: strong peak near 1710 cm^{-1}; nuclear magnetic resonance: doublet at 1.10 ppm (6H), singlet at 2.10 ppm (3H), and a septet; ^1H: 2.50 ppm. Which compound agrees best with these data?

A. 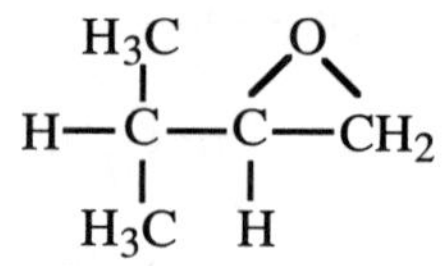

B. 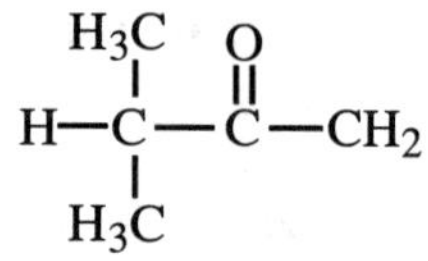

C. 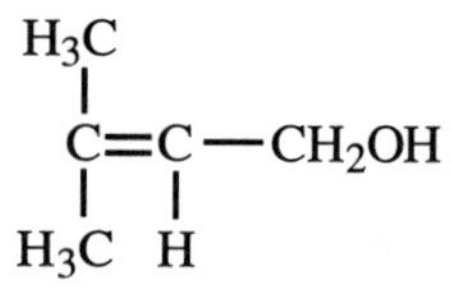

D. 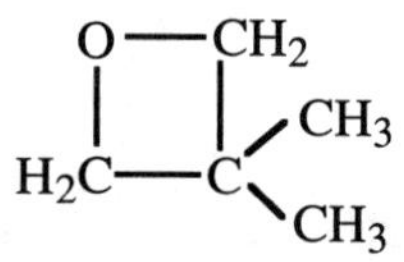

52. What is the major product of the following reaction?

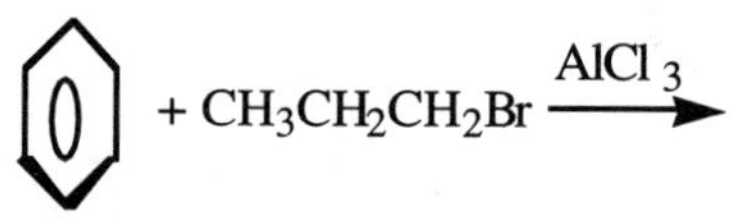

A. 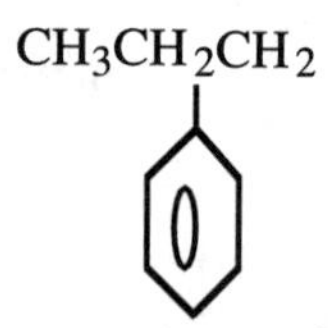

B. 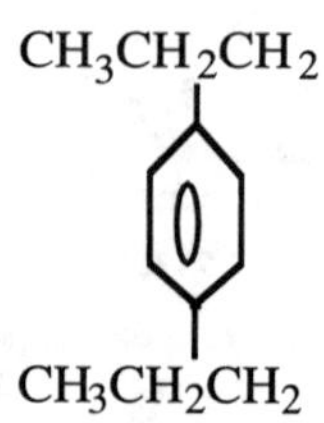

C. 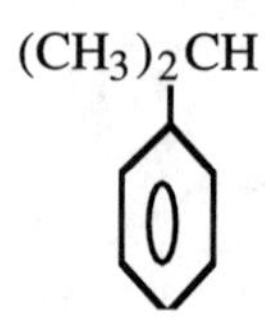

D. 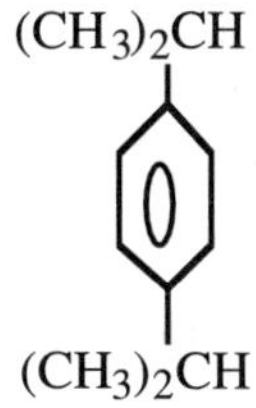

D. 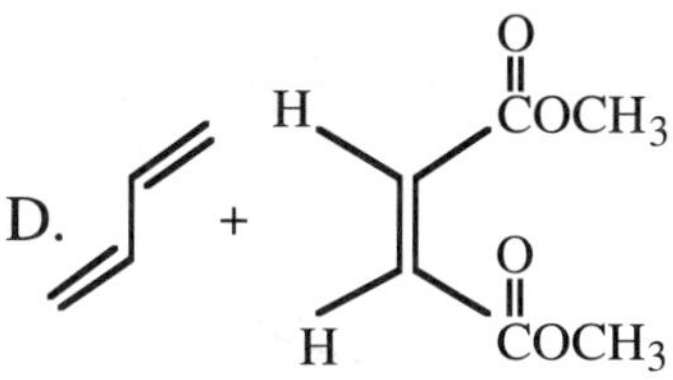

53. Which substituent group functions as a meta-director on electrophilic aromatic substitution reactions?

- **A.** $-NH_2$
- **B.** $-CH_3$
- **C.** $-CF_3$
- **D.** $-F$

54. Cyclooctatetrene reacts with two equivalents of potassium to yield the stable compound $K_2C_8H_8$. The nuclear magnetic resonance spectrum of this compound indicates that all of the hydrogens are equivalent. Which statement best explains these observations?

- **A.** The compound is ionic
- **B.** The compound is cyclic
- **C.** The compound is planar
- **D.** The compound is aromatic

55. Which set of reactants produces the following?

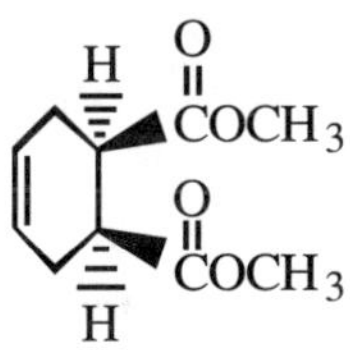

A. 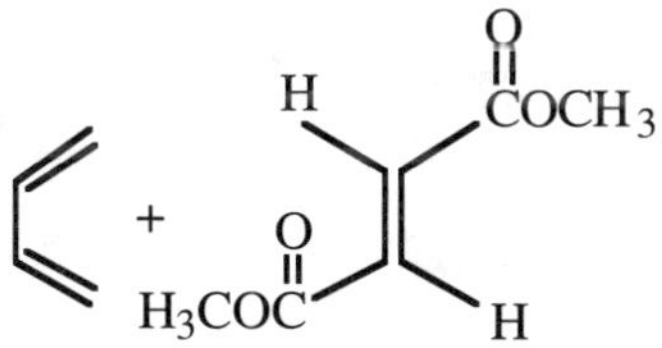

B. 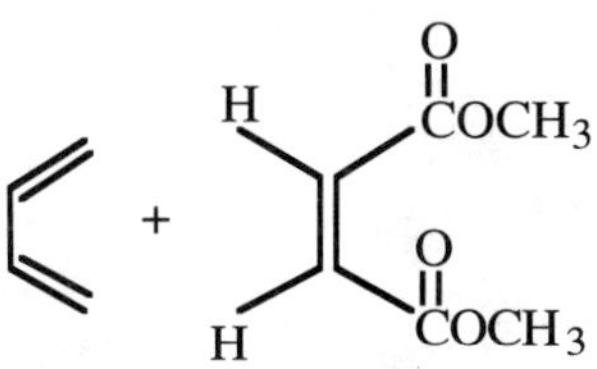

C. 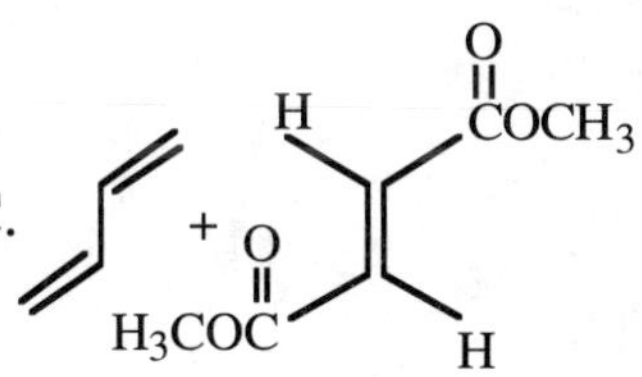

56. Which is the strongest carbon acid?

- **A.** Acetylene
- **B.** Ethene
- **C.** Ethane
- **D.** Methane

57. Which compound is drawn as a trans-isomer?

A. 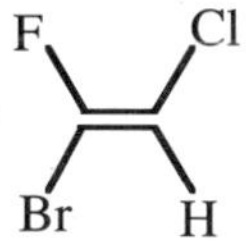

B. 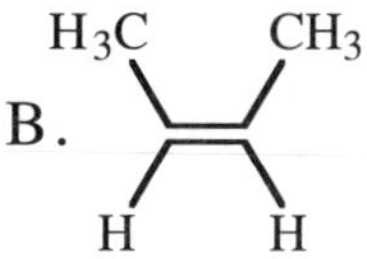

C. 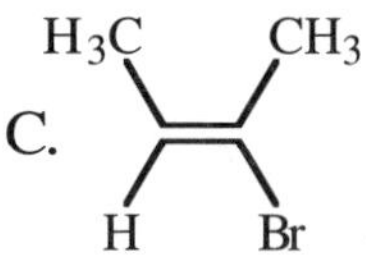

D. 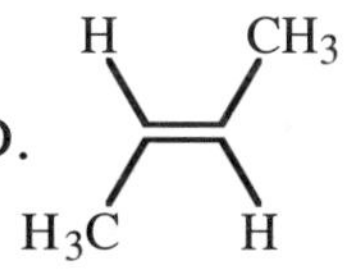

58. In the following reaction, what occurs to the configuration of the chiral carbon?

$$(-)CH_3\underset{\displaystyle OH}{\underset{|}{C}}HCHO + Br_2 \xrightarrow{H_2O} CH_3\underset{\displaystyle OH}{\underset{|}{C}}HCOOH$$

- **A.** Retention
- **B.** Inversion
- **C.** Racemization
- **D.** Loss of chirality

59. Which are cis-isomers?

I. 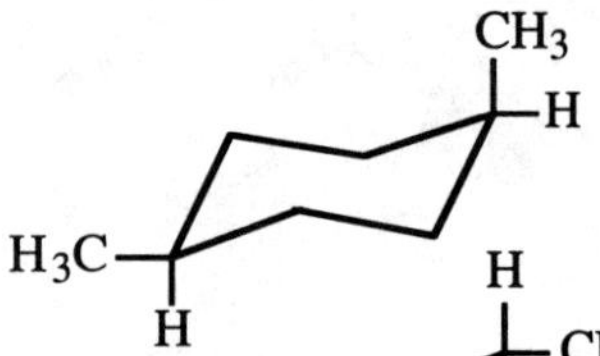

II. 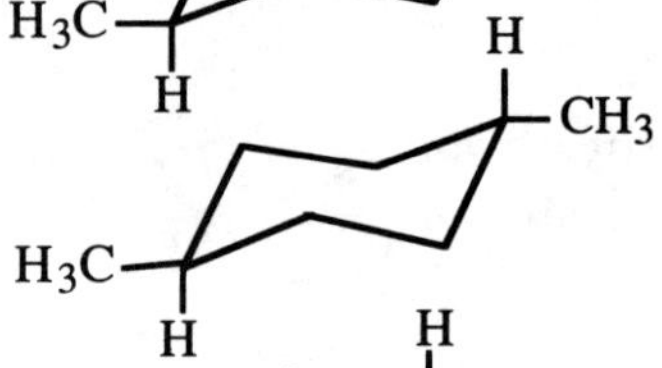

III. 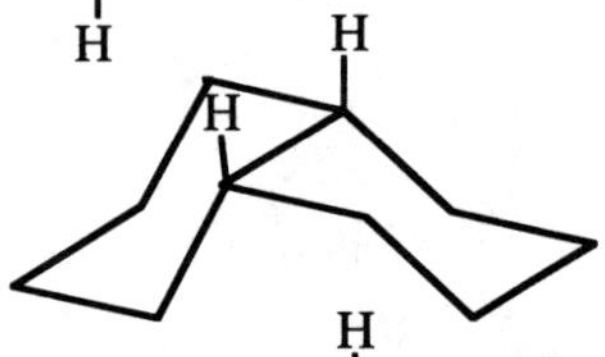

IV. 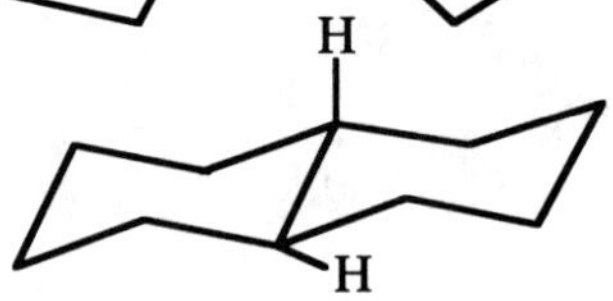

A. I and II
B. I and III
C. I and IV
D. II and III

60. A Grignard reagent reacts with esters to form:

A. primary alcohols.
B. secondary alcohols.
C. tertiary alcohols.
D. ketones.

8.3 READING COMPREHENSION

Read each passage to get an overview of the information. Reread the passage to answer the questions. For each question, read all of the choices carefully. Select the answer that is correct or most nearly correct. Circle the correct answer. This section contains 47 questions.

Time limit: 35 minutes

PASSAGE 1

Computerized transactions of all kinds are becoming ever more pervasive. More than half a dozen countries have developed or are testing chip cards that would replace cash. In Denmark, a consortium of banking, utility and transport companies has announced a card that would replace coins and small bills; in France, the telecommunications authorities have proposed general use of the smart cards now used at pay telephones. The government of Singapore has requested bids for a system that would communicate with cars and charge their smart cards as they pass various points on a road (as opposed to the simple vehicle identification systems already in use in the US and elsewhere). And cable and satellite broadcasters are experimenting with smart cards for delivering pay-per-view television. All these systems, however, are based on cards that identify themselves during every transaction.

If the trend toward identifier-based smart cards continues, personal privacy will be increasingly eroded. But in this conflict between organizational security and individual liberty, neither side emerges as a clear winner. Each round of improved identification techniques, sophisticated data analysis or extended linking can be frustrated by widespread noncompliance or even legislated limits, which in turn may engender attempts at further control.

Meanwhile, in a system based on representatives and observers, organizations stand to gain competitive and political advantages from increased public confidence (in addition to the lower costs of pseudonymous record-keeping). And individuals, by maintaining their own cryptographically guaranteed records and making only necessary disclosures, will be able to protect their privacy without infringing on the legitimate needs of those with whom they do business.

Adapted with permission from Chaum D: Achieving electronic privacy. Scientific American *August: 96, 1992.*

1. The passage suggests that chip cards are being developed because:
   A. they are easier to handle than cash.
   B. they provide greater privacy.
   C. they generate sophisticated data to analyze.
   D. the technology exists and should be used.

2. How does the author characterize the trend toward identifier-based smart cards?
   A. As a technologic advance
   B. As a potential threat to personal privacy
   C. As providing a competitive edge for innovative corporations
   D. As offering greater choices to consumers

3. It can be inferred from the passage that the key technologic innovation that made smart cards possible was:
   A. sophisticated data analysis.
   B. miniaturization of computer components.
   C. sophisticated security systems.
   D. advances in telecommunications.

4. According to the passage, all of the following are advantages of a system based on representatives EXCEPT:
   A. competitive advantages for organizations.
   B. protection of individual privacy.
   C. increased public confidence.
   D. improved identification systems.

5. All of the following could potentially gather data generated by identifier-based smart cards EXCEPT:
   A. businesses.
   B. governments.
   C. individuals.
   D. organizations.

6. In the context of the passage, what does the term cryptographically mean?
   A. Simple
   B. Complex
   C. Coded
   D. Anonymous

7. What does the author suggest is the difference between identifier-based systems and systems based on representatives and observers?
   A. Identifier-based systems are more economical
   B. Systems based on representatives and observers threaten organizational security
   C. Systems based on representatives and observers can better protect individuals
   D. Identifier-based systems can deliver a larger range of services

PASSAGE 2

Hebb's long and close observation of the many chimpanzees in the primate laboratory taught him that experience was not the only factor in the development of personality, including pathological manifestations such as phobias. He showed, for example, that young chimpanzees, born in the laboratory and known never to have seen a snake before, are frightened the first time they are shown one. Chimpanzees are also frightened by models of chimpanzee or human heads or other isolated body parts or of familiar caretakers wearing unusual clothing. Moreover, Hebb was one of the first to observe the social behavior of captive porpoises and to suggest that it implied a level of intelligence comparable to that of the apes. His observations may have influenced his later conclusion that level of play provides a good index of intelligence.

Lashley's interest in the ways the brain categorizes perceptions into knowledge about the world rekindled Hebb's curiosity about concepts and thinking. The problem can be rephrased as a question: How does the brain learn to lump one triangle, car or dog with another, even though no two triangles, cars or dogs produce the same pattern of stimulation on sensory receptors?

The turning point came when Hebb read about the work of Rafael Lorente de Nó, a neurophysiologist at the Rockefeller Institute for Medical Research, who had discovered neural loops, or feedback paths, in the brain. Up to that point, all psychological theories, whether physiological or not, assumed that information passed through the organism along a one-way track, like food through the digestive system. Hebb recognized that Lorente's looping paths were just what he needed to develop a more realistic theory of the mind.

Feedback was not entirely new in learning theory. Almost all models assumed that the output of the organism influences the input in some way, for instance, enabling the animal to receive a reinforcing stimulus. Unfortunately, a feedback proceeding in this way, through a single path, would operate slowly and often unreliably. But with millions of internally connected feedback paths, it would clearly be possible to establish internal models of the environment that might predict the effects of possible responses without having to move a muscle.

8. What was Donald Hebb's profession?
   A. Physiologist
   B. Medical doctor
   C. Psychologist
   D. Anatomist

9. What did experiments with chimpanzees prove to Hebb about behavior?
   A. Experience was not the only factor in shaping behavior
   B. Chimpanzees were frightened by snakes
   C. Chimpanzees were frightened by their caretakers under certain conditions
   D. Primates are very intelligent

10. What evidence does the passage present to support the conclusion that level of play provides a good index of intelligence?
   A. Observations of chimpanzee behavior
   B. Observations of porpoise behavior
   C. No direct evidence
   D. Observation of neural pathways in humans

11. What was the importance of the work of Rafael Lorente de Nó?
   A. He discovered neural loops
   B. He discovered that information passes through the organism along a one-way track
   C. He linked physiology to psychology
   D. He proved the pathologic manifestations of phobias

12. The passage suggests that although the idea of feedback was not new to learning theorists, it had proved of little value. Why?
   A. They assumed that information moves like food through a digestive tract
   B. They suggested that output of an organism affected input
   C. Single-path feedback was too slow and unreliable
   D. It was impossible to construct internal models of the environment

13. Of what use were Lorente's paths to Hebb?
   A. They were of no use
   B. They allowed him to develop a more realistic theory of the mind
   C. They allowed him to construct a single-pathway feedback model of the mind
   D. They allowed him to dismiss the behavioral model of the mind

14. The passage implies that the reaction of laboratory-born chimpanzees to snakes and chimpanzee models was caused by:
   A. conditioning.
   B. experience.
   C. intelligence.
   D. innate factors.

15. What was significant about Hebb's observations of captive porpoises?
   A. He was the first to speculate about the role of play
   B. He was among the first to suggest that porpoises are comparable in intelligence to apes
   C. They influenced his ideas of perception patterns
   D. They allowed him to construct a model of internally connected feedback paths

PASSAGE 3

Unlike any other mammal, a naked mole rat's body temperature fluctuates with ambient temperature. Rochelle Buffenstein and Shlomo Yahav of the University of Witwatersrand in South Africa found that as a result of high heat exchange, small body size and low rates of metabolic heat production, naked mole rats are poikilothermic, or cold-blooded. In nature, the animals live in a relatively thermostable environment: temperatures in the deep tunnels, which are about 50 centimeters underground, remain close to 30 degrees Celsius year-round. Naked mole rats regulate their body temperature behaviorally by basking in warm soil near the surface or by huddling during cold snaps.

The naked mole rat is a prodigious digger. Robert A. Brett, now at the Kenya Wildlife Service, studied a colony of 87 naked mole rats in Kenya's Tsavo West National Park. He recorded that in an average month the colony excavated more than 200 meters of burrows that were four to seven centimeters in diameter. In the process, the animals ejected more than 350 kilograms of soil through some 40 surface openings. All this digging results in intricate systems of interconnected tunnels and multiple nest chambers that are as big as footballs. The animals move among the nests, using the one closest to their current food source.

A burrow system can be astonishingly large. Brett put small radio transmitters on a number of individuals in his study colony and tracked them underground. He discovered that the network was more than 3.0 kilometers long and occupied an area greater than 100,000 square meters, about the size of 20 football fields. Colonies carve out these extensive burrow systems in the reddish, iron- and aluminum-rich soils of the semideserts of Kenya, Ethiopia and Somalia. Although they are not rare, naked mole rats are seldom seen. Small volcano-shaped mounds of earth offer the only clues about their presence. In the cooler parts of the day, these miniature volcanoes "erupt," as the animals kick out soil from recent excavations.

Digging is generally a cooperative endeavor. The animals line up head-to-tail behind an individual who is gnawing on the earth at the end of a developing tunnel. Once a pile of soil has accumulated behind the digger, the next mole rat in line begins transporting it through the tunnel system, often by sweeping it backward with its hind feet. Colony mates stand on tiptoe and allow the earthmover to pass underneath them; then, in turn, they each take their place at the end of the line. When the earthmover finally arrives at a surface opening, it sweeps its load to a large colony mate that has stationed itself there. This "volcanoer" ejects the dirt in a fine spray with powerful kicks of its hind feet, while the smaller worker rejoins the living conveyer belt.

Much of the mole rats' tunneling is done to find food. They eat the succulent tubers of many different geophytes—perennial plants that store water, sugar and starch in swollen roots to enable them to survive the biannual African dry seasons. Most geophytes have irregular or patchy distributions. Mole rats forage for them by tunneling blindly, apparently unable to detect the plants through the baked soil. Brett observed that mole rats sometimes eat only the central parts of large tubers and leave the outer layers alone. They then pack the hollowed-out part with soil. In time, the tuber regenerates, and the colony forages from it again.

Adapted with permission from Sherman PW, Jarvis JUM, Braude SH: Naked mole rats. Scientific American *August: 72, 1992.*

16. What is a poikilothermic animal?
   A. A mammal
   B. An animal that lives in a climate with a steady temperature
   C. A cold-blooded animal
   D. An animal that lives underground

17. The passage suggests that for naked mole rats, the primary function of digging is to:
   A. regulate body temperature
   B. forage for food
   C. build a system of tunnels as protection from predators
   D. engage in social behavior

18. The passage suggests that naked mole rats are indigenous to:
   A. Africa.
   B. unstable environments.
   C. relatively cold climates.
   D. North America.

19. What does the passage imply about the digging behavior of naked mole rats?
   A. It is random
   B. It indicates a structured society
   C. It shows that there is little cooperation
   D. It demonstrates the competitive nature of the animals

20. Naked mole rats regulate their body temperature in all of the following ways EXCEPT by:
   A. living in a relatively thermostable environment.
   B. huddling together.
   C. basking in warm soil.
   D. constantly working.

21. What characterizes the volcanoer rat?
   A. It is larger than the worker rats
   B. It does not function as a member of the colony
   C. It performs only one task
   D. It has powerful front legs

22. What do naked mole rats primarily eat?
   A. Starches
   B. Small insects
   C. Nuts
   D. Geophytes

23. How does the author characterize digging by the naked mole rats?
   A. Planned
   B. A systematic search for warmer soil
   C. A living conveyer belt
   D. A search for nesting chambers

PASSAGE 4

In theory at least, software can be made that is free of defects. Unlike materials and machines, software does not wear out. All design defects are present from the time the software is loaded into the computer. In principle, these faults could be removed once and for all. Furthermore, mathematical proof should enable programmers to guarantee correctness.

Yet the goal of perfect software remains elusive. Despite rigorous and systematic testing, most large programs contain some residual bugs when delivered. The reason for this is the complexity of the source code. A program of only a few hundred lines may contain tons of decisions, allowing for thousands of alternative paths of execution (programs for fairly critical applications vary between tens and millions of lines of code). A program can make the wrong decision because the particular inputs that triggered the problem had not been used during the test phase, when defects could be corrected. The situation responsible for such inputs may even have been misunderstood or unanticipated: the designer either "correctly" programmed the wrong reaction or failed to take the situation into account altogether. This type of bug is the most difficult to eradicate.

In addition, specifications often change during system development, as the intended purpose of the system is modified or becomes better understood. Such changes may have implications that ripple through all parts of the system, making the previous design inadequate. Furthermore, real use may still differ from intended purpose. Failures of Patriot missiles to intercept Scud missiles have been attributed to an accumulation of inaccuracies in the internal time keeping of a computer. Yet the computer was performing according to specifications: the system was meant to be turned off and restarted often enough for the accumulated error never to become dangerous. Because the system was used in an unintended way, a minor inaccuracy became a serious problem.

The intrinsic behavior of digital systems also hinders the creation of completely reliable software. Many physical systems are fundamentally continuous in that they are described by "well-behaved" functions—that is, very small changes in stimuli produce very small differences in responses. In contrast, the smallest possible perturbation to the state of a digital computer (changing a bit from 0 to 1, for instance) may produce a radical response. A single incorrect character in the specification of a control program for an Atlas rocket carrying the first interplanetary spacecraft, Mariner 1, ultimately caused the vehicle to veer off course. Both rocket and spacecraft had to be destroyed shortly after launch.

Adapted with permission from Littlewood B, Strigini L: The risks of software. Scientific American *November: 62, 1992.*

24. Why does the goal of perfect software remain elusive?
- **A.** The complexity of the source code
- **B.** Testing is neither rigorous nor systematic enough
- **C.** Software, unlike hardware, does not wear out
- **D.** Programs make wrong decisions

25. If the computers were operating according to specifications, why did Patriot missiles often fail?
- **A.** The system was not turned off and on enough
- **B.** There was another primary purpose for the missiles
- **C.** Scud missiles were better designed
- **D.** Internal inaccuracies accumulated

26. The failure of the Atlas rocket is attributed to:
- **A.** a small programming error that was greatly magnified by a digital system.
- **B.** the intrinsic behavior of digital systems.
- **C.** specifications that were changed during system development.
- **D.** programmers who did not provide sufficient math proof.

27. In the context of the passage, what is important about a program that contains many decisions?
- **A.** It is complex
- **B.** It contains residual bugs
- **C.** It may have several critical applications
- **D.** Because there are many paths, problems occur that were not anticipated during testing

28. The author cites all of the following as problems resulting from changing specifications EXCEPT:
- **A.** the previous design may prove inadequate.
- **B.** real use may differ from the intended purpose.
- **C.** the software may simply wear out.
- **D.** the system may be used in a way that magnifies inaccuracies.

29. What are the most difficult types of bug to eliminate?
- **A.** Those that result from failure to test a particular input
- **B.** Those that result from the intrinsic behavior of digital systems
- **C.** Those in which the designer correctly programmed the wrong reaction
- **D.** Those that result from changing system specifications

30. In the passage, what purpose is served by the description of well-behaved functions?
- **A.** Contrast with digital systems in terms of the effects of errors
- **B.** A description of most physical systems and their importance
- **C.** An example of continuous physical systems
- **D.** The importance of not changing specifications

31. In the context of the passage, what does the term perturbation mean?
- **A.** A major flaw
- **B.** An upset
- **C.** A slight change
- **D.** A radical change

PASSAGE 5

The specificity and power of the immune system have not escaped the notice of cancer researchers. Assuming that T lymphocytes might be able to eradicate cancer cells as effectively as they lyse virus-infected cells, investigators have long hoped to identify tumor-rejection antigens: structures that T lymphocytes can recognize on tumor cells in the body. These workers reasoned that antigens appearing exclusively (or almost exclusively) on cancer cells could be manipulated in ways that would trigger or amplify a patient's insufficient immune reactions to those targets.

Definitive evidence that tumor-rejection antigens exist on human tumors has been elusive. Yet in the past few years, my colleagues and I . . . have gathered unequivocal proof that many, perhaps most, tumors do indeed display such antigens. Equally important, we have developed ways to isolate genes that specify the structure of these antigens. Moreover, we and others have seen indications that T lymphocytes that normally ignore existing tumor-rejection antigens can be prodded to respond to them. Hence, the design of therapies to generate such T-cell responses to well-defined tumor-rejection antigens has finally become feasible.

The first clues that tumor-rejection antigens sometimes arise on tumors were uncovered in the 1950s, before the distinct roles of antibodies and T cells were elucidated. Several researchers . . . had generated cancers in mice by treating the animals with large doses of a carcinogenic compound. When the mice were freed of their tumors by surgery and subsequently injected with cells of the same tumor, they did not suffer a recurrence. The mice did acquire cancer after being injected with cells from other tumors, however. These observations suggested that cells of carcinogen-induced tumors carry antigens that can elicit a response by the immune system.

For about 20 years after those pioneering experiments were completed, hope ran high that human cancers, too, might bear tumor-rejection antigens. The prospect for antigen-based therapy seemed even better when, toward the end of that period, T lymphocytes were found to be particularly important for ridding the body of abnormal cells. Jean-Charles Cerottini and K. Theodor Brunner of the Swiss Institute for Experimental Cancer Research in Lusanne showed that when mice reject tissue transplanted from an unrelated donor, the animals produce cytolytic T lymphocytes that can destroy cells from the transplant. By then it was apparent as well that when the specialized antigen receptors on cytolytic T lymphocytes bind to foreign antigens on a cell, the lymphocytes both lyse the cell and multiply, amplifying the immune reaction. These discoveries intimated that cancer researchers might make major strides if they concentrated on finding the antigenic targets of cytolytic T lymphocytes and on augmenting the activity of the cytolytic cells.

Adapted with permission from Boon T: Teaching the immune system to fight cancer. Scientific American *March: 82, 1993.*

32. What is the main idea of the passage?
   A. Tumor-rejection antigens sometimes arise on tumors
   B. Many human tumors possess tumor-rejection antigens
   C. T lymphocytes play a vital role in ridding the body of abnormal cells
   D. Antibodies and T lymphocytes have distinct roles

33. What is the role of T lymphocytes in the immune system?
   A. They recognize and eradicate abnormal cells
   B. They destroy tumors in humans
   C. They prevent the recurrence of tumors
   D. They mute the immune system in the presence of tumor antigens

34. In the context of the passage, what is the meaning of the term lyse?
   A. Augment
   B. Nurture
   C. Trigger
   D. Destroy

35. In the context of the passage, what is the significance of antigens?
   A. They are structures on cancer cells that allow T lymphocytes to bind to those cells
   B. They are molecules that extend from cells that kill abnormal cells
   C. They amplify the immune system
   D. They destroy tumors

36. What was the significance of the studies in which mice were injected with carcinogenic compounds?
   A. The mice had a high incidence of tumor recurrence
   B. The studies suggested that cells of carcinogen-induced tumors carry antigens
   C. The studies helped to distinguish between antibodies and T cells
   D. The studies were not successfully replicated in humans

37. Experiments in the transplantation of mouse organs suggested all of the following EXCEPT:
   A. researchers might concentrate on augmenting the activities of cytolytic cells.
   B. lymphocytes multiply when they bind to foreign antigens on cells.
   C. mice produced cytolytic T lymphocytes.
   D. lymphocytes did not lyse foreign cells.

38. The author claims to have gathered unequivocal proof that:
   A. all tumors display antigens.
   B. most tumors display antigens.
   C. many human tumors display antigens.
   D. antigens appear exclusively on cancer cells.

39. The tone of the passage could best be described as:
   A. pessimistic.
   B. optimistic.
   C. cautious.
   D. frustrated.

PASSAGE 6

How, then, do wasps detect their victims within the complex environment, particularly when the caterpillars evade their attackers by hiding, moving or otherwise remaining concealed? Random searching alone certainly seems an implausible way to achieve such a literally vital goal; field studies suggest that a wasp might spend its entire lifetime searching for a single host if the wasp had to find it by chance. For the past 10 years, our research groups have been collaborating in pursuit of the answer. We think we have found it. Furthermore, the basic principles we have discovered seem to apply to other kinds of parasitic wasps, including species that parasitize eggs or other insect stages of development.

Briefly, the answer is this: the wasps home in on unique volatile compounds that they can detect over substantial distances. These chemicals come from the caterpillar's feces and, perhaps more surprising, from the plants on which the caterpillar feeds. Our quest led us into two areas that had been relatively unexplored with respect to these animals. The first was the ability of wasps to learn. They decipher many indirect and frequently changing cues that indicate the location of hosts. This ability represents a level of sophistication previously unexpected in these insects. The second area is the interaction between the wasps and the plants. When attacked by a caterpillar, a plant produces signals that wasps home in on. Research suggests that investigators can exploit the learning abilities of wasps and the wasp–plant conspiracy to control caterpillar pests in the field.

Our findings about the complicated interactions among the parasites, hosts and plants began with the assumption that a specific set of odors from the hosts would guide the wasps to their victims. This supposition was rooted in many studies that indicated that parasitic wasps respond to certain chemical cues. Early efforts identified and synthesized several kinds of chemicals that can act as guides. Such compounds belong to a classs of chemical mediators called kairomones. These substances, which come predominantly from the oral secretions and feces of the caterpillar, act at close range as trail odors or searching stimulants.

These kinds of kairomones, however, could not be the whole story. Because they are nonvolatile, they do not disperse well in the atmosphere. Thus, they cannot be detected over long distances. If wasps had to rely solely on short-range cues from their hosts, their success in finding caterpillars would only be slightly better than chance.

Adapted with permission from Tumlinson JH, Lewis WJ, Vet LEM: How parasitic wasps find their hosts. Scientific American *March: 100, 1993.*

40. In what way does the passage suggest that caterpillars serve as hosts?
   A. For wasp eggs
   B. For nutrients
   C. For chemical compounds
   D. For chemical mediators

41. According to the passage, what is the function of kairomones?
   A. They widely disperse nonvolatile chemicals
   B. They provide long-range cues
   C. They act as searching stimulants
   D. They protect plants

42. What is the key component of the plant–wasp conspiracy?
   A. Plants signal wasps when attacked by caterpillars
   B. Plants and wasps show unexpected interaction
   C. Wasps have the ability to learn
   D. Direct and indirect cues are used

43. What do wasps use to home in on caterpillar hosts?
   A. Random searching
   B. Kairomones
   C. Unique chemical cues
   D. Nonvolatile chemicals

44. According to the passage, what are the implications of learning more about wasp and plant interactions?
   A. Caterpillar pests in agriculture might be controlled
   B. Learning about the behavior of these in insects may improve the understanding of the behavior of other parasitic insects
   C. The relations between hosts, parasites, and plants will be better understood
   D. A greater understanding of chemical dispersion mechanisms will be achieved

45. How do caterpillars act as beacons for parasitic wasps?
   A. They attempt to evade them by hiding and moving
   B. They give off nonvolatile chemical cues
   C. They secrete volatile and complex chemical compounds
   D. Oral secretions and feces act as chemical guides

46. The cues provided by caterpillar kairomones are NOT sufficient to guide parasitic wasps because they:
   A. are volatile.
   B. provide short-range cues.
   C. disperse well in the atmosphere.
   D. are detected over substantial distances.

47. The authors make all of the following observations EXCEPT:
   A. wasps have an ability to learn.
   B. wasps interact with plants.
   C. wasps can decipher many indirect cues.
   D. wasps single out caterpillars as hosts.

8.4 QUANTITATIVE REASONING

Each question or incomplete statement is followed by suggested answers or completions. Read each item, decide which choice is best, and circle your answer. This section contains 40 questions.

Time limit: 35 minutes

1. The largest of four consecutive even integers is two less than twice the smallest. Which of the following is the largest?

A. 8
B. 10
C. 6
D. 14

2. Which line is perpendicular to the y-axis?

A. $y = 3$
B. $x = 3$
C. $x = y$
D. $y = 1 - x$

3. $\left(\frac{1}{x}\right)^6 + \left(\frac{2}{x^2}\right)^3 = ?$

A. $\frac{3}{x^2}$
B. $\frac{9}{x^6}$
C. $\frac{12}{x^6}$
D. $2x^6$

4. What is the probability of obtaining either tails or heads in five tosses of a fair coin?

A. $\frac{1}{2}$
B. $\frac{3}{5}$
C. $\frac{2}{5}$
D. $\frac{5}{8}$

5. What is the slope of a line containing the points (−2, 4) and (1, 3)?

A. 3
B. $\frac{1}{3}$
C. −3
D. $-\frac{1}{3}$

6. $\frac{2}{3} + \frac{1}{4} - \frac{1}{2} = ?$

A. $\frac{-1}{2}$
B. $\frac{1}{12}$
C. $\frac{1}{6}$
D. $\frac{5}{12}$

7. $\frac{2}{3} \times \frac{3}{4} \times \frac{4}{5} = ?$

A. $\frac{9}{12}$
B. $\frac{2}{5}$
C. $\frac{1}{4}$
D. $\frac{3}{8}$

8. If $ax^2 = 2y$, then $\frac{a}{y} = ?$

A. 2
B. $2x^2$
C. $\frac{2}{x^2}$
D. $\frac{x^2}{2}$

9. $\frac{\sqrt{15}\sqrt{3}}{\sqrt{10}} = ?$

A. $\frac{3}{2}$
B. $2\sqrt{5}$
C. $9\sqrt{5}$
D. $\frac{3\sqrt{2}}{2}$

10. If $2^{x/3} = 16$, then $x = ?$

A. −2
B. 4
C. 6
D. 12

11. If the perimeter of a square is 5.2, what is the area?

A. 1.3
B. 1.69
C. 52
D. 13

12. If an ordinary coin is tossed four times, what is the probability that the four tosses will be either all heads or all tails?

A. $\frac{1}{16}$

B. $\frac{1}{4}$

C. $\frac{1}{2}$

D. $\frac{1}{8}$

13. Which of the following is equal to (tan θ) (csc θ)?

A. sin θ
B. cos θ
C. sec θ
D. csc θ

14. Find the perimeter of the composite figure. Use 3.14 for π.

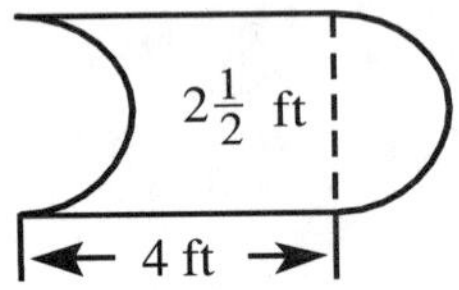

A. 15.85 feet
B. 13.25 feet
C. 10.5 feet
D. 13 feet

15. The angles of a triangle are in the ratio of 2:3:5. What is the measure of the smallest angle?

A. 48°
B. 36°
C. 90°
D. 45°

16. If the area of triangle BCE is 32, what is the area of square ABCD?

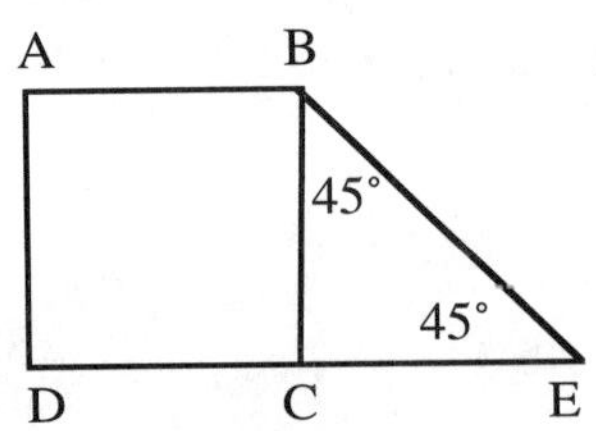

A. 64
B. 32
C. 16
D. 8

17. Nick withdraws from his piggy bank 20% of the original sum. If he must add 80¢ to restore the amount in the bank to the original sum, what was the original sum?

A. \$1.00
B. \$1.80
C. \$2.60
D. \$4.00

18. $-4 - 3\{2 + 1[3 - (2 + 3) + 2] + 2\} + 4 = ?$

A. -12
B. 0
C. 2
D. 8

19. 0.01% of 10 = ?

A. 1
B. 0.1
C. 0.01
D. 0.001

20. If $2x - y = 7$ and $x + y = 2$, then $x - y = ?$

A. 6
B. 4
C. $\frac{3}{2}$
D. 0

21. The distance between Joel's house and the zoo is 12 miles. Joel rode his bicycle from his house to the zoo at an average speed of 12 mph. He walked home from the zoo at an average speed of 6 mph. He took the same route in both directions. What was his average speed for both trips?

A. 8 mph
B. 12 mph
C. 16 mph
D. 20 mph

22. Ned is 3 years older than Jeremy, who is twice as old as Lucy. If the ages of the three total 28 years, how old is Jeremy?

A. 5 years old
B. 8 years old
C. 9 years old
D. 10 years old

23. Randy drove his car until the gas tank was 1/6 full. He stopped to refill the tank to capacity by putting in 20 gallons. What is the capacity of the gas tank?
   A. 20
   B. 21
   C. 24
   D. 28

24. The heights of two children are in the ratio of 2:5. If the first child is 5 feet tall, how tall is the second child?
   A. 1 foot
   B. 2 feet
   C. 5 feet
   D. 6 feet

25. Simplify $\sqrt{\frac{3x^2}{9} + \frac{4x^2}{36}}$
   A. $\frac{3x}{4}$
   B. $\frac{2x}{3}$
   C. $4x$
   D. $\frac{2x^2}{3}$

26. Three times the first of three consecutive odd integers is five more than twice the third. Find the third integer.
   A. 11
   B. 13
   C. 15
   D. 17

27. Maria invests $3600 in the Security National Bank at 5%. How much additional money must she invest at 10% so that the total annual interest income will be equal to 8% of her entire investment?
   A. $3600
   B. $1200
   C. $3000
   D. $5400

28. A plane traveling at 800 mph is 40 miles from Kennedy Airport at 5:58 P.M. When will it arrive at the airport?
   A. 6:00 P.M.
   B. 6:01 P.M.
   C. 6:02 P.M.
   D. 6:03 P.M.

29. William can wash his car in 30 minutes. His son Jack takes twice as long to wash the car. If they work together, how long will it take to wash the car?
   A. 5 minutes
   B. 10 minutes
   C. 20 minutes
   D. 28 minutes

30. The sum of a number and eight equals four less than the product of four and the number. Find the number.
   A. $x = 3$
   B. $x = 2$
   C. $x = 6$
   D. $x = 4$

31. Because of a decrease in sales, a department store reduces its output by 25%. By what percent must the reduced sales be increased for production to return to normal?
   A. 33.3%
   B. 50.0%
   C. 66.7%
   D. 75.0%

32. Dennis leaves home for work, driving at 24 mph. Fifteen minutes later, his wife, Diane, notices that he has forgotten his briefcase. She decides to catch him on the road. If Diane drives at 40 mph, how far must she drive before she catches up with him?
   A. 15 miles
   B. 30 miles
   C. 45 miles
   D. 60 miles

33. There are three consecutive even integers such that the third integer is eight more than the sum of the first and second integers. Find the third even integer.
   A. −8
   B. −6
   C. −4
   D. −2

34. Elizabeth has $5.50 in nickels and dimes. She has five more nickels than dimes. How many dimes does she have?
   A. 35
   B. 30
   C. 25
   D. 20

35. If the ratio of P to Q is 3:4 and the ratio of Q to R is 12:19, what is the ratio of P to R?
   A. 9:19
   B. 1:4
   C. 17:19
   D. 3:19

36. Find the equation of the line that contains the point $(-1, 0)$ and has slope 2.

A. $y = 2x - 1$
B. $y = 2x + 2$
C. $y = 2x$
D. $y = 2x - 3$

37. The following right triangles ABC and DEF are similar. How long is DF?

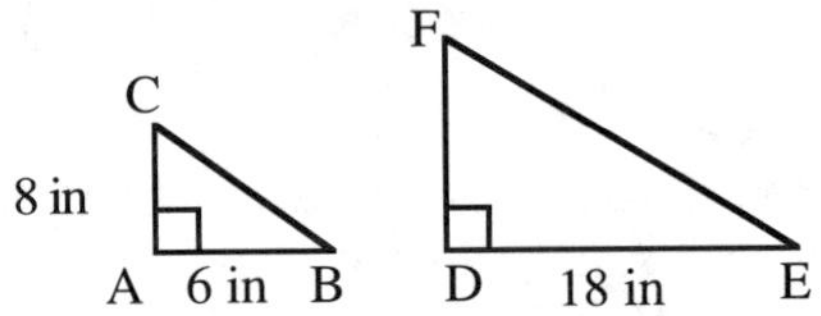

A. 24 inches
B. 20 inches
C. 16 inches
D. 12 inches

38. Which of the following is equal to

$-2 < \frac{x}{3} \leq 2$?

A. $-3 < x \leq 3$
B. $-4 < x \leq 4$
C. $-9 < x \leq 9$
D. $-6 < x \leq 6$

39. Which of the following is equal to sin 2A?

A. $1 - \cos^2 2A$
B. $2 \sin A \cos A$
C. $\frac{1}{\sec 2A}$
D. $2 \sin A$

40. If $\sin \theta = 1/3$, then $\cos \theta = ?$

A. $-\frac{1}{3}$
B. $-\sqrt{\frac{2}{3}}$
C. $\sqrt{\frac{2}{3}}$
D. $\frac{\pm 2\sqrt{2}}{3}$

8.5 VERBAL ABILITY

For antonym questions, choose the word that is most nearly opposite in meaning to the given word. For analogy questions, choose the word that best completes the word pair. This section contains 30 antonym questions and 30 analogy questions.

Time limit: 35 minutes

8.5.1 Antonyms

1. TANTAMOUNT
- **A.** biased
- **B.** equivalent
- **C.** paramount
- **D.** indistinct

2. ABRIDGE
- **A.** elongate
- **B.** abut
- **C.** curtail
- **D.** sever

3. INDIGENT
- **A.** foreign
- **B.** delighted
- **C.** destitute
- **D.** affluent

4. BANE
- **A.** woe
- **B.** solace
- **C.** permission
- **D.** mirth

5. MITIGATE
- **A.** augment
- **B.** assuage
- **C.** highlight
- **D.** settle

6. IMBUE
- **A.** pervade
- **B.** eradicate
- **C.** abstain
- **D.** inculcate

7. CORDIAL
- **A.** upbraid
- **B.** sincere
- **C.** frigid
- **D.** nonalcoholic

8. NONCHALANT
- **A.** accidental
- **B.** lethargic
- **C.** vague
- **D.** anxious

9. MORTIFY
- **A.** decay
- **B.** appall
- **C.** esteem
- **D.** enliven

10. INCLINATION
- **A.** penchant
- **B.** slope
- **C.** abhorrence
- **D.** yen

11. DELUSION
- **A.** explanation
- **B.** misconception
- **C.** pretense
- **D.** appearance

12. METTLE
- **A.** assistance
- **B.** courage
- **C.** timidity
- **D.** order

13. OBSEQUIOUS
- **A.** vigilant
- **B.** deferential
- **C.** conscious
- **D.** imprudent

14. BEDLAM
- **A.** chaos
- **B.** order
- **C.** demise
- **D.** truth

15. CONGEAL
- **A.** soften
- **B.** agree
- **C.** curdle
- **D.** enlighten

16. GARRULOUS
- **A.** taciturn
- **B.** unspeakable
- **C.** aggressive
- **D.** powerful

17. SOPORIFIC
- **A.** pacifying
- **B.** repugnant
- **C.** invigorating
- **D.** elusive

18. IMPORTUNE
  A. exacerbate
  B. acquiesce
  C. prioritize
  D. placate

19. EQUIVOCATE
  A. envision
  B. clarify
  C. verify
  D. announce

20. PERIPHERAL
  A. focal
  B. casual
  C. ambiguous
  D. ethereal

21. INSENSATE
  A. angry
  B. vibrant
  C. quiet
  D. unimaginative

22. AMORPHOUS
  A. liquid
  B. circumspect
  C. particular
  D. obligatory

23. PROSCRIPTION
  A. engraving
  B. recommendation
  C. indictment
  D. accolade

24. CONCOMITANT
  A. controversial
  B. prerequisite
  C. disassociated
  D. judicial

25. PROGENITOR
  A. heir
  B. advocate
  C. representative
  D. prophet

26. IMMUTABLE
  A. tractable
  B. unspeakable
  C. remarkable
  D. stolid

27. ABECEDARIAN
  A. bibliographer
  B. hypnotic
  C. exegete
  D. lexical

28. ANAMNESTIC
  A. recital
  B. nostalgic
  C. insensate
  D. forgotten

29. APODICTIC
  A. proposal
  B. interpretive
  C. axiomatic
  D. given

30. BASILISK
  A. benign
  B. ornamental
  C. mortal
  D. essential

8.5.2 Analogies

1. SILK:WORM :: LINEN:
  A. flax
  B. cotton
  C. sisal
  D. millet

2. BIANNUAL:ONE HALF ::BIENNIAL :
  A. two
  B. one
  C. yearly
  D. every

3. CARPENTER:JIGSAW :: BUTCHER:
  A. meat hook
  B. mallet
  C. conveyor
  D. cleaver

4. EGG:LARVA ::CHRYSALIS:
  A. cocoon
  B. imago
  C. cygnet
  D. pupae

5. PALM:COCONUT ::PINE :
  A. cone
  B. nut
  C. tree
  D. squirrel

6. BIORHYTHM:INNATE ::IMPRINTING:
  A. instinctive
  B. learned
  C. symbiotic
  D. habituated

7. INERTIA:ROCK ::FLUX:
   A. bluff
   B. sand
   C. river
   D. tributary

8. BRANCH:PLIABLE ::ACROBAT :
   A. ossified
   B. slight
   C. flagrant
   D. lithe

9. OWL:SAGACIOUS ::OAK:
   A. foliated
   B. gnarled
   C. stalwart
   D. yielding

10. PALEONTOLOGY:DINOSAURS ::MYCOLOGY :
   A. bacteria
   B. cells
   C. mushrooms
   D. fish

11. OCHER:EARTH :: CERULEAN:
   A. sky
   B. pasture
   C. star
   D. clay

12. MOLD:PENICILLIN ::CELLULOSE :
   A. adhesive
   B. margarine
   C. rayon
   D. metabolism

13. LAMB:WOLF ::PACIFIC :
   A. liminal
   B. oceanic
   C. bucolic
   D. bellicose

14. INDIGO:NAVY ::HENNA:
   A. lupine
   B. auburn
   C. ash
   D. cocoa

15. WHEELWRIGHT:WAGON ::COOPER :
   A. barrel
   B. harness
   C. wool
   D. cage

16. MNEMONIC:EIDETIC ::AURAL:
   A. ocular
   B. spectral
   C. vestigial
   D. redolent

17. TOUCH:SENSE ::SKIN:
   A. organ
   B. drum
   C. shell
   D. membrane

18. ETIOLOGY:PROPHYLAXIS ::EXCISION:
   A. hypertrophy
   B. prognosis
   C. anamnesis
   D. metastasis

19. POLLUTANT:PANDEMIC ::OXYGEN:
   A. occasional
   B. ubiquitous
   C. scattered
   D. interlaced

20. SUILLINE:PORCINE ::CABALLINE :
   A. equine
   B. murine
   C. bovine
   D. ovine

21. MORPHOLOGY:STRUCTURE ::ETYMOLOGY:
   A. grammar
   B. syntax
   C. spelling
   D. inflection

22. WARY:AWRY ::APT :
   A. pet
   B. opt
   C. pat
   D. tip

23. RECLUSE:SECLUDE :: HERMIT:
   A. solitary
   B. contorted
   C. lonely
   D. captive

24. LUPINE:MAMMAL ::FORMICINE :
   A. oceanography
   B. graphology
   C. entomology
   D. herpetology

25. TRIDENT:POSEIDON ::CADUCEUS :
   A. Athena
   B. Zeus
   C. Hermes
   D. Echo

26. HARE:HAIR :: HEIR:
   A. air
   B. err
   C. hair
   D. ere

27. OCEAN:ROIL :: SKY:
- **A.** turbid
- **B.** turgid
- **C.** drizzle
- **D.** iridian

28. RATIOCINATE:REIFY ::DELIBERATE :
- **A.** rectify
- **B.** reproportion
- **C.** negotiate
- **D.** resolve

29. EFFABLE:CONCEIVABLE ::RESTIVE:
- **A.** obtuse
- **B.** obstreperous
- **C.** obtrusive
- **D.** obstructionist

30. ARTIFACT:EXCAVATION ::SCARAB :
- **A.** sarcophagus
- **B.** hieroglyph
- **C.** characteristic
- **D.** ceremony

8.6 ANSWER KEY

8.6.1 Biology

1. A	**10.** D	**19.** B	**28.** C	**37.** C	**46.** D
2. B	**11.** D	**20.** D	**29.** C	**38.** C	**47.** D
3. A	**12.** B	**21.** C	**30.** A	**39.** D	**48.** B
4. B	**13.** A	**22.** D	**31.** C	**40.** A	**49.** D
5. C	**14.** A	**23.** A	**32.** C	**41.** D	**50.** C
6. C	**15.** D	**24.** C	**33.** D	**42.** D	**51.** B
7. B	**16.** B	**25.** A	**34.** D	**43.** D	**52.** D
8. B	**17.** A	**26.** D	**35.** D	**44.** B	**53.** B
9. A	**18.** B	**27.** C	**36.** B	**45.** C	

8.6.2 Chemistry

1. C	**11.** D	**21.** B	**31.** B	**41.** A	**51.** B
2. B	**12.** B	**22.** B	**32.** A	**42.** D	**52.** C
3. C	**13.** D	**23.** C	**33.** D	**43.** D	**53.** C
4. D	**14.** B	**24.** C	**34.** B	**44.** B	**54.** D
5. C	**15.** D	**25.** D	**35.** D	**45.** B	**55.** B
6. A	**16.** A	**26.** D	**36.** D	**46.** B	**56.** A
7. A	**17.** D	**27.** B	**37.** A	**47.** A	**57.** D
8. B	**18.** C	**28.** D	**38.** C	**48.** A	**58.** A
9. A	**19.** C	**29.** B	**39.** D	**49.** D	**59.** B
10. B	**20.** B	**30.** D	**40.** C	**50.** A	**60.** C

8.6.3 Reading Comprehension

1. [A] See paragraph 1.
2. [B] See paragraph 2.
3. [B] See paragraph 1.
4. [D] See paragraph 3.
5. [C] See paragraph 3.
6. [C] The answer is based on context; the terms coded and cryptographic are synonyms.
7. [C] See paragraph 3.
8. [C] The answer is not stated in the passage, but is suggested by the references to psychological theory.
9. [A] See paragraph 1.
10. [C] Paragraph 1 mentions Hebb's conclusion about play and intelligence, but offers no explicit evidence.
11. [A] See paragraph 3.
12. [C] The answer demands an inferential understanding of the last paragraph. The passage suggests that Hebb was involved in postulating a more complex and useful idea of feedback.

13. [B] See paragraph 3.
14. [D] The answer is inferred from the example of young laboratory-born chimpanzees that were frightened by objects that they had never seen before.
15. [B] See paragraph 1.
16. [C] See paragraph 1.
17. [B] See the last paragraph.
18. [A] The passage does not state the geographic range of naked mole rats, but relies on data from a study in Kenya.
19. [B] A vital clue to the answer is found in paragraph 3.
20. [D] Unlike the other answers, D is not mentioned in terms of body temperature.
21. [A] See paragraph 4.
22. [D] See the last paragraph.
23. [C] The question requires recognition of figurative language, such as that found in paragraph 4.
24. [A] See paragraph 2.
25. [D] Answer A is tempting, but D better answers the question.
26. [A] See paragraph 4.
27. [D] Answer D best addresses the broad context of the passage.
28. [C] The passage states that software does not wear out.
29. [C] See paragraph 2.
30. [A] See the last paragraph.
31. [C] Context clues lead to the correct response.
32. [B] Answers A, C, and D are too specific.
33. [A] See paragraph 4.
34. [D] Context clues in the first and last paragraphs indicate the answer.
35. [A] The first paragraph points to the relation between antigens and T cells.
36. [B] See paragraph 3.
37. [D] See the last paragraph.
38. [C] See paragraph 2.
39. [B] The use of such terms as feasible, major strides, and long hoped point to the answer.
40. [A] Paragraph 1 suggests how the wasps use the caterpillars, but it is helpful to understand what the tems parasitic and host mean.
41. [C] See paragraph 3.
42. [A] Only answer A directly addresses the question.
43. [C] Kairomones operate over short distances only. The wider category of answer C is correct.
44. [A] See paragraph 2.
45. [D] See paragraph 3.
46. [B] See the last paragraph.
47. [D] Although the passage discusses caterpillars as hosts, it does not specify that they are the only hosts sought out by wasps.

8.6.4 Quantitative Reasoning

1. D	**8.** C	**15.** B	**22.** D	**29.** C	**36.** B
2. A	**9.** D	**16.** A	**23.** C	**30.** D	**37.** A
3. B	**10.** D	**17.** D	**24.** B	**31.** A	**38.** D
4. A	**11.** B	**18.** A	**25.** B	**32.** B	**39.** B
5. D	**12.** A	**19.** D	**26.** D	**33.** D	**40.** D
6. D	**13.** C	**20.** B	**27.** D	**34.** A	
7. B	**14.** A	**21.** A	**28.** B	**35.** A	

8.6.5 Verbal Ability: Antonyms

1. A. biased
2. A. elongate
3. D. affluent
4. B. solace
5. A. augment
6. B. eradicate
7. C. frigid
8. D. anxious
9. C. esteem
10. C. abhorrence
11. A. explanation
12. C. timidity
13. D. imprudent
14. B. order
15. A. soften
16. A. taciturn
17. C. invigorating
18. D. placate
19. B. clarify
20. A. focal
21. B. vibrant
22. C. particular
23. D. accolade
24. C. disassociated
25. A. heir
26. A. tractable
27. C. exegete
28. D. forgotten
29. B. interpretive
30. A. benign

8.6.6 Verbal Ability: Analogies

1. A. flax
2. A. two
3. D. cleaver
4. B. imago
5. A. cone
6. B. learned
7. C. river
8. D. lithe
9. C. stalwart
10. C. mushrooms
11. A. sky
12. C. rayon
13. D. bellicose
14. B. auburn
15. A. barrel
16. A. ocular
17. A. organ
18. D. metastasis
19. B. ubiquitous
20. A. equine
21. B. syntax
22. C. pat
23. D. captive
24. C. entomology
25. C. Hermes
26. A. air
27. A. turbid
28. D. resolve
29. B. obstreperous
30. A. sarcophagus

8.7 REFERENCE

The Psychological Corporation: *Veterinary College Admission Testing Program* candidate information booklet. San Antonio, TX, The Psychological Corporation, 1995.

APPENDIX A

VCAT Outline

I. Verbal Ability
   A. Antonyms (50%)
   B. Analogies (50%)

II. Reading Comprehension
   A. Literal comprehension
   B. Inferential comprehension
   C. Evaluative comprehension

III. Quantitative Ability
   A. Arithmetic concepts (18%)
      1. Summation
      2. Graphs
      3. Factorials
      4. Inequalities
      5. Reciprocals
      6. Fractions
   B. Discrete mathematics (10%)
      1. Number concepts
      2. Sets
      3. Probabilities
   C. Ratio, proportion, percent, and rate (14%)
      1. Ratio and proportion
      2. Percent
      3. Rate
         a. Speed
         b. Growth
   D. Powers and logarithms (18%)
      1. Exponents
      2. Radicals
      3. Logarithms
   E. Algebra and analytic geometry (20%)
      1. Algebra
      2. Linear algebra
      3. Functions
   F. Euclidean geometry and trigonometry (20%)
      1. Geometry
      2. Trigonometry

IV. Biology
   A. Molecular and cellular (35%)
      1. Bioenergetics
      2. Other molecular biology
      3. Biosynthesis
      4. Cell structure and function
   B. Organismal (40%)
      1. Nutrient processing
      2. Regulation
      3. Gas exchange
      4. Internal transport
      5. Chemical control
      6. Nervous and sensory systems
      7. Movement
      8. Reproduction and development
   C. Population (25%)
      1. Genetics
      2. Behavior
      3. Ecology
      4. Evolution
      5. Patterns of life

V. Chemistry
   A. Inorganic (50%)
      1. Atomic theory
         a. Structure
         b. Nuclear chemistry
         c. Thermodynamics
         d. Periodic table
      2. Bonding theory
         a. Molecules and compounds
         b. Chemical reactions
         c. Oxidation–reduction
         d. Acids and bases
      3. Physical theory
         a. Phases
         b. Solutions
         c. Kinetics
         d. Electrochemistry
   B. Organic (50%)
      1. Structure and mechanism
      2. Simple functional groups
         a. Hydrocarbons
         b. Oxygen-containing groups
         c. Nitrogen-containing groups
      3. Analysis

B

APPENDIX

GRE Subject Test: Biology

I. Cellular and Molecular Biology (33%–34%)
  A. Cellular structure and function (16%–17%)
    1. Biologic compounds
      a. Macromolecular structure and bonding
      b. Abiotic origin of macromolecules (i.e., origin of life)
    2. Enzyme activity, receptor binding, and regulation
    3. Major metabolic pathways and regulation
      a. Respiration, fermentation, and photosynthesis
      b. Synthesis and degradation of macromolecules
      c. Hormonal control and intracellular messengers
    4. Membrane dynamics and cell surfaces
      a. Transport, endocytosis, and exocytosis
      b. Electric potentials and transmitter substances
      c. Mechanisms of cell recognition, cell junctions, and plasmodesmata
      d. Cell wall and extracellular matrix
    5. Organelles
      a. Structure, function, synthesis, and targeting
      b. Nucleus, mitochondria, and plastids
      c. Endoplasmic reticulum and ribosomes
      d. Golgi apparatus and secretory vesicles
      e. Lysosomes, peroxisomes, and vacuoles
    6. Cytoskeleton, motility, and shape
      a. Actin-based systems
      b. Microtubule-based systems
      c. Intermediate filaments
      d. Bacterial flagella and movement
    7. Cell cycle
      a. Growth
      b. Division
      c. Regulation

B. Molecular biology and molecular genetics (16%–17%)
   1. Genetic foundations
      a. Mendelian inheritance
      b. Pedigree analysis
      c. Prokaryotic genetics
         (1) Transformation
         (2) Transduction
         (3) Conjugation
      d. Genetic mapping
   2. Chromatin and chromosomes
      a. Nucleosomes
      b. Karyotypes
      c. Chromosomal aberrations
      d. Polytene chromosomes
   3. Genome sequence organization
      a. Introns and exons
      b. Single-copy and repetitive DNA
      c. Transposable elements
   4. Genome maintenance
      a. DNA replication
      b. DNA point mutation and repair
   5. Gene expression and regulation in prokaryotes and eukaryotes
      a. Mechanisms
      b. The operon
      c. Promoters and enhancers
      d. RNA and protein synthesis
      e. Processing and modifications
   6. Gene expression and regulation
      a. Effects
      b. Control of normal development
      c. Cancer and oncogenes
   7. Immunobiology
      a. Cellular basis of immunity
      b. Antibody diversity and synthesis
      c. Antigen–antibody interaction
   8. Bacteriophages, animal viruses, and plant viruses
      a. Viral genome
      b. Assembly
   9. Recombinant DNA methods
      a. Restriction endonucleases
      b. Blotting and hybridization
      c. Restriction fragment length polymorphisms
      d. DNA cloning, sequencing, and analysis
      e. Polymerase chain reaction

II. Organismal Biology (33%–34%)
   A. Animal structure, function, and organization (9%–10%)
      1. Exchange with environment
         a. Digestion and nutrition
         b. Uptake and excretion
         c. Gas exchange
         d. Energy
      2. Internal transport and exchange (e.g., circulatory system, gastrovascular system)
      3. Support and movement
         a. Support systems (i.e., external, internal, hydrostatic)
         b. Movement systems (i.e., flagellar, ciliary, muscular)

4. Integration and control mechanisms
    a. Nervous system
    b. Endocrine system
5. Behavior (e.g., communication, orientation, learning)
6. Metabolic rate (i.e., temperature, body size, activity)

B. Animal reproduction and development (5%–6%)
1. Reproductive structures
2. Meiosis, gametogenesis, and fertilization
3. Early development (e.g., polarity, cleavage, gastrulation)
4. Developmental processes (e.g., induction, differentiation, morphogenesis)
5. External control mechanisms (e.g., photoperiod)

C. Plant structure, function, and organization, with emphasis on flowering plants (6%–7%)
1. Organs, tissue systems, and tissues
2. Water transport, including absorption and transpiration
3. Phloem transport and storage
4. Mineral nutrition
5. Plant energetics (e.g., respiration, photosynthesis)

D. Plant reproduction, growth, and development, with emphasis on flowering plants (4%–5%)
1. Reproductive structures
2. Meiosis and sporogenesis
3. Gametogenesis and fertilization
4. Embryogeny and seed development
5. Meristems, growth, morphogenesis, and differentiation
6. Control mechanisms (e.g., hormones, photoperiod, tropisms)

E. Diversity of life (6%–7%)
1. Monera (e.g., Archaebacteria, bacteria, cyanobacteria)
    a. Morphology
    b. Physiology
    c. Pathology
    d. Methods of identification
2. Protista
    a. Protozoa (e.g., Mastigophora, Sarcodina, Sporozoa)
        (1) Morphology
        (2) Locomotion
        (3) Physiology
        (4) Importance
    b. Other heterotrophic Protista
    c. Development of cellular slime molds
    d. Importance of Oomycota (i.e., decomposition, biodegradation, pathogenicity)
    e. Autotrophic Protista (i.e., algae)
    f. Distinctive features of Chlorophyta, Rhodophyta, and Chrysophyta
    g. Patterns of cell division in Chlorophyta
    h. Importance (e.g., role in nature, economic uses)
3. Fungi
    a. Distinctive features of Zygomycota, Ascomycota, and Basidiomycota (i.e., vegetative, asexual, and sexual reproduction)
    b. Generalized life cycles
    c. Importance (e.g., decomposition, biodegradation, pathogenicity)
    d. Lichens
4. Animalia, with emphasis on Porifera, Cnidaria, Platyhelminthes, Nematoda, Mollusca, Annelida, Arthropoda, Echinodermata, and Chordata
    a. Major distinguishing characteristics
    b. Phylogenetic relationships

5. Plantae with emphasis on Bryophyta, Pterophyta, Gymnosperms, and Angiosperms
    a. Alternation of generations
    b. Major distinguishing characteristics
    c. Phylogenetic relationships

III. Ecology and Evolution (33%–34%)

This section deals with the interactions of organisms and their environment, emphasizing biological principles at levels above the individual. Ecological and evolutionary topics are given equal weight. Ecological questions range from physiological adaptations to the functioning of ecosystems. Although principles are emphasized, some questions may consider applications to current environmental problems. Questions in evolution range from its genetic foundations through evolutionary processes to their consequences. Evolution is considered at the molecular, individual, and higher levels. Principles of ecology, genetics, and evolution are interrelated in many questions. Some questions may require quantitative skills, including the interpretation of simple mathematical models.

A. Ecology (16%–17%)
1. Environment/organism interaction
    a. Biogeographic patterns
    b. Adaptations to environment
    c. Temporal patterns
2. Behavioral ecology
    a. Habitat selection
    b. Mating systems
    c. Social systems
    d. Resource acquisition
3. Population structure and function
    a. Population dynamics/regulation
    b. Demography and life history strategies
4. Communities
    a. Interspecific relationships
    b. Community structure and diversity
    c. Change and succession
5. Ecosystems
    a. Productivity and energy flow
    b. Chemical cycling

B. Evolution (16%–17%)
1. Genetic variability
    a. Origins (mutations, linkage, recombination, and chromosomal alterations)
    b. Levels (e.g., polymorphism and heritability)
    c. Spatial patterns (e.g., clines and ecotypes)
    d. Hardy-Weinberg equilibrium
2. Evolutionary processes
    a. Gene flow and genetic drift
    b. Natural selection
    c. Levels of selection (e.g., individual and group)
3. Evolutionary consequences
    a. Fitness and adaptation
    b. Speciation
    c. Systematics and phylogeny
    d. Convergence, divergence, and extinction

C

APPENDIX

GRE Subject Test: Chemistry

I. Analytical Chemistry
   A. Classic quantitative analysis
      1. Titrimetry
      2. Separations, including theory and applications of chromatography as well as gravimetry
      3. Data handling, including statistical tests (e.g., t, Q, χ^2)
      4. Standards and standardization techniques
   B. Instrumental analysis
      1. Basic electronics
      2. Electrochemical methods
      3. Spectroscopic methods
      4. Chromatographic methods

II. Inorganic Chemistry
   A. Basic descriptive chemistry of the elements
      1. General chemistry
         a. Properties
         b. Preparations
         c. Reactions of representative elements
         d. Transition metals
         e. Lanthanides and actinides
      2. Behavior as related to periodic trends and electronic structures
   B. Periodic and family trends
      1. Size
      2. Ionization energy
      3. Electron affinity
      4. Period 2 elements versus period 3 elements
      5. Oxidation states
      6. Electronic configurations
      7. Reactivity
      8. Melting and boiling points
      9. Magnetic properties

C. Electronic and nuclear structure
   1. Atomic theory
      a. Fundamental particles
      b. Atomic structure
      c. Electronic configuration
   2. Isotopes
      a. Abundance
      b. Stability of nuclei
   3. Relation to reactivity, spectra, and periodic classifications
D. Transition metal–coordination chemistry
   1. Synthesis
      a. Reactions
      b. Structure
      c. Theory
      d. Reaction mechanisms
      e. Spectra
      f. Bonding isomerism
   2. Organometallic compounds
      a. Synthesis
      b. Structure
      c. Bonding
      d. Reaction pathways
      e. Catalytic processes
E. Special topics
   1. Theories of acids and bases
   2. Inorganic polymers
   3. Ion separations
   4. Ionic solids

III. Organic Chemistry
   A. Conversion of functional groups
      1. Alkenes
      2. Acetylenes
      3. Dienes
      4. Alkyl halides
      5. Alcohols
      6. Aldehydes and ketones
      7. Carboxylic acids and derivatives
      8. Amines
      9. Aromatic compounds
   B. Reactive intermediates and reaction mechanisms
      1. Nucleophilic displacement reactions
      2. Eliminations
      3. Carbonium ions and other cations
      4. Benzyne
      5. Reactions involving carbene or dichlorocarbene
      6. Carbonyl group reactions
      7. Radical reactions
      8. Tools of mechanism chemists
   C. Molecular structure
      1. Isomerism and related topics
      2. Bonding
      3. Stereochemistry
      4. Chemical and spectral methods of determination

D. Special topics
   1. Special reagents
   2. Rearrangements
   3. Structural features of natural products
   4. Synthesis problems
   5. Separations
   6. Chromatography

IV. Physical Chemistry
   A. General chemistry
      1. Acid–base theories
      2. Colligative properties
      3. Gas laws
      4. Electrochemistry
   B. Classic and statistical thermodynamics
      1. Variables
         a. Moles
         b. Pressure
         c. Volume
         d. Temperature
         e. Heat and work
         f. Heat capacity
         g. Energy
         h. Entropy
         i. Gibbs' free energy theory
      2. Equations of state
      3. First, second, and third laws
      4. Phase, chemical, and electrochemical equilibria
      5. Boltzmann's relation and partition functions
   C. Quantum and structural chemistry
      1. Nuclei
      2. Atomic structure
      3. Molecular and crystal structure
      4. Quantization of energy
      5. Basic principles of spectroscopy
   D. Kinetics
      1. Kinetic theory of gases
      2. Chemical kinetics
      3. Collision theory
      4. Absolute rate theory
      5. Rate laws
      6. Reaction mechanisms

D
APPENDIX

MCAT Outline

I. Verbal Reasoning
   A. Comprehension
      1. Identifying the central concern, or thesis, of the passage
      2. Identifying the evidence offered to support the thesis
      3. Identifying background information that is relevant to a specific interpretation
      4. Determining from the context the meaning of significant terms
      5. Recognizing an accurate paraphrase of complex information
      6. Identifying comparative relations among ideas
      7. Identifying stated or unstated assumptions
      8. Recognizing appropriate questions for clarification
   B. Evaluation
      1. Judging the soundness of an argument or a step of reasoning presented in the passage
      2. Judging the credibility of a source
      3. Judging whether a conclusion follows necessarily from the reasons given
      4. Appraising the strength of the evidence for a generalization, conclusion, or claim
      5. Distinguishing between supported and unsupported claims
      6. Judging the relevance of information to an argument or a claim
   C. Application
      1. Predicting a result based on passage content and details about a hypothetical situation
      2. Using the information given to solve a specific problem
      3. Identifying the probable cause of a specific event or result based on the information presented
      4. Determining the implications of conclusions or results for real-world situations
      5. Recognizing the scope of application of hypotheses, explanations, and conclusions
      6. Identifying a general theory or model
   D. Incorporation of new information
      1. Judging the bearing of new evidence on conclusions presented in the passage
      2. Recognizing methods or results that would challenge hypotheses, models, or theories
      3. Determining how a conclusion can be modified to accommodate additional information
      4. Recognizing plausible alternative hypotheses or solutions

E. Content
   1. The Verbal Reasoning section is drawn from the humanities, social sciences, and natural sciences, excluding the subjects covered in the Physical and Biological Sciences sections of the MCAT.
   2. Humanities passages discuss architecture, art and art history, dance, ethics, literary criticism, music, philosophy, religion, or theater.
   3. Social sciences passages come from the fields of anthropology, archaeology, business, economics, government, history, political science, psychology, or sociology.
   4. Natural sciences passages cover astronomy, botany, computer science, ecology, geology, meteorology, natural history, or technology.

II. Mathematics
   A. Performing arithmetic calculations, including proportion, ratio, percentage, and estimation of square root
   B. Understanding second-year high school algebra topics, including exponents and logarithms, both natural and base 10; scientific notation; quadratic and simultaneous equations; and graphic representations of data and functions, including terminology (i.e., abscissa, ordinate), slope, reciprocals, and various scales (i.e., arithmetic, semilog, and log–log)
   C. Knowing the definitions of the basic trigonometric functions (sine, cosine, tangent); the values of the sines and cosines of 0°, 90°, and 180°; the relations between the lengths of sides of right triangles containing angles of 30°, 45°, and 60°; and the inverse trigonometric functions (i.e., $\sin^{-1}$, $\cos^{-1}$, $\tan^{-1}$)
   D. Applying metric units and balancing equations containing physical units. Conversion factors between metric and British systems are provided when needed.
   E. Understanding the relative magnitude of experimental error, the effect of propagation of error, reasonable estimates, and the significant digits of a measurement
   F. Calculating the mathematical probability of an event
   G. Understanding vector addition, vector subtraction, and the right-hand rule. Dot and cross products are not required.
   H. Calculating the arithmetic mean, or average, and range of a set of numbers and understanding statistical association and correlation. Calculation of statistics, such as standard deviation and correlation coefficient, is not required.
   I. An understanding of calculus is not required.

III. Physical Sciences
   A. Chemistry
      1. Stoichiometry
         a. Molecular weight
         b. Empirical formula versus molecular formula
         c. Metric units
         d. Description of composition by percent mass
         e. Mole concept and Avogadro's number
         f. Density
         g. Oxidation number
            (1) Common oxidizing and reducing agents
            (2) Redox titration
         h. Description of reactions by chemical equations
            (1) Conventions for writing chemical equations
            (2) Balancing equations, including oxidation–reduction equations
      2. Electronic structure and the periodic table
         a. Electronic structure
            (1) Orbital structure of the hydrogen atom, principal quantum number *n*, and the number of electrons per orbital
            (2) Ground state versus excited state
            (3) Conventional notation for electronic structure

b. Classification of elements and chemical properties of groups and rows
    (1) Valence electrons of the common groups
    (2) First and second ionization energies and trends
    (3) Electron affinity and variation of properties within groups and rows
    (4) Electronegativity
3. Bonding
    a. Ionic bonds (i.e., electrostatic forces between ions)
    b. Covalent bonds
        (1) Lewis electron dot formulas
            (a) Resonance structures
            (b) Formal charge
            (c) Lewis acids and bases
            (d) Valence shell electron pair repulsion and predicting the shapes of molecules
        (2) Partial ionic character
            (a) Role of electronegativity in determining charge distribution
            (b) Dipole moment
4. Phases and phase equilibria
    a. Gas phase
        (1) Standard temperature and pressure and standard molar volume
        (2) Ideal gas
            (a) Ideal gas law ($PV = nRT$)
            (b) Boyle's law
            (c) Charles' law
        (3) Kinetic molecular theory of gases
        (4) Qualitative aspects of deviation of real gas behavior from ideal gas law
        (5) Partial pressure and mole fraction
        (6) Dalton's law relating partial pressure to composition
    b. Liquid phase (i.e., intermolecular and intramolecular forces)
        (1) Hydrogen bonding
        (2) Dipole interactions
        (3) Van der Waals forces
    c. Phase equilibria (i.e., solids, liquids, gases)
        (1) Phase changes and phase diagrams
        (2) Freezing point, melting point, and boiling point
        (3) Molality
        (4) Colligative properties
            (a) Reducing vapor pressure (i.e., Raoult's law)
            (b) Elevating boiling point ($\Delta T_b = K_b m$)
            (c) Depressing freezing point ($\Delta T_f = K_f m$)
            (d) Osmotic pressure
5. Solution chemistry
    a. Ions in solution
        (1) Anion
        (2) Cation
        (3) Common names, formulas, and charges for familiar ions
    b. Solubility
        (1) Units of concentration (e.g., molarity)
        (2) Solubility product constant and the equilibrium expression
        (3) Common-ion effect
6. Acids and bases
    a. Acid–base equilibria
        (1) Bronsted definition of acids and bases
        (2) Ionization of water
            (a) K_w and its approximate value ($K_w = [H^+][OH^-] = 10^{-14}$ at standard temperature and pressure)

(b) Definition of pH
(c) pH of pure water
(3) Conjugate acids and bases (e.g., amino acids)
(4) Strong acids and bases (e.g., nitric, sulfuric)
(5) Weak acids and bases (e.g., acetic, benzoic)
(a) Dissociation of weak acids and bases, with or without added salt
(b) Hydrolysis of salts of weak acids or bases
(c) Calculation of pH of solutions of salts of weak acids or bases
(6) Equilibrium constants K_a and K_b, pK_a, and pK_b
(7) Buffers
(a) Common buffer systems
(b) Influence and titration curves
b. Acid–base titrations
(1) Indicators
(2) Neutralization
(3) Interpretation of titration curves
7. Thermodynamics and thermochemistry
a. Thermochemistry
(1) Thermodynamic system and state function
(2) Conservation of energy
(3) Endothermic versus exothermic reactions
(a) Enthalpy ΔH and standard heats of reaction
(b) Hess's law of heat summation
(4) Bond dissociation energy as related to heat of formation
(5) Measurement of heat changes (i.e., calorimetry)
(a) Heat capacity
(b) Specific heat (e.g., specific heat of water = 1 cal/°C)
(6) Entropy as a measure of disorder and relative entropy for gas, liquid, and crystal states
(7) Free energy G
(8) Spontaneous reactions and $\Delta G°$
b. Thermodynamics
(1) First law ($\Delta E = Q - W$)
(2) Equivalence of mechanical, chemical, and thermal energy units
(3) Temperature scales
(4) Heat transfer
(a) Conduction
(b) Convection
(c) Radiation
(5) Coefficient of expansion
(6) Heats of fusion and vaporization
8. Rate processes in chemical reactions
a. Kinetics
b. Equilibrium
c. Reaction rate
d. Dependence of reaction rate on concentration of reactants
(1) Rate law
(2) Rate constant
(3) Reaction order
e. Rate-determining step
f. Dependence of reaction rate on temperature; activation energy
(1) Activated complex or transition state
(2) Interpretation of energy profiles showing energies of reactants and products, activation energy, and ΔH for the reaction

g. Kinetic versus thermodynamic control of a reaction
h. Catalysts and enzyme catalysis
i. Equilibrium in reversible chemical reactions
(1) Law of mass action
(2) Equilibrium constant
(3) Application of Le Chatelier principle
j. Relation of the equilibrium constant and ΔG°

9. Electrochemistry
a. Electrolytic cell
(1) Electrolysis
(2) Anodes and cathodes
(3) Electrolytes
(4) Faraday's law relating the amount of elements deposited or gas liberated at an electrode to the current
(5) Electron flow; oxidation and reduction at the electrodes
b. Galvanic cell
(1) Half-cell reactions
(2) Reduction potential; cell potential
(3) Direction of electron flow
c. Concentration cell and direction of electron flow

B. Physics
1. Translational motion
a. Units and dimensions
b. Vectors
c. Speed, velocity, and acceleration
d. Uniformly accelerated motion
e. Freely falling bodies
f. Projectiles
2. Force and motion; gravitation
a. Mass, center of mass, and weight
b. Newton's second law
c. Newton's third law
d. Law of gravitation
e. Uniform circular motion and centripetal force
f. Friction
g. Inclined planes
h. Pulley systems
3. Equilibrium and momentum
a. Equilibrium
(1) Translational equilibrium
(2) Rotational equilibrium, torques, and lever arms
(3) Newton's first law; inertia
b. Momentum
(1) Impulse
(2) Conservation of linear momentum
(3) Elastic and inelastic collisions
4. Work and energy
a. Work
b. Kinetic energy
c. Potential energy
d. Conservation of energy
e. Conservative forces
f. Power

5. Wave characteristics and periodic motion
   a. Wave characteristics
      (1) Transverse and longitudinal motion
      (2) Wavelength, frequency, velocity, amplitude, and intensity
      (3) Superposition of waves, phase, interference, and addition
      (4) Resonance
      (5) Standing waves and nodes
      (6) Beats
   b. Periodic motion
      (1) Hooke's law
      (2) Simple harmonic motion
      (3) Pendulum motion
6. Sound
   a. Production of sound
   b. Relative speed of sound in solids, liquids, and gases
   c. Intensity and pitch
   d. Doppler effect
   e. Resonance in pipes and strings
   f. Harmonics
7. Fluids and solids
   a. Fluids
      (1) Density and specific gravity
      (2) Buoyancy and Archimedes' principle
      (3) Hydrostatic pressure
      (4) Viscosity
      (5) Continuity equation
      (6) Bernoulli's equation
      (7) Turbulence
      (8) Surface tension
   b. Solids
      (1) Density
      (2) Elastic properties
8. Electrostatics and electromagnetism
   a. Electrostatics
      (1) Charge, charge conservation, conductors, and insulators
      (2) Coulomb's law and electric force
      (3) Electric field
         (a) Field lines
         (b) Field as a result of charge distribution
      (4) Potential difference and absolute potential
      (5) Electric dipoles
   b. Electromagnetism
      (1) Magnetic fields
      (2) Electromagnetic spectrum and x-rays
9. Electric circuits
   a. Current
   b. Batteries
   c. Resistance, Ohm's law, series and parallel circuits, and resistivity
   d. Capacitors and dielectrics
   e. Electric power
   f. Root-mean-square current voltage
10. Light and geometric optics
   a. Visual spectrum and color
   b. Polarization
   c. Reflection, mirrors, and total internal reflection

d. Refraction, refractive index, and Snell's law
e. Dispersion
f. Thin lenses, combination lenses, diopters, and lens aberrations
11. Atomic and nuclear structure
a. Atomic number and atomic weight
b. Neutrons, protons, and isotopes
c. Radioactive decay and half-life
d. Quantized energy levels for electrons
e. Fluorescence

IV. Writing Sample
A. Developing a central idea
B. Synthesizing concepts and ideas
C. Presenting ideas cohesively and logically
D. Writing clearly, following accepted practices of grammar, syntax, and punctuation consistent with timed, first-draft composition

V. Biology
A. Molecular biology
1. Enzymes and cellular metabolism
a. Structure and function of enzymes
b. Control of enzyme activity
c. Feedback inhibition
d. Glycolysis
(1) Anaerobic
(2) Aerobic
e. Krebs, or citric acid, cycle
f. Electron transport chain and oxidative phosphorylation
2. DNA and protein synthesis
a. DNA
(1) Structure and composition
(a) Watson-Crick model
(b) Double helix
(c) Base-pair specificity
(2) Transmission of genetic information (i.e., the genetic code)
(3) Replication
b. Protein synthesis
(1) Transcription
(a) Mechanism
(b) Regulation
(2) Translation
(a) Codons and anticodons
(b) Role of mRNA, tRNA, and rRNA
(c) Structure and function of ribosomes
B. Microbiology
1. Structure and life history of viruses
a. Nucleic acid (i.e., DNA, RNA) and protein components
b. Structure and function of bacteriophages
c. Size relative to bacteria and eukaryotic cells
d. Life cycles of phages and animal viruses
2. Prokaryotic cells
a. Structure and physiology
b. Bacterial life history
3. Fungi
a. Major structural types
b. Life history and physiology

- C. Generalized eukaryotic cells
    1. Structure and function of the nucleus
        a. Nucleolus
        b. Nuclear envelope and pores
    2. Structure and function of membrane-bound organelles
        a. Mitochondria
        b. Lysosomes
        c. Endoplasmic reticulum
        d. Golgi apparatus
    3. Structure and function of plasma membranes
        a. Protein and lipid components
        b. Fluid mosaic model and membrane traffic
        c. Movement across membranes
            (1) Osmosis
            (2) Passive and active transport
            (3) Endocytosis and exocytosis
        d. Membrane channels, sodium–potassium pump, and membrane potential
        e. Membrane receptors
        f. Cellular adhesion
    4. Structure and function of the cytoskeleton
        a. Microfilaments, microtubules, and intermediate filaments
        b. Cilia and flagella
        c. Centrioles
    5. Mitosis
        a. Mitotic process and phases of the cell cycle
        b. Mitotic structures
            (1) Centrioles, asters, and spindles
            (2) Chromatids, centromeres, telomeres, and kinetochores
        c. Breakdown and reorganization of the nuclear membrane
        d. Mechanisms of chromosome movement
- D. Specialized eukaryotic cells and tissues
    1. Neural cells and tissues
        a. Structures
            (1) Cell body
            (2) Axon
            (3) Dendrites
            (4) Myelin sheath and Schwann's cells
            (5) Ranvier's nodes
        b. Synapse
        c. Resting potential and action potential
    2. Contractile cells and tissues
        a. Striated, smooth, and cardiac muscle
        b. Sarcomeres
        c. Calcium regulation of contraction
    3. Epithelial cells and tissues
        a. Simple epithelium
        b. Stratified epithelium
    4. Connective cells and tissues
        a. Major cell and fiber types
        b. Loose versus dense connective tissue
        c. Cartilage
        d. Extracellular matrix
- E. Nervous and endocrine systems
    1. Structure and function of the nervous system
        a. Organization of the vertebrate nervous system

b. Sensor and effector neurons
c. Sympathetic and parasympathetic nervous systems
2. Sensory reception and processing
a. Skin, proprioceptive, and somatic sensors
b. Olfaction and taste
c. Hearing
(1) Structure of the ear
(2) Mechanism of hearing
d. Vision
(1) Structure of the eye
(2) Light receptors
3. Endocrine systems
a. Hormones and their sources
b. Function of the endocrine system
c. Major endocrine glands
(1) Hormones
(2) Specificity
(3) Target tissues
d. Cellular mechanisms of hormone action
e. Transport of hormones

F. Circulatory, lymphatic, and immune systems
1. Circulatory system
a. Functions, including its role in thermoregulation
b. Four-chambered heart, pulmonary and systemic circulation
c. Arterial and venous systems and capillary beds
d. Systolic and diastolic pressure
e. Composition of blood
f. Role of hemoglobin in oxygen transport
2. Structure and function of the lymphatic system
3. Immune system
a. Cells
(1) T lymphocytes
(2) B lymphocytes
b. Tissues
(1) Bone marrow
(2) Spleen
(3) Thymus
(4) Lymph nodes
c. Antigens, antibodies, and antigen–antibody reactions

G. Digestive and excretory systems
1. Digestive system
a. Ingestion
b. Stomach
c. Digestive glands, including the liver and pancreas; bile production
d. Small and large intestines
e. Muscular control of digestion
2. Excretory system
a. Role in body homeostasis
b. Structure and function of the kidney
c. Structure and function of the nephron
d. Formation of urine
e. Storage and elimination of wastes

H. Muscle and skeletal systems
1. Muscle system
a. Function
b. Basic muscle types and locations

c. Nervous control of muscles
    (1) Motor and sensory control
    (2) Voluntary and involuntary muscles
2. Skeletal system
    a. Function
    b. Bone structure and the calcium–protein matrix
    c. Skeletal structure
        (1) Specialization of bone types and structures
        (2) Joint structure
    d. Structure and function of cartilage
        (1) Ligaments
        (2) Tendons

I. Respiratory and skin systems
1. Respiratory system
    a. Function
        (1) Gas exchange and the role of alveoli
        (2) Thermoregulation
        (3) Protection against disease and particulate matter
    b. Breathing structures and mechanisms
        (1) Diaphragm
        (2) Rib cage
        (3) Differential pressure
2. Skin system
    a. Function
        (1) Homeostasis and osmoregulation
        (2) Thermoregulation
        (3) Physical protection
    b. Structure

J. Reproductive system and development
1. Reproduction
    a. Male and female gonads and genitalia
    b. Gametogenesis by meiosis
        (1) Ovum
        (2) Sperm
    c. Reproductive sequence
    d. Structure and function of the placenta
2. Embryogenesis
    a. Fertilization
    b. Cleavage
    c. Blastulation
    d. Gastrulation
    e. Neurulation
    f. Major structures that arise out of the primary germ layers
3. Mechanisms of development
    a. Cell specialization
        (1) Determination
        (2) Differentiation
    b. Induction

K. Genetics and evolution
1. Genetics
    a. Mendelian concepts and their application
    b. Hardy-Weinberg principle and population genetics
    c. Meiosis and genetic variability
    d. Sex-linked characteristics
    e. Mutations

2. Evolution
    a. Natural selection
        (1) Fitness
        (2) Differential reproduction
        (3) Group selection
    b. Species and speciation
    c. Origin of life
    d. Comparative anatomy
        (1) Chordate features
        (2) Vertebrate body plan

VI. Organic Chemistry
  A. Biologic molecules
    1. Amino acids and proteins
      a. Description
        (1) Absolute configuration at the α-position
        (2) Amino acids as dipolar ions
        (3) Classification
          (a) Acidic or basic
          (b) Hydrophobic or hydrophilic
      b. Reactions
        (1) Sulfur linkage for cysteine and cystine
        (2) Peptide linkage
        (3) Hydrolysis
      c. General principles
        (1) Primary structure of proteins
        (2) Secondary structure of proteins
        (3) Tertiary structure of proteins
          (a) Role of proline and cystine
          (b) Hydrophobic bonding
        (4) Isoelectric point
    2. Carbohydrates
      a. Nomenclature and classification; common names
      b. Absolute configuration
      c. Cyclic structure and conformation of hexoses
      d. Epimers and anomers
      e. Oxidation of monosaccharides
      f. Hydrolysis of glycoside linkage
    3. Lipids
      a. Structure
      b. Free fatty acids
      c. Triacylglycerols
      d. Steroids
    4. Phosphorus compounds
  B. Oxygen-containing compounds
    1. Alcohols
      a. Important reactions
        (1) Dehydrations (i.e., formation of carbocations)
        (2) Substitution reactions (i.e., S_N1 or S_N2, depending on alcohol and the derived product)
      b. Hydrogen bonding
      c. Effect of chain branching on physical properties
    2. Aldehydes and ketones
      a. Important reactions

(1) Nucleophilic addition reactions at C = O bonds
(a) Acetal, ketal, hemiacetal, and hemiketal
(b) Imine and enamine
(2) Reactions at adjacent positions
(a) Aldol condensation
(b) Enol–keto tautomerism
b. Effect of substituents on the reactivity of C = O
c. Steric hindrance
d. Acidity of α-H
e. Carbanions
f. α-, ß-unsaturated carbonyls
3. Carboxylic acids
a. Important carboxyl group reactions
(1) Decarboxylation
(2) Esterification
b. Hydrogen bonding
c. Inductive effect of substituents
d. Resonance stability of the carboxylate anion
4. Common acid derivatives (i.e., acid chlorides, anhydrides, amides, esters, keto acids)
a. Important reactions
(1) Hydrolysis of fats and glycerides (i.e., saponification)
(2) Hydrolysis of amides
b. Relative reactivity of acid derivatives
c. Steric effects
5. Ethers
a. Cleavage by acid
b. Weak basicity of ethers
6. Phenols
a. Effects of substituents on acidity
b. Hydrogen bonding
C. Amines
1. Stereochemistry and physical properties
2. Major reactions
a. Amide formation
b. Alkylation
3. Basicity
4. Stabilization of adjacent carbonium ions (i.e., carbocations)
5. Effect of substituents on the basicity of aromatic amines
6. Quaternary salts and solubility
D. Hydrocarbons
1. Saturated (i.e., alkanes)
a. Physical properties
b. Important reactions
(1) Combustion
(2) Substitution reactions with halogens
c. Stability of free radicals
d. Chain reactions
e. Inhibition
f. Ring strain in cyclic compounds
2. Unsaturated (i.e., alkenes)
a. Structure and isomerization
b. Physical properties
c. Electrophilic addition (e.g., HBr, H_2O)
3. Aromatic (i.e., benzene)
a. Resonance stability
b. Delocalization of electrons

E. Molecular structure of organic compounds
   1. Sigma and pi bonds
      a. Hybrid orbitals (sp^3, sp^2, sp, and respective geometries)
      b. Structural formulas for molecules involving H, C, N, O, F, S, P, Si, or Cl
      c. Delocalized electrons and resonance in ions and molecules
   2. Multiple bonding
      a. Effect on length and energy of bonds
      b. Rigidity in molecular structure
   3. Stereochemistry of covalently bonded molecules
      a. Isomers
         (1) Structural isomers
         (2) Stereoisomers (e.g., diastereomers, enantiomers, cis–trans isomers)
         (3) Conformational isomers
      b. Polarization of light and specific rotation
      c. Absolute and relative configuration
      d. Conventions for writing R and S forms
      e. Racemic mixtures

F. Separations and purifications
   1. Extraction (i.e., distribution of solute between two immiscible solvents)
   2. Chromatography
      a. Gas–liquid chromatography
      b. Thin-layer chromatography
   3. Distillation
   4. Recrystallization
   5. Solvent choice from solubility data

G. Use of spectroscopy in structural identification
   1. Infrared region
      a. Intramolecular vibrations and rotations
      b. Recognizing common characteristic group absorptions
   2. Nuclear magnetic resonance spectroscopy
      a. Protons in a magnetic field; equivalent protons
      b. Spin–spin splitting

E

APPENDIX

GRE General Test

VERBAL ABILITY

The verbal ability measure tests the ability to reason with words in solving problems. The verbal ability measure consists of four question types: analogies, antonyms, sentence completions, and reading comprehension sets.

Analogies

Analogy questions test the ability to recognize relations among words and the concepts they represent and to recognize when these relations are parallel. Eliminating the four incorrect answer choices requires the ability to formulate and then analyze the relation linking six pairs of words (i.e., the given pair and the five answer choices) and to recognize which answer pair is most nearly analogous to the given pair. Types of relations found in analogy questions include size, contiguity, and degree.

Antonyms

Antonym questions test knowledge of vocabulary more directly than do any of the other verbal question types. Antonym questions measure both vocabulary and the ability to reason from a given concept to its opposite. Antonyms are generally confined to nouns, verbs, and adjectives. Answer choices may be single words or phrases.

Sentence Completions

Sentence completion questions measure the ability to recognize words or phrases that both logically and stylistically complete the meaning of a sentence. Sentence completion questions provide a context within which to analyze the functions of words as they relate to and combine with one another to form a meaningful unit of discourse.

Reading Comprehension Sets

Reading comprehension questions measure the ability to read with understanding, insight, and discrimination. Answering these questions requires the ability to recognize explicitly stated elements in the passage, assumptions underlying statements or arguments in the passage, and the implications of those statements or arguments.

The six types of reading comprehension questions focus on: (1) the main idea, or primary purpose, of the passage; (2) information explicitly stated in the passage; (3) information or ideas implied or suggested; (4) possible application of the author's ideas to other situations; (5) the author's logic, reasoning, or persuasive techniques; and (6) the tone of the passage, or the author's attitude as it is expressed through the language used in the passage.

The test contains two long and two short reading comprehension passages. Each long passage is followed by seven or eight questions, and each short passage is followed by three or four questions. The four passages are drawn from different subject areas in the humanities, social sciences, biologic sciences, and physical sciences.

QUANTITATIVE ABILITY

The quantitative ability section measures basic mathematical skills, understanding of elementary mathematical concepts, and the ability to reason quantitatively and solve problems with numbers. The mathematics knowledge required is assumed to be common to the background of all examinees. The questions include three broad content areas: arithmetic, algebra, and geometry.

Arithmetic

Arithmetic topics include arithmetic operations (i.e., addition, subtraction, multiplication, division, and nonnegative powers) on rational numbers; estimation; percent; average; interpretation of graphs and tables; properties of numbers (i.e., those relating to odd and even integers, primes, and divisibility); factoring; and elementary counting and probability.

Algebra

Algebra questions involve operations with radical expressions, factoring and simplifying of algebraic expressions, equations and inequalities, and absolute value. These questions measure the ability to solve first- and second-degree equations and inequalities and simultaneous equations; the ability to read a word problem and set up the necessary equations or inequalities to solve it; and the ability to use basic algebraic skills to solve unfamiliar problems.

Geometry

Geometry questions involve properties associated with parallel lines, circles and their inscribed and central angles, triangles, rectangles, other polygons, measurement-related concepts of area, perimeter, volume, the Pythagorean theorem, and angle measure in area degrees. This section tests the ability to perform simple coordinate geometry as well as knowledge of special triangles, such as isosceles, equilateral, and 30°–60°–90°. The ability to construct proofs is not measured.

QUANTITATIVE COMPARISON

Quantitative comparison questions test the ability to reason quickly and accurately about the relative sizes of two quantities or to perceive that not enough information is provided to make such a decision.

DATA INTERPRETATION

Data interpretation questions, like the reading comprehension questions in the verbal measure, usually appear in sets. These questions are based on data shown in tables or graphs. They test the ability to synthesize information and select the appropriate data to answer a question or determine that sufficient information is not provided.

ANALYTICAL ABILITY

Each analytical section includes two types of questions: analytical and logical. Analytical reasoning questions appear in groups of three or more, with each group based on a different set of conditions describing a fictional situation. Each logical reasoning question is usually based on a separate short passage; however, sometimes two or three questions are based on the same passage.

LOGICAL REASONING

Logical reasoning questions test the ability to understand, analyze, and evaluate arguments. Some of the abilities tested by specific questions include recognizing the point of an argument, recognizing assumptions on which an argument is based, drawing conclusions and forming hypotheses, identifying methods of argument, evaluating arguments and counterarguments, and analyzing evidence.